ATTENTION DEFICIT HYPERACTIVITY DISORDER (ADHD) RESEARCH

ATTENTION DEFICIT HYPERACTIVITY DISORDER (ADHD) RESEARCH

MICHELLE P. LARIMER
EDITOR

Nova Biomedical Books
New York

Production Coordinator: Donna Dennis
Editorial Production Manager: Donna Dennis
Senior Production Editor: Susan Boriotti
Office Manager: Annette Hellinger
Graphics: Andrea Charles, Magdalena Nuñez and Annemarie VanDeWater
Editorial Production: Marius Andronie, Maya Columbus, Keti Datunashvili, Melissa Diaz, Andrew Kallio, Vladimir Klestov, Lorna Loperfido, Joann Overton and Rusudan Razmadze
Circulation: Ave Maria Gonzalez, Vera Popovic, Luis Aviles, Alexandra Columbus, Raymond Davis, Cathy DeGregory, Marlene Nuñez, Jeannie Pappas, Lauren Perl and Katie Sutherland

Library of Congress Cataloging-in-Publication Data
Available Upon Request

ISBN: 1-59454-156-6

An Imprint of Nova Science Publishers, Inc.
400 Oser Ave, Suite 1600
Hauppauge, New York 11788-3619
Tel. 631-231-7269 Fax 631-231-8175
e-mail: Novascience@earthlink.net
Web Site: http://www.novapublishers.com

Printed in the United States of America

Contents

Preface

ADHD is characterized by learning and behavioral problems including short attention span, impulsivity, hyperactivity and impairments in perceptual, language and motor skills. Between 4-10% of school-age children are believed to have it with boys outnumbering girls 2-3 to one. An adult form is also now recognized. The symptoms of Attention Deficit Disorder are caused by a neurological dysfunction within the brain. The underlying physiological mechanism which causes Attention Deficit Disorder is still not thoroughly understood and remains under intense scientific study. It is presumed that brain chemistry is out of balance and that specific chemicals called neurotransmitters may be lacking in individuals with Attention Deficit Disorder. Leading-edge research from around the world is presented in this new volume.

ADHD is best viewed as the extreme of certain behavioral traits that vary genetically throughout the entire population. However, there has been little research into genetic brain differences that may predispose certain children to be diagnosed with ADHD. Most human studies have examined subjects only after ADHD has taken its toll. Chapter I reviews the use of one animal model, the Naples High and Low excitability rats, to investigate the neural basis of ADHD vulnerability. Chapter II is not a survey of new findings but a very different way to view old ones. It extends Barkley's 1997 theory that ADHD is a neurological disorder of impaired executive functions and (1) suggests that ADHD produces many difficulties in small-world social networks, networks where so much is done not only through a friend but also through friends of that friend, and (2) reviews (a) the challenges of a male fetus to his depressed or otherwise less than robust mother and (b) the screening, whether in ADHD assessments of sons or when sizing up prospective husbands, by females of males for the social dependability that is so critical in networks. The association of oppositional defiant disorder with increased rates of ADHD, combined type (ADHD-CT), anxiety disorders and depressive disorders are replicated findings. However, to date, the specific associations between oppositional defiant disorder, ADHD-CT, anxiety disorders and dysthymic disorder symptoms have not been studied in primary school age children with ADHD-CT. Chapter III deals with these issues.

Research indicates that children with ADHD suffer from frontal striatal and right hemisphere dysfunction. As would be expected, children with ADHD have been found to be deficient on measures of executive functioning and are more likely to exhibit nonrighthandedness. Chapter IV discusses implications for further research and how lateralization/perceptual bias findings may, potentially, affect treatment of the neuropsychological deficits associated with ADHD. Children with attention deficit hyperactivity disorder (ADHD) are at risk for significant academic difficulties. Although academic problems are well documented for these children, there is little information about specific ways in which children with ADHD may differ from comparison children in their comprehension of and memory for complex, interconnected information such as that represented in stories. Chapter V explores such issues.

Twenty seven children and adolescents, ages 4 to 18 years, fullfiling the DSM-IV diagnostic criteria for attention deficit hyperactivity disorder were included in a study discussed in Chapter VI. Transcranial magnetic stimulation was performed on all subjects, with recording of the motor evoked potential at the biceps brachii. Central motor conduction time was calculated by the method of cervical root stimulation. Due to the shape variability, the amplitude of the motor responses was not measured in the study.

Attention Deficit/Hyperactivity Disorder (ADHD) is the most common developmental disorder of childhood, affecting 3 - 5% of children in the United States, and often continuing into adulthood. ADHD is associated with multiple serious complications, including poor school achievement, substance abuse, automobile accidents, etc. Chapter VII presents several recently developed computational procedures that have been shown to improve the assessment of ADHD. Chapter VIII reports several findings that support the model of a multisystem dysfunction underlying ADHD pathophysiology: low dopaminergic tone could mediate overall symptom severity, abnormal noradrenergic tone impairment in attention, and serotoninergic activity impulsivity. In addition, studies have reported abnormal MAO activity in children with ADHD and in individuals with high impulsivity, ADHD with conduct disorder, and thrill-seeking personality characteristics. The authors review the literature on the efficacy of stimulants in adults, particularly in relation to dose. The pharmacokinetics and behavioural pharmacology of stimulants are examined in order to better identify factors that may assist in determine an appropriate stimulant dose for adults. The potential risks of using high doses of stimulant are explored in Chapter IX.

In: Attention Deficit Hyperactivity Disorder Research
Editor: Michelle P. Larimer, pp. 1-18
ISBN 1-59454-156-6

Chapter I

Cortical and Limbic Systems Mediating the Predisposition to Attention Deficit and Hyperactivity

F. Gonzalez-Lima[1]
University of Texas at Austin, Austin, Texas

Abstract

ADHD is best viewed as the extreme of certain behavioral traits that vary genetically throughout the entire population. However, there has been little research into genetic brain differences that may predispose certain children to be diagnosed with ADHD. Most human studies have examined subjects only after ADHD has taken its toll. But without biomarkers that determine ADHD onset, it is impossible to distinguish primary etiological factors from what may be compensatory factors. Although human studies could address this question; in practice the necessary studies are difficult to do. Identical twins discordant for ADHD are rare, and longitudinal research is time consuming and costly. Animal models become necessary for understanding the predisposing biological factors for attention deficit and hyperactivity given these practical limitations and the ethical constraints to selectively breed humans diagnosed with ADHD. This chapter reviews the use of one animal model, the Naples High and Low excitability rats, to investigate the neural basis of ADHD vulnerability. The Naples rats are two genetic strains of selectively bred rats. The High and Low excitability strains are hyper-reactive and hypo-reactive to spatial novelty, respectively. These strains also display differences in the duration of non-selective (orienting) attention, which is reduced in the High strain and increased in the Low strain. These two strains were compared to randomly-bred rats that show average attention and motor reactivity to spatial novelty tasks to determine differences in their brain metabolic capacity. Differences in cytochrome oxidase activity, a marker of metabolic capacity, between the High and Low strains and randomly-bred

[1] Contact address: Prof. Dr. F. Gonzalez-Lima The University of Texas at Austin, 1 University Station A8000, Austin, TX 78712-0187, USA. Phone (512) 471-5895, Fax (512) 471-4728.email: gonzalez-lima@psy.utexas.edu

rats were found in specific regions of the cerebral cortex and limbic system. The differences in the brain metabolic capacity of High excitability rats are presumed to model the ADHD attention deficit and hyperactive-impulsive type; whereas the neural differences in Low excitability rats model the ADHD predominantly inattentive type. Observed prefrontal cortex differences may underlie the differences in behavioral inhibition in the two strains. Posterior parietal cortex differences may underlie the differences in goal-directed attention. Other changes in cortical amygdala and limbic cortices were linked to poor emotional control in the High excitability strain. The dentate granule cells of the hippocampus also showed metabolic differences, which may underlie strain differences in spatial exploration. Selective breeding of rats to vary behavioral traits such as attention and reactivity to novelty resulted in genetic strains that allowed identification of the specific metabolic differences in cortical and limbic regions mediating these behaviors.

Introduction

Attention Deficit Hyperactivity Disorder (ADHD) is regarded by many clinicians and scientists as the most prevalent psychiatric disorder in children, which by some estimates affects 5-10% of school-age children worldwide, mostly boys (Wilens, Biederman and Spencer, 2002). However, other scientists engaged in heredity studies argue that ADHD is best viewed as the extreme of certain behavioral traits that vary genetically throughout the entire population (Levy, Hay, McStephen, Wood, and Waldman, 1997). For example, novelty-seeking is a behavioral trait that shows marked individual differences. Novelty may be sought externally by increasing interactions with new environmental stimuli (individual is hyper-reactive) or internally by engaging in "day dreaming" (individual is hypo-reactive to external stimuli). The predominantly hyper-reactive individual may be hyperkinetic and impulsive, whereas the predominantly hypo-reactive individual may be regarded as inattentive to external stimuli. While novelty-seeking is a positive trait from an adaptive viewpoint, it may lead to disruptive behavior under certain settings such as in the traditional classroom where children are required to sit quietly and pay attention to a teacher or work in a task that may be repetitive or boring. At any given time most school children have difficulty in remaining still, concentrating and staying on task. According to our behavior genetic view, in a small percentage of the population these traits are extreme enough to interfere seriously with school activities, but most children with these traits are manifesting individual brain-behavior differences rather than being mentally ill.

Children with these behavioral traits are usually identified in the classroom by teachers, some of whom are less tolerant than others, and then teachers and counselors often request psychological evaluation for ADHD and often pressure parents to put these children on medication to manage the disruptive behavior. Cultural variations in the diagnosis of ADHD are also strong (Taylor, 1998). The same behavior may be culturally constructed as normal or may lead to a diagnosis of a psychiatric disorder. Adults from different cultures have widely different degrees of tolerance for children's disruptive behavior and rough and tumble play that result in different rates of diagnosis of ADHD (Leung, Luk, Ho, Taylor, Mark and Bacon-Shone, 1996).

About ten years ago a group of researchers broadened the ADHD diagnostic criteria from DSM-III to DSM-IV, which have resulted in a greater number of children diagnosed as mentally ill because the old criteria were focused on hyperactivity and the new criteria include hyperactive-impulsive and inattentive subtypes (Carlson and Mann, 2000). For example, in 1990-1992 in the USA and Germany, there were reports of less than 5% ADHD prevalence among school age children. By 1995, using the broadened DSM-IV criteria, these estimates in the USA and Germany jumped to 12-18% (Elia, Ambrosini, and Rapoport, 1999). While it is obviously impossible for the number of mentally ill children to double or triple in a few years, it is also true that the behavioral traits of inattention, hyperactivity and impulsivity that lead to a diagnosis of ADHD are a leading cause of learning and behavioral problems for children in schools around the world.

There is mounting evidence that heredity plays a significant role in the susceptibility for the behavioral traits that qualify for a diagnosis of ADHD based on family and twin studies (Faraone and Biederman, 1994; Levy, Hay, McStephen, Wood, and Waldman, 1997). For example, parents diagnosed with ADHD are more likely to have children with ADHD than parents without this diagnosis, and children with an identical twin having ADHD are much more likely to have it too (Epstein, Conners, Erhardt, Arnold, Hechtman, Hinshaw, Hoza, Newcorn, Swanson, and Vitiello, 2000). The heritability of ADHD is about 80 (70-95% of trait variation in the population), which is close to the heritability of human height. Various genes involved in dopaminergic neurotransmission have been reported to show differences in individuals with ADHD. Genes encoding D2 and D4 dopamine receptors and the dopamine transporter gene, for example, appear to show mutations in ADHD (Swanson, Flodman, Kennedy, Spence, Moyzis, Schuck, Murias, Moriarity, Barr, Smith, and Posner, 2000).

But genetic predispositions are manifested in interaction with the environment. It is likely that there are also non-genetic factors involved, especially due to insults to the brain during fetal or early postnatal development. Animal models have also shown that parental separation during early postnatal development results in hyperactive young animals with increased impulsiveness and attention deficits (Braun, Kremz, Wetzel, Wagner, and Poeggel, 2003). Therefore, while there is high heritability which increases the risk for an ADHD diagnosis, other factors such as early brain injury and postnatal care may also contribute to ADHD.

ADHD causes great suffering to those afflicted and their families as evidenced by the high rates of school failures and learning difficulties, greater than that of the general population (Willens, Biederman, and Spencer, 2002). Since ADHD is a major public health concern due to its high prevalence, educational impact, and personal cost to children and their caregivers, a great amount of research has been devoted to it recently. However, in spite of this great effort, the neurological basis of ADHD remains poorly understood. One reason for this limited understanding has been a relative lack of research into the neurobiological factors that predispose certain children to become victims of ADHD.

Most human studies have examined their subjects only after ADHD has taken its biological and psychological toll, and these studies have amassed numerous biological and psychological markers linked to the behavioral syndromes of ADHD. But without biological markers determined before ADHD onset, it is not possible to dissect out the primary etiological factors of ADHD from what may be compensatory factors that are the consequence rather than the cause of ADHD. Although human studies could in theory address this question using, for example, identical twins discordant for ADHD or their healthy relatives or conducting longitudinal studies of at-risk children; in practice the necessary studies would be very difficult to carry out. Identical twins discordant for ADHD are rare; and longitudinal research is time consuming, requires large amounts of funding and personnel, and invariably has high rates of drop-outs. Given these practical limitations and the ethical constraints to selectively breed or clone humans with ADHD, then animal models become crucially necessary for understanding the predisposing biological factors for attention deficit and hyperactivity. This chapter reviews the use of an animal model, the Naples High and Low excitability rats, which has been used successfully to investigate the functional neuroanatomical basis for ADHD vulnerability.

Animal Models of Attention Deficit and Hyperactivity

To model differences in the genetic predisposition to react to novel environments is important to address questions related to ADHD, which is characterized by attention impairment with or without impulsiveness, hyperkinesis, and restlessness (Sagvolden and Sergeant, 1998). The use of animals as research models allows investigators to answer some research questions addressing the neurobiological mechanisms of attention and hyperactivity that cannot be studied in humans (Papa, Sadile, Sergeant, Shumake, and Gonzalez-Lima, 1998).

In animals, attention deficits and hyperactivity have been produced mainly through deprivation models, lesion models and genetic models. In the deprivation models, rats may be reared in social isolation (Hall, Humby, Wilkinson, and Robbins, 1997) or undergo prolonged parental separation as infants (Braun, Kremz, Wetzel, Wagner, and Poeggel, 2003). Under certain conditions, these social manipulations during maturation lead to attention deficits and hyperactivity.

The lesion approach consists on damaging the brain through surgical or toxicological interventions. For example, a number of neural regions regarded to be critically involved in attention may be render inoperative and then the lesioned group is compared to a control group on measures that are presumed to reflect attention (Roberts, De Salvia, Wilkinson, Collins, Muir, Everitt, and Robbins, 1994). Infant rats have also been exposed to X-ray radiation of the hippocampal formation which results in granular cell degeneration and deficits linked to ADHD (Diaz-Granados, Greene and Amsel, 1994). One problem with these models is that a priori knowledge of the brain regions implicated is necessary to select the regions investigated.

Genetic models have also been developed in mice and rats. Mice models are based on the proposal that existing mouse strains or experimental mutants with defects in dopamine transmission show differences in motor activity. For example, the acallosal mouse strain (Magara, Ricceri, Wolfer, and Lipp, 2000) and the coloboma mouse mutant (Wilson, 2000) have been proposed as ADHD models. However, these and related mice strains have other physiological and brain abnormalities, such as lack of a corpus callosum, that are clearly unrelated to humans with ADHD. In the case of mice with mutations of the dopamine system, a difficulty with these models is that a priori knowledge of the dopamine genes implicated in ADHD is necessary to select the mutations investigated. There are reports of several dopamine-related genes believed to be abnormal in ADHD patients, such as the D4 and D2 dopamine receptor genes and the dopamine transporter genes (Swanson, Flodman, Kennedy, Spence, Moyzis, Schuck, Murias, Moriarity, Barr, Smith, and Posner, 2000). However it is likely that the predisposition to ADHD has several complex etiologies, with different genetic contributions to the different ADHD subtypes and with many genes affected. This inherent complexity would minimize the impact of any single gene mutation, as it is currently investigated in the mice mutant models.

However, it is not necessary to wait for all the genes implicated in ADHD to be discovered to be able to model genetic predisposition in animals. Even though the specific genes for ADHD may not be known, the behavioral traits of the ADHD subtypes are well characterized. Thus, one readily available genetic approach is to selectively breed rats showing specific behavioral traits relevant to ADHD. The spontaneously hypertensive rat (SHR) is the oldest and most frequently used rat model based on the selective breeding strategy. The SHR strain was originally developed to study hypertension, but it was found that these rats also show hyperactivity in the open field test, deficient sustained attention, and motor impulsiveness (Sagvolden, 2000). These behavioral abnormalities resembling ADHD developed as an unintended effect of the inbreeding process used to generate the SHR strain. However, a great disadvantage of using SHR as a model for ADHD is that these rats are hypertensive in addition to their behavioral defects. Moreover, the SHR hypertension as well as their behavioral alterations is of neurological origin, which compromises the ability to isolate the genetic effects on the brain that are responsible for ADHD-like behavior.

Two related rat models have avoided the problem of hypertension found in the SHR strain, and are therefore more promising genetic models of ADHD. One is the Wistar-Kyoto Hyperactive (WKHA) rats, and the other is the Naples High and Low excitability rat strains. The WKHA rats were developed by a cross of Wistar-Kyoto rats having normal blood pressure with the SHR strain. After successive selective breeding, the traits of hyperactivity and hypertension were separated. The WKHA rats obtained show hyperactivity to a novel environment as the SHR strain, but they have normal blood pressure (Hendley, 2000). While there has been progress in separating the traits for hyperactivity and hypertension in the WKHA rats, there is no information on the brain differences responsible for their hyperactivity. In contrast, there are mapping studies available on the brain systems linked to ADHD-like behavioral traits in the Naples strains (Gonzalez-Lima and Sadile, 2000; Gallo, Gonzalez-Lima and Sadile, 2002).

The Naples rats are two genetic strains of selectively bred Sprague-Dawley rats developed in Naples, Italy, which have been proposed as putative animal models of ADHD (Aspide, Gironi-Carnevale, Sergeant and Sadile, 1998). Using mazes such as the Lat maze, hexagonal tunnel maze, and asymmetric radial arm maze, rats that were vulnerable to display high or low exploratory behavior to spatial novelty tasks were selectively bred together. The different reactivity to novelty in these two rat strains cannot be explained by differences in general motor activity because they do not display significant differences in their baseline motor activity (Cerbone, Pellicano, and Sadile 1993). As compared to randomly-bred rats, the

Naples High and Low excitability rat strains are hyper-reactive and hypo-reactive to spatial novelty, respectively. High excitability rats show an increase in the frequency of locomotion (horizontal activity) and in rearing (vertical activity), but the duration of each rearing episode was reduced in the High excitability rats. Conversely, Low excitability rats show a decrease in the frequency of locomotion and rearing, but the duration of each rearing episode lasted longer. Hence, these genetic strains display alterations in non-selective attention as measured by the duration of rearing episodes, which is reduced to 82% of the random-bred level (assumed as 100%) in the High excitability strain and increased to 147% in the Low excitability strain (Aspide, Gironi-Carnevale, Sergeant and Sadile, 1998). The Naples strains do not differ in learning abilities per se, but rather in motor reactivity to spatial novelty (i.e., frequency of crossings and rearings in mazes), non-selective attention or orienting in maze (i.e., duration of each rearing episode), and inattention to reinforcement in low motivational level (i.e., consumption of chocolate in baited arm of maze when not food-deprived).

The Naples High excitability rats are presumed to model the "ADHD-plus" variant (combined attention deficit hyperactive-impulsive type) where rapid attention shifts and hyper-reactivity prevail, whereas the Naples Low excitability rats model the "ADHD-minus" variant (predominantly inattentive type) with sluggish attention and hypo-reactivity (Gallo, Gonzalez-Lima and Sadile, 2002). These two genetic strains can be compared to randomly-bred rats that show average attention and motor reactivity to spatial novelty tasks to determine differences in their brain metabolic capacity.

Brain Mapping Using Cytochrome Oxidase Histochemistry

Regional brain metabolic capacity can be mapped using cytochrome oxidase, a mitochondrial enzyme that can be used as an endogenous neurometabolic marker because of its key role in neuronal respiration (Gonzalez-Lima and Cada, 1998). The functional activity of regional and cellular compartments of nervous tissue is tightly coupled with oxidative energy metabolism. Cytochrome oxidase is the oxygen-activating enzyme for the respiration of all animal and plant cells (eukaryotes), and it is the site of oxidative phosphorylation where energy is conserved for synthesis of ATP (Wikström, Krab, and Saraste, 1981). ATP is used for all energy-consuming functions of neurons. The main consumer of ATP in neurons is the Na^+/K^+ pump that upholds ion balance, sustaining the resting membrane potential that is depolarized in the electrical firing of neurons (Hevner, Duff and Wong-Riley, 1992). For a steady resting membrane potential, the ionic gradients across the membrane must be maintained using metabolic energy derived from the hydrolysis of ATP. Since the Na^+/K^+ pump moves these ions against their electrochemical gradients, ATP must be hydrolyzed to provide the energy to actively transport these ions to maintain the charge separation across the membrane constant. An increased neuronal electrical activity will ultimately lead to increased cellular aerobic respiration and obligatory cytochrome oxidase activity to generate ATP.

This coupling between cytochrome oxidase activity and the energy-demanding ionic pumps related to the electrical activity of neurons is what led Wong-Riley (1989) to postulate that the level of cytochrome oxidase activity within neurons should be coupled with their functional level of activity. Thus the more active neurons in a brain region have increased cytochrome oxidase content in their mitochondria (Hevner, Liu, and Wong-Riley, 1995). Increased neuronal electrical activity leads to increased cellular respiration and cytochrome oxidase activity to produce more ATP. Tonically active neurons are those with more cytochrome oxidase activity to maintain a greater capacity for energy production needed to fuel ionic pumps and other ATP-dependent processes required for proper electrical activity. Experimental manipulations that increase or decrease the activity of neurons over days produce corresponding increases or decreases of cytochrome oxidase activity inside their mitochondria (Wong-Riley, Nie, Hevner, and Liu, 1998). The precise location of cytochrome oxidase reactivity can be determined at regional, cellular, and subcellular compartments using light and electron microscopy. Therefore, there is anatomical certainty of how an increase in cytochrome oxidase activity is represented subcellularly in response to physiological neuronal activity (Hevner, Liu, and Wong-Riley, 1995).

Cytochrome oxidase histochemistry has shown that the metabolic capacity of the brain can change in response to alterations in neuronal functional activity. For example, cytochrome oxidase has been applied as a metabolic marker in the auditory system (Gonzalez-Lima and Cada, 1994, 1998), the visual system (Wong-Riley, Nie, Hevner, and Liu, 1998), and brain regions outside primary sensory systems (Hevner, Liu, and Wong-Riley, 1995). Although most experimental manipulations have focused on invasive procedures aimed at decreasing cytochrome oxidase levels, there is also evidence of increases in cytochrome oxidase activity (Nobrega, Raymond, DiStefano and Burnham, 1993). Using our studies as examples, regional cerebral cytochrome oxidase activity has been increased with various genetic (Papa, Sadile, Sergaent and Gonzalez-Lima, 1998; Shumake and Gonzalez-Lima, 2003), hormonal (Crews, Coomber, Baldwin, Azad and Gonzalez-Lima, 1996; Jones, Gonzalez-Lima, Crews, Galef and Clark, 1997), environmental (Coomber, Crews and Gonzalez-Lima, 1997), and behavioral manipulations (Poremba, Jones and Gonzalez-Lima, 1997; Crews, Coomber and Gonzalez-Lima, 1997). We have been able to demonstrate that some learning-related increases in neuronal memory functions are related to increases in cytochrome oxidase activity (Poremba, Jones and Gonzalez-Lima, 1998) using the same sensitive histochemical and quantitative imaging procedures applied to the Naples genetic strains. Mapping of cytochrome oxidase activity in nervous tissue is based on specific methodological considerations that determine the sensitivity as well as the possibility of quantification of the cytochrome oxidase staining method in terms of enzyme activity units. When cytochrome oxidase histochemistry is quantitatively measured to obtain enzyme activity, it offers a major advantage over other cytochrome oxidase measuring techniques. Bicgon and Wolff (1986) introduced the use of computerized image analysis with internal standards of known enzymatic activity as a method to achieve quantification of acetylcholinesterase activity from histochemically stained brain sections. A similar approach has been developed by Gonzalez-Lima and Garrosa (1991) to quantify cytochrome oxidase activity by histochemical staining using a technique that is compatible with autoradiography. Gonzalez-Lima and Cada (1994) adopted a cytochrome oxidase procedure that was found more sensitive than the other available protocols, and incorporated the use of internal standards and quantitative densitometry. The present level of sensitivity and quantification of our technique can successfully detect genetic effects on the brain produced by selective breeding (Gonzalez-Lima and Sadile, 2000; Shumake and Gonzalez-Lima, 2003). Cytochrome oxidase methods with higher threshold for detecting cytochrome oxidase reactivity may be adequate for other applications but may fail to detect subtle neural activity changes that are demonstrated by our more sensitive quantitative method.

Brain Metabolic Differences in the Naples Models of Attention Deficit and Hyperactivity

Only a subset of the brain regions in ADHD-diagnosed individuals may be responsible for their genetic predisposition to be classified within one of the ADHD subtypes. The functional neuroanatomical basis for the genetic predisposition to attention deficit and hyperactivity has been successfully investigated using cytochrome oxidase histochemistry in naïve rats of the Naples High and Low excitability strains (Gonzalez-Lima and Sadile, 2000; Gallo, Gonzalez-Lima and Sadile, 2002). Metabolic differences in cytochrome oxidase activity between the High and Low excitability strains and randomly bred control rats were found in specific regions of the prefrontal and parietal cerebral cortex, the hippocampal formation and parahippocampal cortex, and the amygdala and periamygdaline cortex (Gonzalez-Lima and Sadile, 2000). The specific regions affected are listed in Table 1, which also indicates the direction of the metabolic difference. These regions are illustrated in Figure 1, which shows sections of the rat brain stained with cytochrome oxidase histochemistry. Below we explain each of the neuroanatomical systems modified in High and Low excitability strains and propose the functional relevance of these neural differences to behaviors associated with the ADHD subtypes with and without hyperactivity.

Table 1. Cortical and limbic regions with different metabolic activity in Naples strains as compared to randomly-bred rats (baseline).

Region	Low Excitability Rats	High Excitability Rats
Medial prefrontal cortex	Increased	Baseline
Posterior parietal cortex	Baseline	Decreased
Dentate granule cells	Decreased	Baseline
Entorhinal cortex	Increased	Increased
Cortical amygdala	Baseline	Decreased
Perirhinal cortex, ventral	Baseline	Decreased
Perirhinal cortex, dorsal	Decreased	Decreased

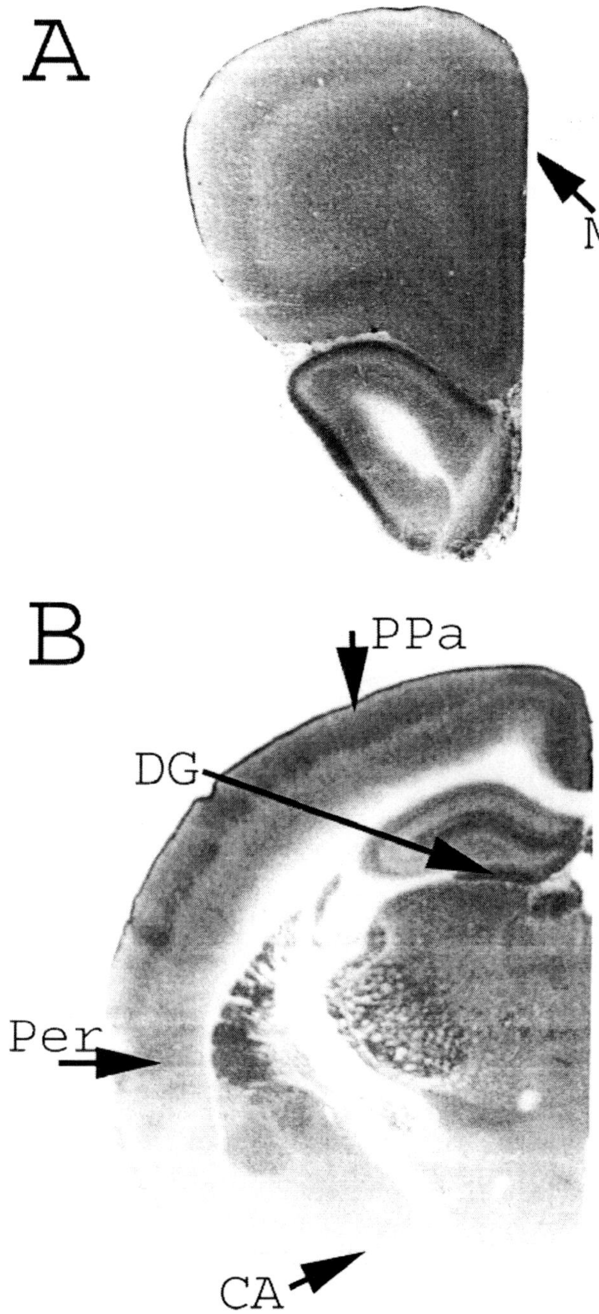

Figure 1: Cortical and limbic regions showing significant metabolic differences between the Naples rats and randomly-bred rats. A. Anterior section at the level of the medial prefrontal cortex (MPF). B. Posterior section at the level of the posterior parietal cortex (PPa), dentate gyrus (DG), perirhinal cortex (Per), and cortical amygdala (CA). Cytochrome oxidase histochemical staining (Gonzalez-Lima and Cada, 1998).

Prefrontal Cortex

The prefrontal cortex is found anterior to the primary sensorimotor cortical areas in all mammals. It is small in rodents as compared to humans where it constitutes about a quarter of the cerebral cortex. The cortical region at the anteromedial end of the frontal cortex is regarded as part of the prefrontal cortex in both rats and humans. This region is traditionally called the medial prefrontal cortex in the rat (Sullivan and Brake, 2003) and its boundaries are delimited by the projection field it receives from the dorsomedial nucleus of the thalamus. Low excitability rats show an increased metabolism in the medial prefrontal cortex that may explain their behavioral hypo-reactivity but normal baseline motor activity (Cerbone, Patacchioli and Sadile, 1993). Increased metabolic activity of this medial prefrontal cortical region in normal rodents is correlated with the inhibition of behavior during extinction of instrumental goal-seeking behavior (Nair, Berndt, Barrett and Gonzalez-Lima, 2001) and extinction of Pavlovian conditioned responses (Barrett, Shumake, Jones and Gonzalez-Lima, 2003). Subjects with higher medial prefrontal cortex activity are more successful at inhibiting their behavior. Indeed, the medial prefrontal cortex in mice showed a 0.99 correlation between cortical metabolic activity and extinction of conditioned emotional behavior (Barrett, Shumake, Jones and Gonzalez-Lima, 2003). Therefore, increased baseline metabolism in this prefrontal cortical region that mediates behavioral inhibition would be expected to contribute to the hypo-reactivity phenotype manifested by the Low excitability rats.

This particular medial prefrontal region is not affected in a genetic animal model of depression, the congenitally helpless rats, which show baseline reduced motor activity (Shumake, Poremba, Edwards and Gonzalez-Lima, 2000). Therefore, the low behavioral reactivity of the Low excitability strain does not appear to be caused by the depressive phenotype found in congenitally helpless rats (Shumake and Gonzalez-Lima, 2003).

Parietal Cortex

The parietal cortex is made of anterior regions related to primary somatosensory systems and posterior regions that have been linked to higher order polymodal sensory integration and attention mechanisms in both rats and humans. Decreased metabolic activity of the posterior parietal cortical region in the High excitability rats may correlate with their particular spatial attention deficit. For example, the posterior parietal cortex showed reduced metabolic capacity in the High excitability rats as compared to normal controls. The posterior parietal cortex is linked to spatial attentional processes in humans (Andersen and Buneo, 2003) and other species, including rats (Kolb and Walkey, 1987).

Humans with posterior parietal cortex lesions have difficulty in attending to visual stimuli. For instance, the integration of visual stimuli with somatosensory information is necessary to be able to correlate the visual environment with the position of the body parts. A form of sensory neglect in which patients ignore the left half of the body and visual field is characteristic of patients with right posterior parietal cortex damage (Andersen and Buneo, 2003). Rats with ischemia leading to decreased cytochrome oxidase activity in the posterior parietal cortex show impaired learning of the Morris water maze, a task that relies on attention to spatial cues and body position (Cada, de la Torre and Gonzalez-Lima, 2000). Although the activity of the posterior parietal cortex is generally regarded as linked to the integration of different types of sensory inputs, its activity is also relevant to motor expression because the output of the posterior parietal cortex is synaptically connected with motor and premotor cortical areas in both rats and humans (Matelli and Luppino, 2001). Therefore, a reduced metabolic capacity in the posterior parietal cortex may underlie the short spatial attention span correlated with the abnormally high rate of body movements in the High excitability rat strain in response to a new environment.

Hippocampal Formation and Parahippocampal Cortex

The only specific region that showed a significant difference in metabolic capacity between the High and Low excitability rats was within the hippocampal formation, supporting the conclusion that these strains differ in hippocampal function (Cerbone, Pellicano and Sadile, 1993). The hippocampal formation in rats and humans is made of three main components: the hippocampus proper, the dentate gyrus and the subiculum. The strain difference was found in the dentate gyrus, which is characterized mainly by a layer of granular cells that are packed densely. The outer granular cell layer of the dentate gyrus showed a lower activity in the Low excitability rats. The granular cells are critical for hippocampal function because they give origin to the mossy fiber system, an important association pathway that connects the dentate gyrus with the hippocampus proper. In particular, mossy fibers convey the activity of the dentate granule cells to the pyramidal cells in the CA3 field of the hippocampus. CA3 pyramidal cells send collaterals to the CA1 pyramidal cells, which in turn send their axons to the subiculum. The subiculum then projects to the entorhinal cortex, which closes the circuit by projecting back to the dentate gyrus. This projection is called the perforant path, which is the main input to the hippocampal formation (van Groen, Kadish, and Wyss, 2002). A reduction in the activity of this pathway would result in the weakening of the main link in an intrinsic neuron circuit thought to underlie the working memory functions of the hippocampal formation. Working memory refers to the retention of information necessary to guide ongoing behaviors, and deficits in working memory can be readily demonstrated in mazes with rats having hippocampal dysfunction (Wan, Pang, and Olton, 1994).

The granular cells of the hippocampal formation are of particular relevance in young children with the ADHD predominantly inattentive type, because the granular cells of the dentate gyrus are actively dividing in infants and are thus more vulnerable to postnatal influences that may affect their metabolic capacity. In rats, the granule cells of the dentate gyrus exhibit postnatal cell division and they are especially vulnerable during infancy to X-rays that disrupt cell division (Diaz-Granados, Greene and Amsel, 1994). Indeed, even before the label ADHD was invented, Altman (1986) proposed that dentate granule cell hypoplasia is a key reason for the brain dysfunction underlying learning disabilities in children, and showed that it could be modeled by X-ray irradiation of infant rats. Therefore, the metabolic mapping of regional cytochrome oxidase activity in the High and Low excitability rats is consistent with previous studies indicating that the dentate granule cells in the hippocampal formation may be critical for the behavioral differences between these two strains.

This conclusion is reinforced by the finding that the entorhinal cortex showed elevated metabolism in both Low and High excitability rats. The entorhinal cortex in the parahippocampal gyrus is the cortical region directly connected with the hippocampal formation in all mammals. The entorhinal cortex receives converging information from sensory cortical areas and then conveys this information to the dentate gyrus through a massive pathway, the perforant path (van Groen, Kadish, and Wyss, 2002). The entorhinal cortex is the main input to the hippocampal formation, and an elevation in entorhinal activity should have elevated dentate activity in both the Low and High excitability rats. However, the Low excitability strain is distinguished by low intrahippocampal dentate circuit activity in spite of high external input activity from the entorhinal cortex.

Amygdala and Periamygdaline Cortex

The amygdala is made of several parts, including a large basolateral nuclear group and a small corticomedial nuclear group. Most subdivisions of the amygdala were unaffected in the Naples rats. The only subdivision with group differences was the cortical amygdala, with lower activity in the High excitability rats. This is a limbic region whose general dysfunction has been linked traditionally to an increase in emotionality that is consistent with the hyper-reactivity shown by the High excitability rats. Increase in metabolic activity in the cortical amygdala has been related to the acquisition of a conditioned bradicardiac response in normal rats (Gonzalez-Lima and Scheich, 1986). Hence a decrease in metabolic capacity in the cortical amygdala may handicap conditioned suppression and disrupt the emotionality of the High excitability rats.

The amygdala is surrounded by periamygdaline cortex. In particular, the cortical amygdala receives its main input from the perirhinal and olfactory cortical areas. The perirhinal cortex also showed reduced metabolic capacity in the High excitability rats as compared to randomly-bred controls. Similarly, aged rats with impaired performance in the water maze have decreased cytochrome oxidase activity in perirhinal cortex as compared to unimpaired rats (Villarreal, Gonzalez-Lima, Berndt and Barea-Rodriguez, 2002). Since posterior parietal and perirhinal metabolism are correlated to spatial learning, it would be expected that reduced baseline metabolic capacity in these cortical regions may impair the spatial attention ability of the High excitability rats.

Interestingly, when maze exploration is done under low and high motivational level (hungry vs. satiated rats in a baited radial arm maze), the High excitability rats show impaired attention toward reinforcement at low motivational level (Gallo, Gonzalez-Lima and Sadile, 2002). Both the Naples hyper-reactive rats and children diagnosed with ADHD show attention deficit mainly at low motivational level (Carlson and Tamm, 2000). Together these findings imply interactions between the motivational (limbic) and spatial attention (neocortical) components of novelty-seeking that are correlated to differences in metabolic capacity of specific brain regions of the High excitability rats.

Conclusions

ADHD is a highly heritable condition, as heritable as height in the human population (Epstein, Conners, Erhardt, Arnold, Hechtman, Hinshaw, Hoza, Newcorn, Swanson, and Vitiello, 2000). But there has been little research into genetic brain differences that may predispose certain individuals to develop the various ADHD subtypes. Human studies with neuroimaging techniques have reported that certain regions in the prefrontal cortex, basal ganglia and cerebellum are smaller or show abnormal metabolism in children diagnosed with ADHD (Anderson, Polcari, Lowen, Renshaw, and Teicher, 2002). While all these reported neural systems may be modified, it is not possible to tell which of the observed brain differences are related to the predisposing genetic causes, which are consequences of living with ADHD, and which are neural correlates of the various behavioral responses seen in people diagnosed with ADHD. There is no way to learn from these human neuroimaging studies which regions may be disrupted as a result of ADHD and which regions may be modified due to genetic causes that make some individuals likely to be diagnosed with ADHD.

This question can be readily addressed in animal models genetically selected to show particular behavioral characteristics of ADHD subtypes. However, one must always bear in mind that animals serve only as simplified models. In this chapter we have described the neocortical and limbic systems modified in the Naples rat strains as a way to highlight the brain systems that may underlie the genetic vulnerability to ADHD-like behaviors. The Naples rat strains are different from randomly-bred control rats in the metabolic capacity of a subset of specific brain areas that mediate spatial attention information and emotional processing, suggesting ADHD-like differences of attentional and motivational aspects of behavior produced by the selective breeding. The reported brain differences in the Naples strains are best viewed as resulting from the selective breeding of certain ADHD-like behavioral traits that vary genetically throughout the rat population rather than as a psychiatric disorder. In the human population, ADHD is also best viewed as the extreme of certain behavioral traits that vary genetically throughout the entire population (Levy, Hay, McStephen, Wood, and Waldman, 1997).

Remarkably, only neocortical and limbic regions showed heredity-linked differences in cytochrome oxidase activity out of over seventy brain regions analyzed in the Naples strains (Gallo, Gonzalez-Lima and Sadile, 2002). No sensory or motor areas or other subcortical structures were differentially affected in the Naples rats. However, we did not examine lower brainstem regions or the cerebellum in the Naples rats. There are reports that the cerebellar vermis of boys diagnosed with ADHD may be affected (Anderson, Polcari, Lowen, Renshaw, and Teicher, 2002).

The medial prefrontal cortex showed higher metabolism in the Low excitability rats relative to the High excitability and control rats. Since increased metabolism of the medial prefrontal cortex underlies the inhibition of behavior in both instrumental and classical conditioning paradigms (Nair, Berndt, Barrett, and Gonzalez-Lima, 2001; Barrett and Gonzalez-Lima, 2003), we interpret this genetic difference in prefrontal metabolism as responsible for the greater behavioral inhibition of Low excitability rats and the lower behavioral inhibition of High excitability rats. Indeed, this neural difference could be related to the similar distinction found in the ADHD subtypes with and without impulsivity. The ADHD impulsive subtype would resemble the High excitability strain in both aspects: lower prefrontal cortex activity and lower capacity for behavioral inhibition (Gallo, Gonzalez-Lima and Sadile, 2002).

The posterior parietal cortex also showed reduced metabolic capacity in the High excitability rats as compared to normal controls. Since the posterior parietal cortex mediates spatial attention processes and its outputs are linked to the motor cortex, we interpret the genetically selected deficiency in parietal metabolism as contributing to the decreased attention span and motor hyper-reactivity shown by High excitability rats during maze exploration.

The hippocampal formation and the amygdala are the two better known components of the limbic system. They are closely related to other areas of the cerebral cortex. As key components of the limbic system, they are generally concerned with emotional behavior and learning functions. Specifically, the Low excitability rats showed lower metabolism in a constituent of the hippocampal formation, the dentate granular cells. In contrast, the High excitability rats showed lower metabolism in a part of the amygdala, the cortical amygdala. Therefore, the observed metabolic reductions in these limbic structures and adjacent cortical areas in the Naples strains suggest functional differences in emotional processing.

The two Naples strains provided specific examples of the utility of measuring regional brain metabolism with cytochrome oxidase as a way to map the neural systems mediating genetic differences between strains with behavioral phenotypes modeling ADHD subtypes with and without hyperactivity. More generally, the studies of the Naples genetic models reviewed here support the conclusion that behavioral phenotype differences can be related to genotype differences in regional brain metabolic capacity.

Acknowledgements

I thank Dr. Erika Gonzalez-Lima for her assistance in the preparation of this chapter. The help of Jason Shumake with the figure is gratefully acknowledged. This work was supported by NIH grant R01 NS37755.

References

Altman J. An animal model of minimal brain dysfunction. In Lewis M. (Ed.). *Learning Disabilities and Prenatal Risk.* Urbana and Chicago: University of Illinois, 1986.

Andersen RA. Buneo CA. Sensorimotor integration in posterior parietal cortex. *Advances in Neurology.* 93:159-77, 2003.

Anderson CM. Polcari A. Lowen SB. Renshaw PF. Teicher MH. Effects of methylphenidate on functional magnetic resonance relaxometry of the cerebellar vermis in boys with ADHD. *American Journal of Psychiatry,* 159: 1322-8, 2002.

Aspide R. Gironi Carnevale UA. Sergeant JA. Sadile AG. Non-selective attention and nitric oxide in putative animal models of Attention deficit Hyperactivity Disorder. *Behavioural Brain Research.* 95(1):123-33, 1998.

Barrett D. Shumake J. Jones D. Gonzalez-Lima F. Metabolic mapping of mouse brain activity after extinction of a conditioned emotional response. *Journal of Neuroscience.* 23(13):5740-9, 2003.

Biegon A. Wolff M. Quantitative histochemistry of acetylcholinesterase in rat and human brain postmortem. *Journal of Neuroscience Methods.* 16(1):39-45, 1986.

Braun K. Kremz P. Wetzel W. Wagner T. Poeggel G. Influence of parental deprivation on the behavioral development in Octodon degus: modulation by maternal vocalizations. *Developmental Psychobiology.* 42(3):237-45, 2003.

Cada A. de la Torre JC. Gonzalez-Lima F. Chronic cerebrovascular ischemia in aged rats: effects on brain metabolic capacity and behavior. *Neurobiology of Aging.* 21(2):225-33, 2000.

Carlson CL. Mann M. Attention deficit/hyperactivity disorder, predominantly inattentive subtype. *Child & Adolescent Psychiatric Clinics of North America.* 9(3):499-510, 2000.

Carlson CL. Tamm L. Responsiveness of children with attention deficit-hyperactivity disorder to reward and response cost: differential impact on performance and motivation. *Journal of Consulting & Clinical Psychology.* 68(1):73-83, 2000.

Cerbone A. Pellicano MP. Sadile AG. Evidence for and against the Naples high- and low-excitability rats as genetic model to study hippocampal functions. *Neuroscience & Biobehavioral Reviews.* 17(3):295-303, 1993.

Coomber P. Crews D. Gonzalez-Lima F. Independent effects of incubation temperature and gonadal sex on the volume and metabolic capacity of brain nuclei in the leopard gecko (Eublepharis macularius), a lizard with temperature-dependent sex determination. *Journal of Comparative Neurology.* 380(3):409-21, 1997.

Crews D. Coomber P. Baldwin R. Azad N. Gonzalez-Lima F. Brain organization in a reptile lacking sex chromosomes: effects of gonadectomy and exogenous testosterone. *Hormones & Behavior.* 30(4):474-86, 1996.

Crews D. Coomber P. Gonzalez-Lima F. Effects of age and sociosexual experience on the morphology and metabolic capacity of brain nuclei in the leopard gecko (Eublepharis macularius), a lizard with temperature-dependent sex determination. *Brain Research.* 758(1-2):169-79, 1997.

Diaz-Granados JL. Greene PL. Amsel A. Selective activity enhancement and persistence in weanling rats after hippocampal X-irradiation in infancy: possible relevance for ADHD. *Behavioral & Neural Biology.* 61(3):251-9, 1994.

Elia J. Ambrosini PJ. Rapoport JL. Treatment of attention deficit-hyperactivity disorder. *New England Journal of Medicine.* 340(10):780-8, 1999.

Epstein JN. Conners CK. Erhardt D. Arnold LE. Hechtman L. Hinshaw SP. Hoza B. Newcorn JH. Swanson JM. Vitiello B. Familial aggregation of ADHD characteristics. *Journal of Abnormal Child Psychology.* 28(6):585-94, 2000.

Faraone SV. Biederman J. Is attention deficit hyperactivity disorder familial? *Harvard Review of Psychiatry.* 1(5):271-87, 1994.

Gallo A. Gonzalez-Lima F. Sadile AG. Impaired metabolic capacity in the perirhinal and posterior parietal cortex lead to dissociation between attentional, motivational and spatial components of exploration in the Naples High-Excitability rat. *Behavioural Brain Research.* 130(1-2):133-40, 2002.

Gonzalez-Lima F. Cada A. Cytochrome oxidase activity in the auditory system of the mouse: a qualitative and quantitative histochemical study. *Neuroscience.* 63(2):559-78, 1994.

Gonzalez-Lima F. Cada A. Quantitative histochemistry of cytochrome oxidase activity: Theory, methods, and regional brain vulnerability. In Gonzalez-Lima F. (Ed.) *Cytochrome Oxidase in Neural Metabolism and Alzheimer's Disease.* New York: Plenum Press, pp. 55-90, 1998.

Gonzalez-Lima F. Garrosa M. Quantitative histochemistry of cytochrome oxidase in rat brain. *Neuroscience Letters* 123: 251-3, 1991.

Gonzalez-Lima F. Sadile AG. Network operations revealed by brain metabolic mapping in a genetic model of hyperactivity and attention deficit: the Naples high- and low-excitability rats. *Neuroscience & Biobehavioral Reviews.* 24(1):157-60, 2000.

Gonzalez-Lima F. Scheich H. Classical conditioning of tone-signaled bradycardia modifies 2-deoxyglucose uptake patterns in cortex, thalamus, habenula, caudate-putamen and hippocampal formation. *Brain Research.* 363(2):239-56, 1986.

Hall FS. Humby T. Wilkinson LS. Robbins TW. The effects of isolation-rearing on preference by rats for a novel environment. *Physiology & Behavior.* 62(2):299-303, 1997.

Hendley ED. WKHA rats with genetic hyperactivity and hyperreactivity to stress: a review. *Neuroscience & Biobehavioral Reviews.* 24(1):41-4, 2000.

Hevner RF. Duff RS. Wong-Riley MT. Coordination of ATP production and consumption in brain: parallel regulation of cytochrome oxidase and Na+, K(+)-ATPase. *Neuroscience Letters.* 138(1):188-92, 1992.

Hevner RF. Liu S. Wong-Riley MT. A metabolic map of cytochrome oxidase in the rat brain: histochemical, densitometric and biochemical studies. *Neuroscience.* 65(2):313-42, 1995.

Jones D. Gonzalez-Lima F. Crews D. Galef BG Jr. Clark MM. Effects of intrauterine position on the metabolic capacity of the hypothalamus of female gerbils. *Physiology & Behavior.* 61(4):513-9, 1997.

Kolb B. Walkey J. Behavioural and anatomical studies of the posterior parietal cortex in the rat. *Behavioural Brain Research.* 23(2):127-45, 1987.

Leung PWL. Luk SL. Ho TP. Taylor E. Mark FL. Bacon-Shone J. The diagnosis and prevalence of hyperactivity in Chinese schoolboys. *Br J Psychiatry,* 168, 486-96, 1996.

Levy F. Hay DA. McStephen M. Wood C. Waldman I. Attention deficit hyperactivity disorder: A category or a continuum? Genetic analysis of a large-scale twin study. *Journal of the American Academy of Child and Adolescent Psychiatry,* 36, 737-44, 1997.

Magara F. Ricceri L. Wolfer DP. Lipp HP. The acallosal mouse strain I/LnJ: a putative model of ADHD? *Neuroscience & Biobehavioral Reviews.* 24(1):45-50, 2000.

Matelli M. Luppino G. Parietofrontal circuits for action and space perception in the macaque monkey. *Neuroimage.* 14(1 Pt 2):S27-32, 2001.

Nair HP. Berndt JD. Barrett D. Gonzalez-Lima F. Maturation of extinction behavior in infant rats: large-scale regional interactions with medial prefrontal cortex, orbitofrontal cortex, and anterior cingulate cortex. *Journal of Neuroscience.* 21(12):4400-7, 2001.

Nobrega JN. Raymond R. DiStefano L. Burnham WM. Long-term changes in regional brain cytochrome oxidase activity induced by electroconvulsive treatment in rats. *Brain Research.* 605(1):1-8, 1993.

Papa M. Sadile A. Sergeant JA. Shumake J. Gonzalez-Lima F. Functional imaging probes to study the neural bases of behavior in genetic animal models of ADHD: A comparative analysis of short and long-term markers of neuronal activity. In Gonzalez-Lima F. (Ed.) *Cytochrome Oxidase in Neural Metabolism and Alzheimer's Disease.* New York: Plenum Press, pp. 145-69, 1998.

Poremba A. Jones D. Gonzalez-Lima F. Metabolic effects of blocking tone conditioning on the rat auditory system. *Neurobiology of Learning & Memory.* 68(2):154-71, 1997.

Poremba A. Jones D. Gonzalez-Lima F. Functional mapping of learning-related metabolic activity with quantitative cytochrome oxidase histochemistry. In Gonzalez-Lima F. (Ed.) *Cytochrome Oxidase in Neural Metabolism and Alzheimer's Disease.* New York: Plenum Press, pp. 109-44, 1998.

Roberts AC. De Salvia MA. Wilkinson LS. Collins P. Muir JL. Everitt BJ. Robbins TW. 6-Hydroxydopamine lesions of the prefrontal cortex in monkeys enhance performance on an analog of the Wisconsin Card Sort Test: possible interactions with subcortical dopamine. *Journal of Neuroscience.* 14:2531-44, 1994.

Sagvolden T. Sergeant JA. Attention deficit/hyperactivity disorder--from brain dysfunctions to behaviour. *Behavioural Brain Research.* 94(1):1-10, 1998.

Shumake J. Poremba A. Edwards E. Gonzalez-Lima F. Congenital helpless rats as a genetic model for cortex metabolism in depression. *Neuroreport.* 11(17):3793-8, 2000.

Shumake J. Gonzalez-Lima F. Brain systems underlying susceptibility to helplessness and depression. *Behavioral and Cognitive Neuroscience Reviews,* 2: 198-221, 2003.

Swanson JM. Flodman P. Kennedy J. Spence MA. Moyzis R. Schuck S. Murias M. Moriarity J. Barr C. Smith M. Posner M. Dopamine genes and ADHD. *Neuroscience and Biobehavioral Reviews.* 24(1):21-5, 2000.

Sullivan RM. Brake WG. What the rodent prefrontal cortex can teach us about attention deficit/hyperactivity disorder: the critical role of early developmental events on prefrontal function. *Behavioural Brain Research.* 146(1-2):43-55, 2003.

Taylor E. Clinical foundations of hyperactivity research. *Behavioural Brain Research.* 94(1):11-24, 1998.

van Groen T. Kadish I. Wyss JM. Species differences in the projections from the entorhinal cortex to the hippocampus. *Brain Research Bulletin.* 57(3-4):553-6, 2002.

Villarreal JS. Gonzalez-Lima F. Berndt J. Barea-Rodriguez EJ. Water maze training in aged rats: effects on brain metabolic capacity and behavior. *Brain Research.* 939(1-2):43-51, 2002.

Wan RQ. Pang K. Olton DS. Hippocampal and amygdaloid involvement in nonspatial and spatial working memory in rats: effects of delay and interference. *Behavioral Neuroscience.* 108(5):866-82, 1994.

Wong-Riley MTT. Nie F. Hevner RF Liu S. Brain cytochrome oxidase: Functional significance and bigenomic regulation in the CNS. In Gonzalez-Lima F. (Ed.) *Cytochrome Oxidase in Neural Metabolism and Alzheimer's Disease.* New York: Plenum Press, pp. 1-54, 1998.

Willens TE. Biederman J. Spencer TJ. Attention deficit/hyperactivity disorder across the lifespan. *Annual Review of Medicine,* 53, 113-131, 2002.

Wikström M. Krab K. Saraste M. *Cytochrome Oxidase: A Synthesis.* New York: Academic Press, 1981.

Wilson MC. Coloboma mouse mutant as an animal model of hyperkinesis and attention deficit hyperactivity disorder. *Neuroscience & Biobehavioral Reviews.* 24(1):51-7, 2000.

In: Attention Deficit Hyperactivity Disorder Research
Editor: Michelle P. Larimer, pp. 19-58
ISBN 1-59454-156-6

Chapter II

ADHD: Inhibition, Emergent Networks, and Maternal Investment

James Brody[1]
Forum Host and Editor for Evolutionary Psychology and Clinical Sociobiology

Abstract

This chapter is not a survey of new findings but a very different way to view old ones. It extends Barkley's 1997 theory that ADHD is a neurological disorder of impaired executive functions and (1) suggests that ADHD produces many difficulties in small-world social networks, networks where so much is done not only through a friend but also through friends of that friend, and (2) reviews (a) the challenges of a male fetus to his depressed or otherwise less than robust mother and (b) the screening, whether in ADHD assessments of sons or when sizing up prospective husbands, by females of males for the social dependability that is so critical in networks.

Language has been proposed as a vital underpinning for executive functions and ADHD individuals often have difficulty with language but obvious parallels exist between human executive functions and even the behavior of plants: thus, we can reinterpret the theoretical importance of language and look for ADHD individuals to have intact executive functions in specific linguistic and non linguistic areas. That is, ADHD may not always be domain general. We can also look less for difficulties with word retrieval in plans and essays but more for problems in adjusting the relative importance of different ideas and appreciating the mutual influences between them.

The chapter explores a few ramifications for how we assess and treat ADHD. That is, we are not handicapped equally in our adaptive strategies, partnerships level irregularities, and we can expect to find intact abilities in some domains of an ADHD mind that compensate families and mates for their extra work. Behavior genetics reminds us that specific talents appear within families for several generations and that every living

[1]1262 West Bridge St., Spring City, PA 19475. Jbrody@compuserve.com; Forum Host and Editor for Evolutionary Psychology and Clinical Sociobiology, sponsored by Behavior Net. (www.behavior.net/forums/evolutionary)

creature arranges its environment: free will becomes our personal will, sometimes producing peace and satisfaction even for ADHD individuals.

"Children who are excessively active, are unable to sustain their attention, and are deficient in their impulse control to a degree that is deviant for their developmental level are now given the clinical diagnosis of attention deficit/hyperactivity disorder." (ADHD: American Psychiatric Association, 1994 Barkley, 1997, p. 3).

"...ADHD is a developmental disorder of behavioral inhibition that impairs the development of effective self-regulation (executive functioning) and is not, as its name implies, chiefly a disorder of attention." (Barkley, 1997, p. 46).

Attention deficit, hyperactivity disorder (ADHD) most often appears when tasks are prolonged, slow-paced, maintained by delayed reinforcement, or intrinsically boring. Associated difficulties often occur in memory, language, time sensitivity, emotional regulation, and problem solving. These annoyances give the appearance of a disorder that impairs performance regardless of task. This disorder is usually associated with interpersonal rejection, social immaturity, and lifetimes of lesser achievement in comparison with siblings who do not have ADHD.[2]

The first definition reflects our interest in hyperactivity and poor sustained attention as markers for ADHD, the second definition directs us to considerations of self control. The difference is profound. Barkley (1996, 1997) spearheads our shift in focus to lapses in behavioral inhibition especially in regard to prepotent, instinctive behavior that is inhibited in mature individuals while ongoing task-relevant behavior is both sustained and protected from interference.

Conjoining Barkley's ADHD Model with Network Theory and Evolutionary Biology

We are a part of nature, not apart from her.

First, emergent nonrandom networks, a gift from statistical physics, describe wide arrays of social organizations, including those in termites (Fewell, 2003), dolphins (Lusseau, 2003), scientists, words, and neural organizations (Barabasi, 2002). The pervasive character, speed, and expandability of such networks and their potential to shift configurations in relation to resource abundance (including the presence or lack of reciprocal inhibition) strongly suggests they were an essential part of the environments in which humans evolved. Failures in network negotiation, however, shadow many of the failures that we already see in ADHD social careers and very likely parallels similar failures in their neural organization.

Second, this chapter presents some basic ideas from biology as expressed by Raff (1996) and Lewontin (2000): many organisms manage themselves and their environments through

[2] The disorders of ADD-inattentive type, Oppositional Defiant Disorder, Conduct Disorder, and Antisocial Personality Disorders are not discussed here. ADD-inattentive type appears to be a separate disorder although it shares part of its name with ADHD (Barkley, 1996, 1997). The latter three disorders are not an essential part of ADHD but ADHD makes them more noticeable and the latter can make an individual with ADHD more socially objectionable.

inhibition, internalization, prolongation, and reconstitution and in ways that resemble not only human executive functions but also the gambits that genetic sequences follow when they evolve. It will be suggested that the strategies that unite genes, behavior, and human planning reflect a selectionist exploratory system (Gerhart & Kirschner, 1997; Kirschner & Gerhart, 1998) that supports variations in gambits and retains those that work. Thorndike and Skinner would not be surprised!

Third, language, pivotal in Barkley's model, is perhaps less of a cause than he believes but more of an outcome and an emergent, one with reproductive and exploratory functions with which reasoning and planning are loosely attached.

Fourth, the evolutionary concept of maternal investment, both physiological (*in utero* and for the months after birth) and social, describes the processes by which mothers assure the survival of males who will, in turn, invest in the rearing of their own children.

The Barkley Schema For ADHD[3]

Barkley (1990; 1996; 1997) presents a case that ADHD:

(1) Reflects a developmental lag that persists across the life span,

(2) Has pervasive effects on social, academic, and vocational success,

(3) Is not a disorder of attention but one of inhibition. That is, prepotent, perhaps instinctive, behaviors are not suppressed in favor of longer term satisfactions. Similarly, we find impairments in the ability to hold on to a task or a plan and implement it after an interruption.

(4) Is accompanied by linguistic impairments that impede the individual's capacity for contemplation, analysis, and invention.

Inspired by Bronowski (1974; 1977), Barkley argues that failures in neural inhibition lead to failures in "executive functions": self-directed behaviors that are mediated by language and that rest on our capacity to (1) internalize events, (2) prolong them in our mind, (3) separate our feelings from facts, and (4) reconstitute events - breaking them into components and reassembling those components into a different order and with a different set of priorities. Because of mental recombination we can design a better mousetrap while we sit under a tree.

(1) *Neural inhibition* lays the foundation for mental internalization, prolongation, objectification, and reconstitution of external events.

[3]This chapter is sexist but surprising, focusing on males but as seen by females. ADHD is noticed, after all, 2-5 times more frequently in males and diagnosed according to the behaviors that annoy mothers, sisters, and their extended phenotype, schoolteachers. I find that difference to be meaningful, not a measurement artifact. Evolutionary theory and empirical research justify our viewing females as defining the standards for male attainment. Nonetheless, there is substantial overlap in our two genders and, sometimes, individual reversals. Please change some of my pronouns from "he" to "she" as it may suit you.

(2) *Internalization* refers to the representation of external events not only on chalk board or stone carvings but also within our minds.

(3) *Objectification* detaches emotionality from factual material. We categorize events by their physical attributes, consequences, and timing rather than how we feel about them. A mental bin specific to "food" probably has selective advantages over one for "things that make me mad."

(4) *Reconstitution* consists of analysis and synthesis. We break apart events from each other and recombine them. For example, should I go to my favorite bank, cafe, and printer in three trips to the same neighborhood or save time and fuel and make only one trip that includes all three destinations?

I suggest that executive functions are also important because they manage our network standing in relation to our social and physical environments: we become more sensitive to indirect influences while retaining awareness of our immediate setting.

Networks: Sociality at any Scale[4]

> "I'm not a big-picture kind of guy and had a lot of trouble in web design where I had to be aware of several projects moving along at the same time. My current job lets me process short transactions, once and done." Anon, 2004.

"Fit(ness)" applies to the match between an organism and its environment (Paul, 1992; Dawkins 1982). A lot of that match depends on the organism's capacity for managing both itself and its settings. Parents, siblings, and peers are a significant aspect of our environment and humans sometimes compete but in a clever way, competing to build cooperation. Our children are assessed in regard to social skills first by females who may or may not be kin and often by non related, dominant females. (Male judgments occur later.) Skillfully connecting and disconnecting social ties may be more salient for survival than the intact ability to see and in living cells or school yards, interactions between genes and network politics influence the fate of each player. After all, losing one participant is less damaging than losing the entire network (Watts & Strogatz, 1998; Barabasi, 2002) and groups of children make this choice every day. I suggest that ADHD can, therefore, be seen as a disorder of connectivity: new options for special situations are not incorporated into the preexisting behavioral routines. Thus, ADHD, an outcome linked to difficulties in behavioral inhibition, also becomes a disorder of organization, one wherein the liabilities within a mind parallel the liabilities found in external social relationships and physical environments. Messy desks do, indeed, reflect messy minds. Emergent nonrandom networks may underlie what happens in our heads, book bags, and homes.

[4]The following paragraphs were adapted from Brody, 2004.

Some Basics of Emergent Random Networks

A video, *ADHD in Adults,* features "Pat" who gives a tour of her home. One room is cluttered behind its closed door: the bed is a storage shelf for fabric, clothing, and sewing materials, several years' of school reports for her son march across the floor, the closet contents moved forever to the open floor after her husband repaired some pipes. Barkley remarks: "For most people with ADHD, life is much like Pat's room - poorly organized and highly random." (Barkley, 1994a)

Emergent network enthusiasts find similar rules in an extraordinary array of events, rules that apply when speed and access are important, fit hand-in-glove not only with modern genetics and physics but also sociology and common sense. The implications are substantial for neurology, psychology, psychiatry, sociology, ecology, and evolutionary biology.[5] Emergent networks have also provoked empirical study by a multitude of independent teams (introductions available in Barabasi, 2002; Buchanan, 2002; Strogatz, 2003).

One important thing about emergent networks is that *similar functional relationships occur between the members of an emergent network and often do so regardless of the nature of those members.* We easily find similar emergent networks in societies of humans (Granovetter, 1973; Watts & Strogatz, 1998), insects (Fewell, 2003), and dolphins (Lusseau, 2003). Emergent networks are also found in cellular biochemistry, assemblies of genes, scientific citation patterns, the ties between actors, computer scientists, mathematicians, or physicists, and even within electrical power grids: a few key individuals link vast numbers of their peers (Barabasi, 2002; Buchanan, 2002).

This section is about *nonrandom emergent* networks that consist of nodes and the links between them (Barabasi, 2002). In contrast to random networks, emergent networks grow (thus, the adjective *emergent*) and incoming nodes are preferentially attached to nodes that already have the most links (therefore, *nonrandom*). In Barabasi's memorable phrase, "the rich get richer," and often, "the first get richer." The outcome is that in many emergent networks, there are a few nodes with many connections and many nodes with only one or two. Three kinds of emergent network are useful for this chapter: clustered, hierarchic, and winner-take-all (Barabasi, 2002; Buchanan, 2002; Strogatz, 2003, Watts, 2002; 2004). These arrangements, taken together, may be states in an oscillator, driven by resource availability (Brody, 2004; Watts, 2004), but for illustrative purposes, I treat them here as distinct events.

Clusters: Independent Neighborhoods

Individuals in clusters are guided by two kinds of local environments: those provided by their nearest conspecific and those provided by their physical environments. The awareness of individual workers is apt to be myopic rather than synoptic: communities result not from a

[5] Emergent networks promise an understanding of (1) the fact of seamless integration between different sensory qualities of color, shape, shade, and even words and odors and their contexts and (2) how such integration is achieved by widely scattered locations in the brain (Gazzaniga, 1992). Edelman (1987), for example, introduced the concept of "reentrant signaling" between separate communities of neural clusters. Each local neural community both influences and is influenced by other communities that manage a slightly different aspect of a sensation, action, or memory (Edelman, 1999; Gazzaniga, 1992; Tononi, 1994; Sporns, 1994; Singer, 1994; Sacks, 1987). Injury sometimes leads to perceptual voids because interconnecting axons are sheared, fragmenting the islands that still function.

master planner but from the compounded interactions between hundreds or thousands of participants, each of whom is guided by his immediate neighbors and setting (Camazine, Deneubourg, Franks, Sneyd, Theraulaz, & Bonabeau, 2001. See also Pinker, 2002 & Sowell, 1987 for application of these concepts to political philosophies). Most connections in the brains of *C elegans*, cats, and rhesus are local: small specialized circuits in a mind allow it to detect and track minute environmental changes (Gazzaniga, 1992; Tononi, 1994; Edelman & Tononi, 2000; Camazine et al, 2001).

The traditional urban neighborhood is composed of clusters, united by family and cultural traits, somewhat independent of the larger neighborhood or city except in festivals, crises, and sporting events. Because of sustained personal contacts and immediate consequences, ADHD individuals should do better in emergent social clusters that exist because of similarities between their members. This prediction matches how ADHD interacts with teacher liveliness and organization, class size, task activity, and immediate reinforcement (Barkley, 1990, 1997).

Small-World Networks

> "Models of dynamical systems with small-world coupling display enhanced signal propagation speed, computational power, and synchronizability." (Watts & Strogatz, 1998, p. 440.)

Speed, power, and interface could be the evolutionary value in small-world organizations. But first, three small-world anecdotes:

(1) Knock on a speakeasy door, whisper "Nick sent me" and the door opened.
(2) My son, his wife, and my grandson, Colin, live near Boston. I feel closer to them when I listen to a Boston radio station late at night.
(3) Russ Barkley's 1997 book, and his arrangements of the data therein, emerged from his nearly accidental reading on a flight Jacob Bronowski's 1977 book, *A Sense of the Future*, and a 1974 essay, "On the biological nature of language," included therein.

Clusters are centers of intimacy between immediate neighbors who adjust to each other and to their local environment but separate clusters can also be synchronized into a "small-world network." A cluster of five friends may connect to five other clusters, each one perhaps through a different member of the original cluster. For example, if a New Yorker develops one contact in Tokyo, he also gains second, third, and fourth degree contact with other people in Tokyo. Shortcuts between separate clusters allow (1) average path length in the network to be small, (2) local neighborhoods to retain their specialization, and (3) the total number of participants to be quite large (Watts & Strogatz, 1998).[6] They offer, therefore, advantages of speed, detail, and power. They are also quite resistant to random attacks.

Small-world networks are observed in cellular biochemistry, assemblies of genes, scientific citation patterns, electrical power grid connections, the social ties between actors,

[6]One misleading aspect of clusters is that most of the participants are unaware of the scope of their connections to other individuals: thus, the phrase "small-world phenomenon."

computer scientists, mathematicians, and physicists, and even the spread of sexually transmitted diseases: a few key individuals link vast numbers of their peers. These effects are also seen in language. Cancho and Solé found, based on the 100 million word collection of the *British National Corpus*, that 2.67 steps connect any two words in British English. (Cited in Albert & Barabasi, 2001. See also Strogatz 2003.) Yook, Jeong, & Barabasi (2001) linked words if they were synonyms according to the Merriam-Webster Dictionary. The average path length was 4.5 for a cluster of 22,311 words, the clustering coefficient was 0.7, far larger than the value of 0.0006 for a random network of the same size. (See also Albert & Barabasi, 2001.)[7]

Some language from network physics will help (Barabasi, 2002; Buchanan, 2002, Strogatz, 2003). First, *nodes* can be individuals, a business, a web page, or an amino acid. Second, *links* connect the nodes and may consist of telephone lines, letters,

Internet links, or the metabolic paths in a cell or the feeding relationships in an ecosystem. Finally, nodes with many connections are known as *hubs*.

Even though there are a million participants, small-world connectivity allows any node to be only 3 to 6 steps away from any other node. Thus, small-world networks allow for the rapid collection and distribution of information even when the total network is quite large. (Watts & Strogatz, 1998, graph these relationships. See also Barabasi, 2002.)

By means of sparse connections between clusters, a field of crickets, or a swarm of fireflies chirp, or flash in unison in much the same ways as humans synchronized by the evening news (Watts & Strogatz, 1998; Barabasi, 2002; Buchanan, 2002; Strogatz, 2003). Within our brains, there are massive numbers of clusters but many axons travel a little further within a brain area, and still others make bundles that go to separate nuclei (Barabasi, 2002). Longer connections between distant clusters stitch our many sensations into one fabric. Consciousness evolves and we can drive the car while tuning the radio or thinking about ADHD.

Winner-Take-All Networks

Patterns of inter-connectivity appear to be sensitive to resource availability: dictators and black holes emerge in hard times when one hub sets the pace for all others and network organizations simplify. Early settlers (such as the biochemical, ATP) often collect more links than do later ones. That is, one hub maintains its percentage of the total number of links in a network regardless of competition: the dominant hub is so fit that newcomers cannot displace it (Barabasi, 2002). Barabasi applies the phrase "Winner-take-all" to these networks.

Winner-take-all was also used by Frank & Cook (1995) to describe the economic outcomes of high quality industrial reproduction (each copy is as good as the original), mass familiarity, and market domination by an existing product: one manufacturer or brand then swamps all competitors. Barabasi (2002) compares winner-take-all to black holes and applies the metaphor to Microsoft's dominance of operating systems for personal computers.[8]

---

[7]Gerhart & Kirschner (1997) describe metazoan evolution as the conservation of core metabolic patterns in every cell while adding small differences that manage a specific environment. Power law organizations appear to be consistent with those requirements.

[8]"Black hole" can be misleading to the same degree as other labels such as "the rich get richer" or "winner-take-all." The popular implication is that of an organization that consumes all resources. The meaning is more restricted,

Winner-take-all fits dominance hierarchies when the *alpha* either inhibits reproduction in subordinates or eats their young: the winner really does "take all." These effects have been seen in hens, cows, ponies, fish, crabs, lobsters, crayfish, lizards, frogs, rats, primates, and social insects (See Camazine et al, 2001, p. 456 for references that span from Schjelderup-Ebbe in 1913 to Heinze 1994. Price, 1967, and Stevens & Price, 2000, describe depression as reactions to defeat in dominance contests, an outcome that could result from loss or actually work in favor of an undisputed leader.) We might also expect to find winner-take-all in some human hierarchies such as those in religions, sciences, and artistic traditions. Whatever is first accumulates resources and denies them to whatever is second. Even without growing beaks or fur or buying *Windows*, we can experience black holes when we have obsessions: powerful ideas that direct our lives, resist competition, and consume disproportionate assets. We also find them in communal fads, social movements, or dictatorships. These things, like ADHD, appear through a failure of inhibition. And we might expect ADHD individuals to be more easily fixated within black holes when demands are clear and there is a high ratio of regimented models who also deliver prompt consequences for deviance. These organizations may come from the political left or right, whether communists or brownshirts.

ADHD is Consistent with Failure to Achieve a Stable Small-World Configuration

We find small-world networks everywhere and their abundance hints of their likely importance in our evolutionary history: we would not be what we are if we did not evolve within their boundaries. Furthermore, some of their attraction is that small world networks occur widely in computer simulations and statistical physics: the organizations that we find in our heads follow the same rules that we observe in very tiny worlds or stellar ones. We have a sun surrounded by planets, not by other suns, we can generally think about one or two things at a time. Again, we are a part of nature, not apart from her.[9]

To the extent that ADHD individuals have difficulty with small-world networks, we can expect them to have difficulty not only with external social organizations but also internal ones as when putting ideas in proper sequence in paragraphs or essays or when emphasizing or minimizing concepts in relation to each other. Trivial and major ideas achieve equal importance. Connecting words, the "ands," "buts," and "therefores," and many prepositions may show inconsistent or deviant uses, or will be forgotten entirely, by ADHD writers. Paragraphs may not have suitable endings that connect them to other paragraphs. The difficulty is not simply one of word retrieval, but of adjusting the relationships between the words, sentences, and paragraphs.

Small-world networks follow a power law distribution: that is, a few major hubs have many connections but most participants have only one to three (Watts, 2002; Barabasi, 2002;

---

however, in the less popular sense of one hub's retaining a constant percentage of links, regardless of new arrivals and competition from other hubs. (Bianconi & Barabasi, 2000).

[9] I remember Alessandra Lippucci and I giving talks on phase transitions and politics. We talked afterwards. I was fascinated not only with her but also with my awareness of engaging three conversations at once. I have never before or since been so awake.

Strogatz, 2003, Buchanan, 2002; Murray, 2003).[10] Power laws tell us to expect unlimited numbers of small events but very few large ones in an ecosystem: ants and termites are far more numerous than jaguars, orangutans, or elephants. Michelangelo, Isaac Newton, Albert Einstein, Babe Ruth, and Tiger Woods are rarer than the average dauber, dabbler, sports fan, or handicap player. Google, or, for that matter, major extinctions in mature ecosystems, large earthquakes, or grand mal seizures within the nervous system are comparatively infrequent events (Bak, 1996; Kauffman, 2000; Barabasi, 2002; Strogatz 2003).

The surprising aspect of small-worlds is how closely tied every participant is to all the other participants. For example, despite differences in size and population, elephants and ants are closer neighbors than we might expect because species in large ecosystems are generally connected by two links on food chains. About six links will connect any two Americans, four to six connect most scientists, and 19 links will take you from any web page to any one of a billion others (Barabasi, 2002). These relationships also hold forth in small wet places: forty-three species were mapped for the average number of links between chemicals in their cells. Regardless of species size, the number is approximately three: a few molecules participate in the majority of the reactions but most participate in only one or two (Albert & Barabasi, 2001; Barabasi, 2002).

Hubs collect assets that stabilize both itself and its partners. The network becomes more resilient as new arrivals fill ever smaller niches and refine both energy and raw materials in ever more diverse but efficient ways. Thus, the many small refinements connected to a hub smooth the pace of development as each new specialization handles one or two annoyances but for a couple of hubs and an ever larger collection of other nodes. Unfortunately, ADHD individuals show difficulty with remote antecedents and consequences and should exhibit even greater difficulties with the indirect ones. Lessened participation in small-world networks precludes benefiting from network resilience: The individual, instead alternates from local clusters to winner-take-all as his mind centers only on himself or only on a media event.

First, the ADHD child's immediate neighbors in a work group will have more influence on him than his teacher in the center of the room. The idea in front of him may swamp his awareness of its dominance of or submission to other ideas. Summaries and outlines that depend on those relationships become impossible for him to construct. Rephrasing becomes difficult and we can expect more quoting of more sources and less condensation of those

[10]These organizations have been noticed before. Clustering applies to some of the phenomena managed by Adam Smith's concept of an "invisible hand." (See description of clustering in economics and politics in Sowell, 1987, and Pinker, 2002). Vilfredo Pareto, an Italian economist, noticed that approximately 80% of the wealth is controlled by 20% of the population but the percentages can vary during relative prosperity or collapse. Pareto's observations may be one of the first expressions of a power law. Lotka (1926) used them to compare scientific productivity: bell curve distributions describe performances averaged for many participants but Lotka curves (power laws) rank individuals by their degree of success: a few attain extraordinary influence (Murray, 2003). Sewall Wright in the 1920s used clustering to account for speciation in small herds of farm stock and intermittent crossbreeding (sparse interconnections) to prevent the expression of undesirable recessive traits from too much inbreeding. (Sagan & Druyan, 1992; Provine, 1986/1989). Granovetter (1973) applied the concept to social contacts and job referrals (cited in Barabasi, 2002; Strogatz, 2003). Many social scientists and some biologists (e.g., Fewell, 2003) view "gene" explanations as inadequate for understanding social behavior but now take to network theory which is even more reductionist than genetics.

quotes into a single statement. If they are going to tell one part, they have to tell the entire thing and may prefer not to make the attempt.

Second, we can expect ADHD individuals to have difficulty not only with remote connections between themselves and partners but also with the partners of those partners. This flaw has never been assessed by ADHD researchers. (The advantages of an emergent network lie not with your immediate contacts but with everyone and everything with which your friends are connected. Remember Granovetter (1973): job leads often come not from friends but from friends of friends.) In addition, ADHD individuals should also have difficulty maintaining their property because of the many indirect, delayed, external influences (taxes, zoning, weathering, erosion, weeds, drainage from surrounding developments, contractors, cost of supplies) these are all parallel developmental cascades that impinge on each component of their assets. Messy rooms sometimes have extended rings of confusion that escort their occupant forever.

Third, because of network instability, both internal and cognitive, we can expect ADHD minds to oscillate between the extremes of self-centered participation in a local cluster and being swept up in the fads of a winner-take-all.[11] Small-world stability evolves through the mutual relationships between their participants but individuals with ADHD can be undependable if their likely partners are too remote in time and place. The exclusion, however, works in two directions but for different reasons: other people exclude ADHD individuals as unreliable and ADHD individuals may frequently be unaware of the extended networks one step beyond their friend or supervisor or, if aware, so not sense their importance and want no part of them. We can understand why, on the one hand, ADHD individuals are more successful in the immediacy of self-employment in a job they chose and in "McJobs" wherein there are many brief, immediate contingencies but in seriatum. On the other hand, they are less successful when decisions must be tempered by remote outcomes and participants.

Failures of Inhibition and Winner-Take-All

> "Organisms are extremely internally heterogeneous. Their states and motions are consequences of many intersecting causal pathways, and it is unusual that normal variation in any one of these pathways has a strong effect on the outcome. To be ill is precisely to be dominated by a single causal chain. To be obsessed by an *idée* fixe which motivates all one's actions, or to be convinced that all behavior on the part of others, without distinction, is hostile, is a form of mental illness...Indeed, we may define 'normality' as the condition in which no single pathway controls the organism." (Lewontin, 2000, pp. 93-94).

Lewontin understands ADHD and an array of other stereotypic disorders.

Inhibition modulates the frequency and intensity of current behavior, sets the opportunities for new behavior, or delays, suppresses, or adjusts the priority of primitive, less

[11] Strogatz (2003) is a fascinating, readable discussion of synchrony between similar oscillators: events (no matter how many) that are similar, repetitive, and weakly connected eventually come obey Kuramoto's rule and come into synchrony. Watts (2004) also pursues these phenomena.

mature, all-or-none ones. Disrupt those inhibitory systems and the underlying organizations become more ratcheted and impulsive. Four (of many possible) diverse examples show these effects and hint of an underlying unity that we have seen expressed in Barkley's model for ADHD and Raff's for developmental evolution:[12]

(1) Bipolar (manic depressive) disorder, characterized by sudden, extreme changes in moods, goals, and activity level can emerge after even mild head injuries (Robinson & Jorge, 2002). Such injuries might be expected to disrupt inhibitory connections between neural clusters. Further, both head injuries and repeated bipolar episodes are associated with deterioration in sustained attention (Cavanagh, Van Beck, Muir, & Blackwood, 2002; Clark, Iversen, & Goodwin, 2002; Ferrier & Thompson, 2002). The individual becomes more impulsive, selfish, and immature.

(2) Pennington (1991) observes that executive functions are perhaps the most newly evolved and, therefore, depend most on both the inhibition and synchronization of underlying systems. Disruption should bring stereotypy in both thoughts and conduct.

(3) Kauffman (1993; 1995) finds that chaotic and orderly arrangements differ by the number of interconnections between their participants. An average of fewer than two links characterizes chaotic organizations: there is little or no organization. An average of three or more links produces very orderly structures. The phase transition, wherein power laws operate, lies between an average of 2-3 interconnections. That is, sever constraints and many islands of independent activity appear.[13] Apply more than just a handful of restrictions and every network participant becomes Gulliver in Lilliputia: all tied down and going nowhere.

(4) Bianconi (Bianconi & Barabasi, Barabasi, 2002) converted emergent networks into terms from quantum physics. That is, the fitness of nodes corresponds to quantum energy levels in a Bose gas in a manner also similar to that of electron shells.[14] This translation finds that hubs have lower energy levels but isolated nodes, perhaps analogous to an outer electron shell, have higher. Bianconi's ideas suggest the counterintuitive notion that hub size varies inversely with system energy: *the fewer the resources, the larger but also the simpler the organization.*

Winner-take-all arrangements monopolize system resources: many smaller units pay the organizational cost of the large one. Alternative ideas are both less probable and more expensive, their extra cost no longer paid by their greater sensitivity to local variations in

---

[12]Some of this material was adapted from Brody (2004).

[13] See Brody, 2002, for an application of these ideas to an evolutionary model of psychiatric diagnosis and treatment. Mental disorders can be seen as falling to either side of a phase boundary in networks that separates constraint from mobility.

resources. A winner-take-all situation may reflect the same statistical payoffs that favor *WalMart* over *Sears*, the Internet over real life stores, *Verizon* over your local telephone company, or the Third Reich over the Weimar Republic. Declining wealth predicts dictatorships that may come from the left or right.

The behavior that we see may parallel the organizations that we will find within a mind. Winner-take-all networks could underlie what we observe in Obsessive Compulsive Disorder, Tourette's Syndrome, and Attention deficit, Hyperactivity Disorder as well as explosive or homicidal behaviors, panic or eating disorders, hypochondria, depression, delusions, personality disorders, false memories, or powerful ideas such as those found in hypnotic states, love, religious ecstasy, and scientific quests. The rigidity of these phenomena can also be expected to increase after an injury or during infections, hunger, or fatigue. We can also expect winner-take-all to shadow what we call "strong reciprocity" that emerges in times of declining resources: a social group not only punishes competing beliefs but also any loyalist who fails to punish defectors (Gintis, 2000).

Thus, observations from the study of mutations, psychopathology, learning disorders, network analyses, and quantum physics are mutually consistent and reinforce common sense: choice declines when resources fail. Conversely, behavioral flexibility appears to be rare, expensive, and easily disrupted. As we have seen in other kinds of networks, moderate amounts of cross-talk between distributed clusters may prevent overreactions while supporting the organism's sensitivity to small changes. Increase cross-talk and networks freeze. Reduce cross-talk and behavior becomes more ratcheted when simpler ideas compete with each other in a winner-take-all manner (Brody, 2002).

We can expect ADHD individuals to:

- Become followers in winner-take-all arrangements,
- Be among the first to experience resource erosion during economic slumps,
- Require more explicit reminders of social standing (such as uniforms and rank),
- Function better in the rapid events and immediate consequences in private businesses when the ADHD individual is the hub, and
- When there are commissions rather than salaries.

Female Investment and Impulsiveness[15]

"There are no perfect fruitflies." Lewontin, 1961.

There should be: after all, sexual selection corrects genetic variation and female *Drosophila* have been choosing between their males for a very long time. Developmental noise and genetic variation, however, continually produce new defects or replay the old ones and daughters repeat the decisions of their mothers and once more separate fools from

[14] Bose and Einstein derived predictions that molecules in gases near absolute zero (-273 degrees K) will act as a single molecule. A case can be made that a loss of resources in social systems and in individual participants leads to greater stereotypy: individuals can be treated as identical and interchanged with one another.

[15] Some of this material is from Brody (2001).

geniuses. *Some of the variation in the fitness of sons, however, may arise from variation in the fitness of their mothers in ways that do not relate to any specific DNA sequence.* ADHD may be due not only to genes but also the uterine contexts in which the genes develop.

Mothers and wives sometimes scrimp on what they spend on their males.

In polygamous species such as humans, competing genes from fathers and mothers wrestle in the uterine arena. Females who expect to have several different mates invest less in the fetus fathered by any one of them but males, who can get children from several mothers, want the largest offspring possible regardless of costs to any one mother and the offspring that she might have with a different male. Paternal imprinted genes favor larger placentas and fetuses that take a greater control of maternal blood pressure and glucose (Haig, 1993; 2002). They also produce, if unopposed, nonviable fetuses with small amounts of neocortex but excess hypothalamic and muscle tissue. Maternal imprinted genes, if unopposed in fetal mice, produce neonates with large amounts of neocortex but less hypothalamic and muscle tissue (Keverne, Fundele, Narasimha, Barton, & Surani, 1996).

Maternal investment, particularly in an immature, subordinate, or an older mother is further compromised by stress, drought, or famine. Along similar lines, maternal anxiety, depression, physical immaturity, illness, low intelligence, socioeconomic status, and smoking may be correlated impaired maternal fitness (in both the network and the traditional meanings) and raise the probability of ADHD (Barkley, 1990) and related disorders.[16]

Whether for rhesus, chimp, or human infants, mothers, aunts, and grandmothers exert a quality control function on male social behavior; hyperactive young males who fail to learn are evicted prematurely by the matriline and die (Suomi, 1999. See below.) Young human males are assessed not only by mothers but also by maternal relatives and their extended phenotypes that include teachers and doctors.

We should not be surprised that mothers, more than fathers, and more for sons than for daughters, arrange for doctor visits, tutoring, and special education services. *We should also not be surprised that most diagnoses of ADHD behavior depend on rating scales completed by females.* The cumulative effect on human evolution has been that of a selective "exploratory system": lots of responses are made by a developing entity and some of them are repeated but many others discarded as a function of results (Kirschner & Gerhart, 1998; see below for further discussion of this important idea). Evolution should work in directions that allow more efficiency: that is, less wasted investment on failed attempts. Female scrutiny of lovers and sons by the same criteria works in that direction.

We can expect a mother who has children with several different males to have a higher risk for bearing children with ADHD even if she is not impulsive herself.

Given that having sons exerts greater costs on mothers than having daughters, we can expect the youngest of a series of brothers to be at a greater risk for ADHD.

We might also predict that socially subordinate females and those of lower socioeconomic status (SES), even if not impulsive, will have more ADHD children and for the risk to be even higher for mothers who are both subordinate and of low SES.

---

[16]On the other hand, maternal investment can be amplified by aunts and grandmothers (Suomi, 1999; Lahdenpera, Lummaa, Helle, Tremblay, & Russell, 2004; Hawkes, 2004).

Sons and Lovers: What Women Want

> "With notable exceptions the study of female choice has limited itself to showing that females are selected to decide if a partner is of the right species, of the right sex, and sexually mature. While the adaptive value of such choices is obvious, the adaptive value of subtler discriminations among broadly appropriate males is much more difficult to visualize or document. One needs both theoretical arguments for the adaptive value of such female choice and detailed data on how females choose." Trivers, 1972/2002, pp. 94-95.

> "Where the male invests parental care, female choice...should also involve, perhaps primarily involve, questions of the male's willingness and ability to be a good parent. Will he invest in the offspring? If willing, does he have the ability to contribute much?" (Trivers, 1972/2002, p. 96).

There is a 2-3 times greater occurrence of ADHD in males than in females and suggestions are made that our assessments are gender biased and unfair to an equal number of girls who also have ADHD (Barkley, 1996). *Evolutionary biology suggests, however, that the difference is not an artifact*: mothers of every generation must ask the same questions about her sons and lovers because males vary more and may, indeed, express more ADHD, than females.

Hrdy (1999) describes vitality, plumpness, hairiness, and even a close resemblance to the father as means to pass the first inspections that human mothers make in different cultures. Sons, however, are more variable than daughters for a staggering range of characteristics (Miller, 2000; Pinker, 2002) and bear the greater focus of maternal scrutiny (Trivers, 1972).

More human males are conceived than delivered (1.6-1.2/1 vs. 1.05/1, Spreen, Risser & Edgell ,1995) sometimes due to allergic reactions between mother and her son (Spreen et al, 1995). Infants that pass maternal physiological standards are carried to full term and have fewer developmental impairments, less impulsive behavior, and higher IQs (Spreen et al, 1995).

Human mothers abort children or put them up for adoption in relation to paternal fitness and investment, and economic conditions (Hrdy, 1999) but they abort sons more than daughters in drought, famine, or changes in maternal social dominance (Kruuk, Clutton-Brock, Albon, Pemberton, & Guinness, 1999).

There are other signs of how much males cost for females.[17] In one pre-industrial society, a daughter lengthens the mother's life by an average of 23 weeks, a son shortens it by an average of 34 (Helle, Lummaa, & Jokela. 2002). In other studies, sons have more problems at delivery apart from their larger size (Lieberman, Lang, Cohen, Frigoletto, Acker, & Rao, 1997), often require longer gestation (Divon, Ferber, Nissell, & Westgren, 2003), sometimes trigger immune reactions in mothers (Blanchard, 2001; Spreen et al, 1995), and have higher rates of infant mortality (Spreen et al, 1995). More sons are born in the spring (Cagnacci, Renzi, Arangino, Alessandrini, & Volpe, 2003) and usually to younger mothers (Trivers & Willard, 1973). A series of brothers often predicts that the youngest will have greater

[17]These studies are often preliminary and not systematically replicated. The absence of experimental controls makes it easy to assemble a case from sand as I might have unintentionally done here.

fluctuating asymmetry (Lalumière, Harris, & Rice, 1999), a greater risk for being homosexual (Blanchard, 2001; Cohen, 1999), and some greater risk for psychopathology (Herrell, Goldberg, True, Ramakrishnan, Lyons, Eisen, & Tsuang, 1999; Fergusson, Horwood, & Beautrais,1999). Small males at birth are less likely to marry (Phillips, Handelsman, Eriksson, Forsen, Osmond, & Barker, 2001). Further, children with physical defects are more likely targets for institutionalization and abandonment (Buss, 1999) or parental abuse and infanticide (Daly & Wilson, 1981; 1988). We, again, expect males to show the greater numbers of defects and to die earlier.

There is little recognition, however, that female choices seen at mating are applied again just after birth and are continued for the next three decades. Human females assess both sons and lovers for health, social prowess, and the ability to acquire resources to share them. Males are next examined for economic standing, political skill, strength, and intelligence: all of them foundations for his willingness to invest in children and his ability to do so (Buss, 1998; 2003; La Cerra, 1994).[18]

Male variability is constrained by sexual selection: (1) competitions between males with each other and (2) the choices made by females at mating time (Bateman, 1948; Trivers, 1972; Buss, 1998; 2000, 2003; Judson, 2002). Males, therefore, sometimes have great gifts and sometimes great handicaps or, sometimes, combinations of both. Thus, sons face demands to get along with women who separate the gifted from the bizarre, the dependable from the psychopaths. The one assessment we observe in research on ADHD, the other from mate selection data. That is, *the rating scales for ADHD reflect the mating preferences of women, suggesting that female standards for husbands are also applied to their male offspring as mothers screen them for kindness, cooperation, cleverness, and strength - reasonable predictors for later paternal investment.*

The Big Impairment: Fitness in Networks

> "ADHD should be found to reduce the survival and reproductive advantage conveyed by the executive functions and self-regulation when observed to operate over substantial time periods of an evolutionary scale." Barkley, 1997, p. 304.

> "It's more important that my son have good friends rather than good grades." Anon.

I once asked a mother that if she had to choose, would she opt for academics or peer acceptance for her hyperactive son. I was puzzled for several decades about her preference. What we now know of emergent networks, however, strongly agrees with her position and suggests that she spoke from evolutionary good sense although her husband might have made the opposite choice.

The ADHD literature documents the connectivity problems of preschool, elementary, adolescent, and adult individuals with ADHD. ADHD children may be assessed within 20 minutes by their peers as untrustworthy and unreliable (Barkley, 1997). Sixty percent of

[18]A man feeding an infant is rated as more attractive by women. A woman feeding an infant has no effect on the ratings that she gets from men (La Cerra, 1994).

ADHD children argue with authority and 30 percent develop conduct disorder, associated with fighting and property destruction. ADHD individuals, generally males, are apt to die sooner and experience more accidents (Barkley, 1990). (Rhesus mothers could share stories with their human equivalents.) These impairments appear in preschool, elementary, and secondary school and continue after graduation (Weiss & Hechtman, 1993; Barkley, 1990, 1996). Network theory accommodates these phenomena with a refurbished concept of biological "fitness."

Fitness, however, is one of the most controversial words in evolutionary biology and has meant, at different times, the "fit" between an organism and its environment, the number of years the organism survived, the number of children that it produced, or the number that it reared to adulthood, or the number that it reared to reproduce, or the number of copies of a particular gene in the population (Paul, 1992; Dawkins, 1989). Emergent network theory suggests the first definition can be resurrected and be both useful and less provocative to social egalitarians.

"Fitness" is a composite in network definitions: it first refers to the number of links connected to a node (an environmental feature, whether living or dead). The more connections, the greater the fitness and hubs that have lots of links have a recruiting advantage when new members join the network. There are four implications: (1) connection to a node brings specialized resources that make a hub more adaptable, (2) networks can stabilize relationships between participants, (3) phylogenetically older components have greater power to channel development, and (4) attacks on hubs can be more disruptive than assaults on nodes: three strategic strikes might destroy a network that resists 100 or 1000 random attacks (Watts & Strogatz, 1998; Barabasi, 2002).

There is, second, a *fitness connectivity product*: the number of links at a defined moment is multiplied by the rate at which the node makes new links (Barabasi, 2002) and the payoffs, including winner-take-all outcomes, can be huge for incorporating lots of links. *Google* and *Yahoo* are contemporary examples. A fitness connectivity product describes the marketing success of a new invention or might apply to the growth of a fast-growing attachment, whether a love or a cancer. Palm Pilot displaced Newton, Boeing displaced DeHavilland (Barabasi, 2002) and spooning with Cindy Lou temporarily replaces football with the guys. Fitness varies, then, both in relation to the number of your existing partners and your rate of recruiting new ones.

The network conception of fitness can be applied to relationships between individuals or between any organism and the features of its environment. Most humans are network creatures, stabilized by peers, family, and even total strangers but handicapped when socially isolated even in solitary confinement, asylums, and sensory deprivation experiments. (Maguire & Troisi, 1998; Brody, 2000, 2002). ADHD individuals, if alone, will also be more variable, helpless, and erratic sometimes to the point of being bizarre. ADHD individuals, however, are not only isolated but help to create their isolation in the first place.

ADHD Careers and Network Fitness

> "William Pelham and Mary Bender (1982) estimate that over 50% of ADHD children have significant problems in social relationships with other children. Mothers (Campbell & Paulauskas, 1979), teachers (Barkley, DuPaul, & McMurray, in press-a), and peers (Johnson, Pelham, & Murphy, 1985; Pope, Pierman, & Mumma, 1989) report hyperactive children to be significantly more aggressive, disruptive, domineering, intrusive, noisy, and socially rejected than normal children, especially if they are male hyperactives (Milich & Landau, 1982; Pelham & Bender, 1982). Investigators who have directly observed these peer interactions suggest that the inattentive, disruptive, off-task, immature, and provocative behaviors of ADHD children quickly elicit a pattern of controlling and directive behavior from their peers when they must work together...In their communication patterns, ADHD children in these studies have been found to talk more but to be less efficient in organizing and communicating information to peers with whom they are asked to work. Morever (sic), despite talking more, the ADHD children are less likely to respond to the questions or verbal interactions of their peers. Hence there is less reciprocity in the social exchanges of hyperactive children with their peers..." Barkley (1990, p. 84).

These are network phenomena and there are cross-species similarities.

Suomi (2000; see also 1999) reports careers in young rhesus that resemble ADHD. Infant males are usually reared for two years by matrilines of mother, aunts, and grandmothers as well as dominant, non related females. Males who do not make eye contact but get into endless fights and some of them with larger opponents, and attempt leaps that are beyond their ability are evicted after their first year to death in the jungle. Those who pass the social inspection of their mothers are kept for a second year before graduation to male troops for further selection, ranking, and training. In laboratory studies, Suomi (2000, 1999) curtailed maternal investment, rearing young rhesus with siblings and peers but not with mothers. These youngsters became hyperactive and more easily addicted to alcohol.

In the case of humans:

(1) Young males are reared in groups of female relatives and their extended phenotypes (teachers, counselors, pediatricians, and psychologists).

(2) Maternal/aunt/grandmother/teacher investment can last several decades. Commitment will vary in accord with the child's cleverness, reciprocity, and social consistency as well as with the mother's resources.

(3) Oppositional sons and impaired maternal consistency often occur together. Eviction from maternal protection is associated with reduced social and academic achievement. Socialization is handled by special education and alternative schools that remove disruptive males from mainstream society. Severe externalizing behaviors (defiance, antisocial behavior, and extreme mood swings) are often associated with eviction from day care and eventually from the maternal home.

Impulsive males strain and sever relationships first with adult female authorities (mothers, then teachers) and later with male authorities. These careers are first marked by annoying snippets of disruptive behavior: climbing too high, being out of seats, a reduced awareness of danger, noisiness, failing to adjust activity level to social demands, and interrupting other people. Like Suomi's impulsive rhesus, however, difficult human children elicit maternal scolding, sleep loss, social rejection, and grieving. (Mash & Dozois, 1996). Such children fail to cuddle, return smiles, or sleep or eat with regularity.

In contrast, a preschooler's ability to make eye contact, stick to tasks, and use social skills---albeit for his selfish ends---can insure maternal advocacy even if he annoys her and lots of other people. (He also recruits females who are not relatives.) Clinical observation suggests that mothers of oppositional sons (and sometimes daughters) form a micro environment for their offspring, one that sometimes starts with the child's extended demands for his mother to sleep with him through the night. As he ages, she handles the bi-directional conflicts between him and outsiders in school and sometimes in the courts while he acquires the social inhibition and material resources to pursue his self interests without her. *The difference between maternal advocacy and abandonment may lie not with the child's activity level but with his ability to cling, make eye contact, and maintain reciprocity with her. It can be OK for him to fight if he fights well and is contrite afterwards.*

Investment from a dominant mother or aunt (either related or adoptive) will sometimes move a lively, oppositional, and highly determined young male rhesus into troop leadership (Suomi, 1997). A good friend persistently irritated his primary teacher and was eventually moved by his parents to an experimental school, part of a university school of education. The younger teachers invested in him in the ways that he demanded. He has since written extensively on scientific topics and has made multiple appearances in the electronic media.

The lesson? Not all hyperactive, annoying children have ADHD.

Satisfiability (SAT) Problems[19]

> "You are chief of protocol for the embassy ball. The crown prince instructs you either to invite Peru or to exclude Qatar. The queen asks you to invite either Qatar or Romania or both. The king, in a spiteful mood, wants to snub either Romania or Peru or both. Is there a guest list that will satisfy the whims of the entire royal family?" (Hayes, 1997).

Satisfiability problems (SAT) vary in difficulty: easy problems have a few hypothetical participants and few demands from each one, a small range of more difficult problems have more participants and more demands from each, and finally, a very large range where computers fail and humans walk quickly away from them (Hayes, 1997; Anderson, 1999). Thus, SAT difficulty can be varied in a systematic manner but within a narrow middle range of problem difficulty, research might show progressive increases in the complexity of problem that a child will attempt and solve as he or she gets older. It might also reveal differences in SAT performance in relation to the evolutionary content of the problem.

SAT problems exhibit properties similar to those of physical aggregates: a realm of chaotic disorganization, one of recurring, predictable order, and a narrow boundary between them that consists of growing or shrinking clusters of organization, whether in water that is

[19] Some of this material has been adapted from Brody (2001) and Brody (2002).

beginning to freeze, magnetism, spin glasses, or in electronic decision networks (Hayes, 1997; Anderson, 1999; Monassin, Zecchina, Kirkpatrick, Selman, & Troyansky, 1999). And in a surprising parallel to what we understand of decision networks that also show three phases (order, chaos, and a narrow boundary between them, Kauffman, 1993; 1995), SAT solvability is a function less of the number of participants but more of the number of demands made by each one: an average of three demands freezes the system. SAT problems, therefore, have a fundamental, primal feel to them because they show a phase transition, a pattern that suggests their evolutionary and emergent network importance (Anderson, 1999).

SAT may be more important than they first appear because (1) solutions require balancing competing demands from participants, (2) every one of us has different wishes, (3) managing alliances demands satisfying the participants by carrots and sticks so that mutual exchanges continue, and (4) the example translates into one that involves hunter and gatherer dilemmas such as past resources, profitable search tactics (each member is given tasks that match his or her skills), and competing demands within a group and from competing groups in the same territory. *These types of computations exert previously unrecognized selective pressures in social groups and, like emergent networks, have always been part of our evolutionary environment.*

SAT problems offer promise for assessing ADHD and perhaps distinguishing it from bipolar disorder (Brody, 2001a). We might also expect ADHD individuals to have greater difficulty if time and sequence are factors: that is, do one clause of the problem now, another later. There may also be a way to arrange SAT demands in sequence so that one path leads to a solution that is not possible with a different one.

Executive Functions without Language: *Hox* Origins

Raff and Lewontin on Executive Functions

> "An organism's life consists of constant midcourse corrections." (Lewontin, 2000, p. 93)

> Every day, cats turn fish to fur. Jesus was impressed.

Executive Functions (EF) are behaviors that manage other behaviors, often through the inhibition of an prepotent response until there is a time, place, and manner that deliver greater payoffs for the same effort. The external dilemma and its solutions are internalized, prolonged, subjected to recombination, and finally expressed in a more adaptive form. Language is presumed to be a necessary step in the operation of executive functions that improve the fit between an individual and his setting. While language can help or betray us, it may not be an essential component of self-direction.

There are striking parallels between the ontogeny of gene sequences and those of minds. Selected concepts in evolutionary-developmental biology (evo-devo, Raff and Kaufman,

1983; Raff, 1996; Gould, 1977, 2002) and some of Barkley's descriptions overlap.[20] That is, partial inhibition of ancestral structures allows modifications to develop, most of the older habits continue to work, the new ones lead to new environments, and the overall match improves between an organism and its settings. Thus, Raff (1996) speaks of strategies that apply not only to *Hox* transcriptional genes and embryology but also fit the development of our minds:

(1) Existing gene structures duplicate, (*Drosophila* have four *Hox* genes, humans have 13, many of them copies of the original four)
(2) One member of the pair changes so that it no longer codes exactly the same information as the first member,
(3) New outcomes appear as a function of amplification and constraint between the first and second member, and as parallel developmental cascades realign, and
(4) "Cooption" appears as the modified structure interacts with previously inaccessible opportunities, whether internal or external to the organism.[21]

Thus, we can find inhibition, prolongation, objectification, and reconstitution in every living organization: these are dynamic functions that mediate evolutionary adaptation and that also appear to be impaired in ADHD. Barkley's hypothesis that impaired inhibition underlies the linguistic and social difficulties shown by ADHD individuals is consilient with what we find elsewhere in development. In popular terms, you have to out with some of the old before your can in with the new.

If executive functions are self-directed behaviors that improve the fit between an occupant and its opportunities, then executive functions occur in aggregates of unicellular organisms and in every multicellular creature.

Lewontin (2000) describes executive functions in plants and animals but, like Raff, doesn't use the term "executive function." First, the combination of an organism and its setting is a unitary construction. Environment does not exist unless it is defined by an organism and each partner, within and across generations, modifies the other. And the living partner demonstrates self-regulating processes that improve the fit between him and his elements of his setting, whether living or not. This viewpoint echoes many developmental psychologists and, according to Allport (1955) owes more to Leibnitz than to Locke and can be found not only in Allport (1955), Plomin, DeFries, & Loehlin (1977), Scarr and McCartney (1983); Popper (1984/1992), Plomin (1994), Cohen (1999), Coen (1999), Laland, Odling-Smee, & Feldman, (2000), Plomin, DeFries, McClearn, & McGuffin, (2000), Turner (2000), and Lewontin (2000), Rowe (2001), Brody, Bloom, & Turner (2002), and Pinker (2002).[22]

---

[20]1977: Gould published *Phylogeny and Ontogeny* and Bronowski published *A Sense of the Future*. Raff (1996) extends Gould and resurrects evolutionary-developmental biology; Barkley, that same year, details Bronowski's speculations about human cognitive evolution. Barkley and Raff, however, tell very similar stories. Bronowski's influence on both of them? Or two minds tracing the same script for different actors?

[21]Raff (1996) speculates that ancestral genetic sequences may remain intact for as long as 5 million years after they are suppressed, a hoary example of inhibition, internalization, and prolongation!

[22]"That the cultural approach yields valuable facts we cannot possibly deny, for culture is indeed a major condition in becoming. Yet personal integration is always the more basic fact. While we accept certain cultural values as

Second, we find internalization, prolongation, and reconstitution, sometimes accomplished with feelings and language sometimes without them. Lewontin (2000) explains:

> "... Organisms do not find already existent ecological niches to which they adapt, but are in the constant process of defining and remaking their environments. At every moment natural selection is operating to change the genetic composition of populations in response to the momentary environment, but as that composition changes it forces a concomitant change in the environment itself. Thus organism and environment are both causes and effects in a coevolutionary process." (Emph. added, JB. Lewontin, 2000, pp. 125-126.)

He defines four steps:

> "First, organisms determine which elements of the external world are put together to make their environments and what the relationships are among the elements that are relevant to them." (p. 51)
>
> Second, "...organisms not only determine what aspects of the outside world are relevant to them by the peculiarities of their shape and metabolism, but they actively construct, in the literal sense of the word, a world around themselves." (p. 54)
>
> "Third, organisms not only determine what is relevant and create a set of physical relations among the relevant aspects of the outer world, but they are in a constant process of altering their environment." (pp. 54-55)
>
> Finally, "...organisms modulate the statistical properties of external conditions as those conditions become part of their environment. Living systems can perform time averaging and rate detection. Like mathematicians, they can perform integration and differentiation." (p. 60)

They anticipate the future when they store calories, hibernate, or build nests.

Exploratory Systems and ADHD: Fitting us to Where We Are

> "The charm of history and it enigmatic lesson consist in the fact that, from age to age, nothing changes and yet everything is completely different." A. Huxley, 1952, p. 259.

The same is true for cellular chemistry and for metazoan body plans.

Small-world networks perform "midcourse corrections" (Lewontin, 2000) in particular settings and such networks are associated with greater stability in the partnerships between occupants and settings. Conversely, the difficulties that an ADHD individual has with small-

---

propriate, as important for our own course of becoming, it is equally true that we are all rebels, deviants, and individualists. Some elements in our culture we reject altogether; many we adopt as mere opportunistic habits, and even those elements that we genuinely *appropriate* we refashion to fit our own personal style of life. Culture is a condition of becoming but is not itself the full stencil." (Allport, 1955, p. 82).

world connectivity predicts difficulties when he selects, constructs, or modifies his niche. Exploratory systems are an important concept for understanding the enduring complications of the disrupted small-world networks seen in ADHD.

Great variation in phenotype often emerges from similar ancestral or parental structures. This is an old pattern: metazoans have ancient metabolic and genetic foundations but an infinite variety of add-on features that multiply the niches that can be occupied: millions of species arose from the same basic plan in a manner similar to that of automobile changes from year to year (Gerhart & Kirschner, 1997; Raff, 1996; Carroll, Grenier, & Weatherbee, 2001; Gould, 2002). Even when genes are constant, environment varies in small but significant ways, creating problems of "fit" between an organism and its setting. *Exploratory systems address these problems.*

Exploratory systems include microtubules within cells, angiogenesis, and immune systems (Kirschner & Gerhart, 1998). Cells generate microtubules every few seconds but retain only those that establish useful connections between the nucleus and other parts of the cell. New blood vessels track tissue metabolism. Antibodies spin themselves into many configurations but stabilize and replicate when they connect to an antigen. Callosity, bone growth, and muscle strength also fit within this model. Even the number of our neurons in a particular section of our brain and their activity reflect an exploratory system: resources are selectively invested rather than scattered equally. Exploratory systems organize by selection (also called positive reinforcement or successive approximation by Thorndike or Skinner!): make the same approaches but toward many targets, keep what works, scrap the rest!

Exploratory system also describes nests, parents, schooling, and language as well as psychological adaptations and learning: *it also describes the function of natural selection.* All provide a pliable boundary between a growing organization and its setting, a boundary that cushions the developing child and weaves him into his surroundings. While genetic variation may account for many individual differences, exploratory systems create some of that variation when they interact with very specific environments.[23]

The tactic of retaining core genetic and biochemical foundations but insulating and refining them in small steps eventually (1) produced hominids and our discovery and refinement of social contracts, (2) improved means to detect cheating in those contracts, and (3) continued manufacture of tools and environments that suit us. *Incremental, cumulative mutations in genes and customs, but in a small-world configuration, allow us to have both ancient goals and innovative tools* (Gerhart and Kirschner, 1997; Kirschner & Gerhart, 1998).

---

[23]Core organizations such as *Hox* or *Pax-6* genes, the bilateral body plan, three-dimensional structures of proteins, and cellular metabolism are nearly identical throughout metazoa (Gerhart & Kirschner, 1997; Raff, 1996). They are said to be *highly conserved.* On the other hand, many structures and behavior can be highly variable. For example, the bar-head goose changed one proline to an alanine in its hemoglobin, increasing hemoglobin's affinity for oxygen but without changing its 3D structure. Bar-heads now fly over Mt. Everest perhaps because of one molecular change (Gerhart & Kirschner, 1997). It is as if the metazoa manufacture tools for managing changes in their settings. A tradesman shopping for tools at *Sears* follows the same strategy: finding a link between what he already has and what he needs to accomplish. Once he has identified and obtained a suitable tool, he uses it again and again and hands it on to his son. Exploratory systems are one of five mechanisms that Kirschner and Gerhart (1998) consider important for evolvability. The others are compartmentation, redundancy, robustness, and weak linkage. (See also West-Eberhard, 1998, on the topic of evolvability).

As we have seen, emergent random networks stabilize organisms and settings through selection, organizing them during the ontogeny of an individual or a species. Networks allow a self-adjusting synchrony to develop whether between thoughts or between children in a classroom. These, however, are also the tasks that Barkley refers to as analysis and synthesis and that regularly baffle ADHD individuals who have difficulty managing their links with friends and probably more difficulty managing indirect links with the friends-of-friends. (Barkley sometimes mentions science as a human expression of analysis and synthesis but nature has been performing science for eons.)

Language is a Karaoke Event

The assignment of symbols to events is a variation on gene duplication: information is copied but in a digital form that allows more rapid, reversible reconstitution. A symbol further allows us to carry our version of the original event indefinitely and to share it with our partners who change it as part of adopting it. (See Dawkins, 1979, on "Memes.") Raff's model - duplication, variation, realignment of parallel developmental cascades, and cooption - is again relevant. Language, therefore, accomplishes more quickly the explorations that other species accomplish through mutation and natural selection.

Barkley (1997) views language as an essential step in the formation of executive functions but five considerations suggest a more limited role: (1) we have seen that multicellular organisms show executive functions without language, (2) language supplements older, if slower, systems that accomplish the objective of exploring settings and achieving the best fit to any one of them, (3) key aspects of language may be a fitness display that indicates health and dependability (Miller, 2000), and (4) language can be a "spin doctor" as we sometimes change or defend our beliefs about external events in ways that suit us but are disconnected from the event (Pinker, 2002). Language, therefore, may be less important in some ways but more so in others: ADHD individuals may be handicapped not just when finding words or sequencing ideas in school reports but in pervasive, subtle ways that we are just beginning to notice, ways that influence social standing apart from handicaps in formal reasoning. It's not just what we say but how we say it that influences our social outcomes.

(1) Nonhuman species show evidence of executive functions. As mentioned in the opening argument for this chapter, we find abundant evidence of inhibition, prolongation, affective regulation, and reconstitution in many multicellular organizations. Each leaf on maize adjusts air flow in relation to its height from the ground, and, thereby, influences its temperature and humidity (Lewontin, 2000), worms build extended kidneys, crickets make acoustic chambers to amplify their calls, coral communities redirect ocean currents, and the social insects make large dwellings that surpass the functionality of a Hyatt (Turner, 2000; Camazine et al, 2001). After all, few of us have babies or school them in Hyatts!

Complex executive functions are seen in other species:

> "When the chimpanzees go out on patrol,' notes biologist Christopher Boehm, 'they often maintain a strict silence of hours, during which they manage, nevertheless, to

behave much as a coordinated group." Ghiglieri (1999, p. 171; see also Wrangham and Peterson, 1996).

Chimpanzee patrols are premeditated, highly cooperative ventures between males and impulsive behavior could have lethal consequences. Indeed, the most likely target for a chimpanzee patrol would appear to be an isolated male with a limited sense of the future.

As to human culture, anthropology and biology are clear that, if culture consists of a set of behaviors that are inherited by means of imitation, then (a) many other species have cultures, and (b) acquired characteristics are transmitted across generations in a Lamarckian way (DeWaal, 2001; Whiten, Goodall, McGrew, Nishida, Reynolds, Sugiyama, Tutin, Wrangham, & Boesch, 1999; Odling-Smee, Laland, & Feldman, 2003).

All of these things are accomplished without language.

(2) Language is, nonetheless, an important exploratory system like our immune system, angiogenesis, or growth of bone and muscle (Kirschner & Gerhart, 1998). It creates links between developing individuals and between individuals and their settings, links that span time and distances. As in other exploratory systems, one component (grammar whether in Japanese, Russian, or English) remains comparatively uniform but another (vocabulary) infinitely varies across languages or within a single language over decades (Pinker, 1994; 2002). Vocabulary can be seen as an iterated outcome from particular environments and passed within and between generations: that is, vocabulary connects individuals to both local history and current opportunities. Thus, a strongly conserved, ancient core (whether a *bilaterian* body plan or a grammar) acquires adaptations such as fins, fingers, or claws or limitless numbers of nouns, verbs, and adjectives.

Once we obtain tools (whether from *Sears* or from *Webster*), we establish a link between a situation and a set of solutions. We establish reciprocity when we apply our tools and convert a setting to an environment: the environments that we modify are more useful than those that we cannot and we retain the former and discard the latter. Tit-for-tat emerges during sustained relationships between humans or between humans and property (Axelrod & Hamilton, 1981; Axelrod 1984, 1997; Ridley, 1996).[24] We, therefore, understand the sustained relationships that human individuals groups make with personal and communal property such as water supplies, fishing grounds, and hunting territories (Ridley, 1996). (In these contexts, language should make cultural change less likely rather than more.)

(3) Language may be our most conspicuous and sensitive index of developmental health. Thus, we do not assess inhibition and maturity directly but monitor their broadcast (Pennington, 1991; Miller, 2000). As with other displays of fitness (Zahavi & Zahavi, 1997), the greater the cost, the greater the attractiveness of the individual who can pay it. Rapid word flow, coherent sequences of ideas, and interspersed references to right and wrong may predict healthy children. Further, in humans and other creatures, sexual displays influence

[24]Tit-for-tat is a durable strategy in iterated Prisoners Dilemma contests between two players with opposing interests (Axelrod, 1987; Poundstone, 1992). Selfishness and betrayal pay best during one-time exchanges. Longer term partnerships, however, pay better when each player forgoes the large jackpot in favor of smaller ones that let both of them continue to play. Ridley (1996) contrasts human relationships with environment during sustained or temporary arrangements. Clustered communities, multi-generational ownership, and finite resources are associated with conservation; government ownership with exploitation.

territory and territory influences not only how well we live but also the number of our mates (Trivers, 1972/2002).

Language, correspondingly, may be more easily fractured than our other executive functions and in several ways that involve vocabulary, grammar, and working, recent, and long term memory. As noted earlier, networks failure in cerebral organizations predicts failure when we sequence ideas and adjust their relative importance. We can also expect:

- Prosody to be affected in some individuals with ADHD.
- If language skill is correlated with fitness, then fluctuating asymmetry should be more evident in individuals with ADHD. (See Gangstad & Thornhill, 2003; Gangestad, 2001, in regard to physical symmetry in human males and mate preferences by females.)

Many of these developmental variations become more important under conditions of harsh competition such as those in courtship or gaining executive positions (Frank and Cook, 1995). Small differences in ability then lead to large differences in employment or when attracting marital partners and friends. In highly competitive conditions, more of us congregate in the diner and fewer at the country club.

Assessment and Remediation

Networks, like genes, seek, respond to, and modify environmental opportunities. Treating ADHD under a network concept will be sometimes different from what we do now with immediate, salient consequences. Since executive functions are not strictly dependent on language, we may look for signals and outcomes that bypass lectures and reach more instinctive, perhaps intact skills. The point of intervention is not in a therapist's office but at the dinner table, in a study hall, or on a construction crew. There is a smaller role for what is said and a greater one for prosody, immediacy, speed, and relevance to the task at hand...all signals of a relatively intact set of competencies.

Further, ADHD individuals, like all of us, negotiate between what they want and what the rest of us allow: these differences between shared and nonshared environments, between what is customary and what is desired, drive societies (Krebs, 1998; Wright, 2000; Pinker, 2002; Sowell, 1987). They also drive the partnerships even between ADHD and non ADHD individuals but with less temporal and emotional cushioning between the participants.

Contributions from Emergent Networks to ADHD Theory and Practice

Emergent networks, especially small-world phenomena, suggest that we assess ADHD in regard to "one step beyond" in social networks, time management, problem solving, and even writing essays. Repairing proximal rips in our social fabric may correct those that are more distant. That is, connect with a useful hub and the smaller problems might align themselves accordingly. For example, on Friday or Saturday nights, adolescents and young adults talk to each other, often by cell phone, in order to find out where the party is. The entire circle consists of freeloaders: none of them hosts the party or pays for beer but one member knows someone outside of the immediate circle who won't object to extra guests' drinking from his keg. (These search methods also cover a large list of party sites: it is easy to find a potential host but more difficult to find one whose parents are gone.) Meeting a partner for a date traditionally depends on the friend-of-a-friend process, perhaps brokered by a community *Yenta*. That function now occurs in chat rooms. Drug purchases are not from a friend but from a guy to whom your friend sends you and who changes his location every week.

Can the individual name some friends of friends whom he does not know and what information can he provide about them? What does he know of their income, occupation, and employers? What gossip has he collected about third parties through his immediate contacts? What job leads, repair services, tutoring opportunities, or entertainment has he learned of through indirect links in his network? What has he shared with that network? What is his awareness not only of the developmental paths between the partnerships in past events and future ones but also of the concurrent, parallel cascades that are going on around him? That is, what is his lateral awareness? (More simply, what kind of bridge or poker player is he?) As for his talents, does he perform them on a face-to-face, moment-to-moment basis or can he arrange strategies to manage alternative future outcomes? That is, does he play solitaire or *Nintendo* to beat only the game in front of him or plan ahead for all the situations that might unfold?

Once you have certainty about a diagnosis, whether based on the *Diagnostic and Statistical Manual* (DSM 4, American Psychiatric Assn, 1994, on Barkley's ideas, or on emergent networks, what do you do? Evolutionary psychology and behavior genetics hint of the paths traditionally followed by ADHD individuals and of refinements in our treatment.

Evolutionary Roots for Human Conduct

Twelve-year-old Suzy was failing school and could not concentrate but was passively defiant. She had also saved at least one life in the local swimming pool. She, not the lifeguards, knew the location for each of a dozen children and knew immediately when one of them was missing. She, according to her mother, also was a superior baby sitter. Methylphenidate helped to raise her grades and improve her moods, her caretaker skills led to a nursing career.

Barkley (1992) remarks that ADHD individuals can pay attention when they find the task "interesting." There has been little understanding, however, of why some tasks are interesting but others are not. Evolutionary psychology (Symons, 1979; Buss, 1999; 2003?; Barkow, Cosmides, & Tooby, 1992; Crawford & Krebs, 1998; Pinker, 1997; 2002) tells us why some cues, tasks, and rewards are more salient and why delayed consequences can be fragile in some situations but not in others.

The signs listed in DSM 4 reflect characteristics that we share with many other species but refined during normal human development. Most of our evolutionary siblings have offspring who don't take turns but call out, chatter for many reasons, make melodic noises, climb, run, squirm, often change their seat, and intrude or interrupt adults, siblings, and peers, and are motor-driven in comparison with adults. The youngsters of many species are also less apt to be organized, persistent, and attentive to remote signals from whatever source. They also lose things (young squirrels and robins sometimes fall out of nests) and change tasks often.

Cosmides & Tooby (1992) argue for the existence of a "universal human nature," composed of psychological adaptations and Pinker (2002) gives us a list of about 600 behaviors found in every human culture. Natural selection applies not only to physical traits but also to behavior ones known as "psychological adaptations" that include efficient, modular strategies for becoming a parent, winning a battle, catching food, escaping an enemy, finding your way, or changing your environment (Hess, 1962; Buss, 1999; Miller, 2000; Barkow, Tooby & Cosmides, 1992; Pinker, 2002; Kauffman, 2000; Turner, 2000; Odling-Smee, Laland, & Feldman, 2003). Metazoans have elaborated these strategies, perhaps, for the last 500 million years (Raff, 1996; Gerhart and Kirschner, 1997; Gould, 2002).

Psychological adaptations, like structural ones, are thought to be genetically-based and responsive to a combination of external conditions, past successes, and internal hormonal status but resilient to disruption by social learning. They are hypothesized to characterize every normal human and to have structural and behavior analogs in species that are closely related to us. They are often fun to do and easy to learn as well as modular and hierarchic (Tooby & Cosmides, 1992; Buss, 1999; Miller, 1999, 2000). For example, our tools for seeing, orienting, grasping, and throwing work together as a targeting mechanism. And despite the complicated nature of these tasks, no one has to pay us to throw rocks at a rabbit or swat a fly in midair. When we males are 6 years old, a pretty girl who sits next to us elicits boredom; when we are 14, we glimpse her once again at 100 feet and never get her out of our mind. Thus, psychological adaptations are the things that we humans do when left to ourselves. We may see them on school yards more often than in classrooms and on weekends more than during work hours.

It's possible that ADHD individuals will do all the usual evolutionary things but continue them into later chronological development when compared with non ADHD adults. The details exposed by immaturity, however, may hint not just of annoyances but also of careers and occupations. Barkley (1996; 1997) points out the technical sophistication of modern cultures and the need for its participants to inhibit instinctive behaviors, analyze situations, and reconstitute their elements. In contrast, Barkow et al (1992) is a testament to the ways that culture meets instinctive needs.

There are at least two implications: (1) network theory suggests that ADHD adults occupy similar social positions today that they occupied 10 millennia ago, and (2) not all is hopeless for ADHD individuals in the modern era. Technology becomes ever more adapted to human convenience, not less so. And, the students who interrupt and argue may become radio talk show hosts, thriving stimulation from competition, audiences and fame and define territories on the basis of prosody, guts, and irreverence in ways that a male starling would appreciate. Thus, Pinker's list of 600 adaptations should give us clues to the situations in which we may find relative excellence in ADHD individuals.

On the other hand, not even breathing occurs the same way in every individual and a list of traits found in every culture does not mean those traits will exist to equal degree in every one of its members. The most devastating impairment may be difficulties in managing partnerships: those of us lacking in social perception usually depend on parents, friends, or our wife to compensate for our blindness. Unfortunately, ADHD individuals have difficulty recruiting, maintaining, or profiting from these kinds of relationships. While activity level makes ADHD children noticeable, their failure to find or heed advice get them supervised or excluded.

Max dozed, on his back, black side down, white side up; Madison, the neighbor's cat came to my glass door and ate on the steps where I left food for him. I nudged Max from my side and tossed him toward the door. He spotted our red-haired visitor in midair, landed fully awake, and watched him nonstop for the next 30 minutes. Madison left, Max returned to my couch. Sustained attention would flow in two or three directions if I took Max out to the barn where he and the nesting buzzards could watch each other. And a shared evolutionary history means that a bird and a school boy will give longer sustained attention to a cat than to a history book.

Behavioral Genetics: Things Handed Down

> "If there be such a thing as a natural birthright, I can conceive of none superior to the right of the child to be informed, at first by proxy through his guardian, and afterwards personally, of the life-history, medical and other, of his ancestry." Francis Galton (1883/1911, p. 30.)

We may find that some of the tasks in which an ADHD client persists are composites of talents shared with other family members and revealed in family histories. We may also find that individual pursuit of "nonshared environment" is also a clue, one again to be gleaned by careful inspection of an individual's family lore.

Talents in Family Histories

The concept of psychological adaptations tells us what to expect not only in classrooms but also on the playground; the details of family histories suggest paths for students to explore in consultation with their parents, teachers, and counselors. Clinical anecdotes and biographies are filled with promising examples, so is everyone with whom you speak. Ask them.

"Linda," age 40, sought her natural father after a separation of 39 years (Cohen, 1999). She found that he physically resembled her son but psychologically resembled her. That is, they were both artists, made precise arrangements of books and hearthstone utensils, and had pets named Winston. They both disliked peanut butter and chocolate but loved Snickers bars. Both were intellectual and energetic. They were politically conservative but religious liberals. They also checked out every trail, museum and ruin.

Charles Darwin and his grandfather, Erasmus, had many similarities including their number of children (Erasmus, 12 legitimate and 2 illegitimate; Charles 10) (King-Hele, 1999, pp. 363-364,). Both men were diligent scholars and, despite social anxiety, had large networks of professional colleagues. Both enjoyed rational argument mixed with sweeping speculations about evolution and about plant and animal emotions. Erasmus published 1 million words in 11 volumes; Charles, 2 million in 23 volumes. Charles spent eight years writing four volumes on barnacles, Erasmus, also in 8 years, translated four volumes on plant classifications. Both were fascinated by plant fertilization (Erasmus, one volume; Charles, three), plant movement and sensory abilities (Erasmus, one volume; Charles, three), geology (coral reefs, both men), and animal expression of emotions (even worms). Erasmus published *Zoonomia* in two volumes after hiding it for 24 years, Charles delayed his publication of *On the Origin of Species* for 20 years.[25]

We are all immersed in family resemblance but don't usually talk to doctors about them unless we discuss diabetes, heart disease, or cancer.[26] Very little prompting, however, elicits pages of details about familial resemblance and parental opinions change about their child. (See Steptoe, 1998, on inheritance of genius.) Guilt about bad parenting changes to acceptance of the child; intervention shifts from lectures to acceptance or niche modification.

Labeling individuals globally as "ADHD" also obscures the domains in which they exhibit sustained concentration and organizational skills; it reduces the possibilities of using relatively intact skill areas as platforms for social interventions. The skeptic may reply that a young fisherman would do better without ADHD than with. No doubt. But simply calling him "ADHD" overlooks education and occupations wherein his ADHD is either a smaller handicap or nonexistent. Students eventually find niches where they are less stressed and, sometimes, more prosperous. *Such may, in fact, be the path followed by many ADHD students, both now and before we knew about this disorder.* The job of parents and grandparents is to make those searches less agonizing and more efficient. The behavioral genetics' concept of nonshared environment is consistent with these opportunities.

Nonshared Environment and Personal Will

Every one of us manages two kinds of environments, shared (SE) and nonshared (NSE), that offer clues to the annoyances that we find in ADHD. I suggest that the events wherein ADHD is most evident lie in the imposed environments of schedules and tasks that may be individual or culture-specific. SE favors conformity and, therefore, makes artificial links between individuals and settings. SE is generated by parents of young children, teachers, peers, Marine Corps instructors, police officers, traffic signs, ballet masters, and even country and western bands.

SE has its greatest impact when it is actually present, that is, when rewards and punishments apply immediately to ongoing behavior. Studies of the impact of SE on the variance in long term behavioral traits suggest that its contributions range from 0-10%. Our daughter, a porcelain doll in ballet or church or at her friend's house, will yawn and scratch and whine when she's home. Line dancers move in exact patterns when Garth sings but shuffle, snuffle, and hiccup afterwards, becoming again some of the most rebellious individuals in our culture.

Nonshared environments (also called "unique environments") are those that surround one individual but not another (Plomin, 1994). NSE is an explanatory necessity that explains why genetically identical twins can sometimes be so different. If the kids differ but their genes are

[25] Brody, J. F. (In preparation) We're all twins.

[26] I once asked Aaron Beck about detailed family resemblance. He had noticed them often but didn't "know what to make of them."

the same, their environments must have been *nonshared* or *unique*. That is, parents do not treat two children, not even identical twins, in exactly the same manner.

The unappreciated aspect, however, is that each occupant may define his NSE, rather than accepting whatever is handed to him (Plomin, DeFries, & Loehlin, 1977; Scarr & McCartney, 1983; Bouchard, Lykken, McGue, Segal, & Tellegen, 1990; Bouchard, Lykken, Tellegen, & McGue, 1996; Rowe, 1994; Harris, 1998; Cohen, 1994, 1999; Lewontin, 2000).[27] Two children in the same household effectively occupy two different homes as each child collects and arranges not only his toys but also his memories. NSE often accounts for 35-40% of the variance in long term outcomes. (Genetic factors often contribute about the same portion.)

Interpretation of NSE is difficult because it conflates two aspects of environment: (1) the environments that we each make for ourselves (Lewontin, 2000), and (2) variations in the environments that are provided to us and to no one else (Brody, 2001b). There are hints that the first definition (self-selected NSE) is more influential than the second.[28]

Nonshared environments mean that individuals, guided by genes, make unique arrangements around themselves. Similar genes make similar environments and different genes make different environments: you don't have to compare beavers with flies to see this effect. Identical human twins reared apart from one another often have similar outcomes, as if each twin had nearly identical beacons to guide his development and for some traits such as IQ, the genetic contributions actually increase across the individual's lifetime (Bouchard et al, 1996; Plomin et al, 2000). Adopted children have strong similarities to their natural parents but are no more similar to their adopted parents than to complete strangers (Dunn & Plomin, 1990; Harris, 1998; Cohen, 1999.) Thus, we singletons, even those of us with ADHD, are a "twin" of our individual nature. Given a permissive society and widely distributed assets, resources for a growing middle class imply individual choices in what people do. Even in human societies, a diverse ecosystem offers many opportunities to make a living (Kauffman, 2000).

ADHD individuals build their own worlds but may be less efficient or timely when they must also accommodate the demands from other people. (After all, executive functions make nests and refining them.) Schools, for example, must keep ADHD children for 12 years; the child, therefore, gains leverage in the same manner as any partner with whom you establish an extended relationship; reciprocity emerges. (See Axelrod & Hamilton, 1981; Axelrod 1984, 1997; Poundstone, 1992, on the topic of social cooperation and tit-for-tat.) Teachers without ADHD make nests that the ADHD student cannot make for himself. Such teachers explain lessons a second time, shorten homework assignments, and keep both assignment sheets and homework at school so they won't be lost. Homework is done in learning support class but never at home where it is ignored, or if completed under parental whips, not turned in. (It follows that teachers who have ADHD and who have their own difficulties with

[27]NSE was invented to account for the differences that occur between monozygotic twins (MZ). If G is identical, differences must reflect E. If G, however, arranges E, then we still have a problem. Geneticists will eventually admit that "identical" was a transitional definition that does not apply to identical twins: indeed, such do not exist in nature. MZ will vary, if not in their DNA sequences, then in the regulator decisions that switch structural genes on or off.

planning, timing, emotionality, and problem-solving, are less apt to engage in nest building and problem solving but will follow their own instincts to complain or pass the child on to another teacher.)

Nonshared Environment and Clinical Interventions

> "Dawkins' examples (e. g. beavers' making dams: JB) are undeniably examples of instincts---of stereotyped inherent patterns of behavior...Such instincts are shared by most individuals in a species, but the present topic is individual differences in traits. *Yet the conceptual distance between the human expression of individual differences and the extended phenotype of a species may not be so great.* (italics added, JB)" (Rowe, 1994, p. 91).

The following paragraphs are adapted from a chapter on bipolar disorder (Brody, 2004) and a chapter on statistical physics and psychiatric diagnoses (Brody, 2002). They apply to our treating individuals with ADHD.

(1) No single template defines our clients. Their assets and liabilities will be unique for each of them. No one medicine or behavior trick will work every time.

(2) Each client selects experiences that meet her particular, sometimes peculiar allotment of psychological adaptations and experience-producing drives (Bouchard, et al., 1996). Many of our encounters with ADHD will be arise from a poor fit between our client and his niche of the moment.

(3) Behavioral family histories may reveal how parents and grandparents with similar temperaments and talents found a place to be driven but without being locked up or divorced. These lessons are sobering: take similar genes in similar outcomes and expect similar outcomes. Put similar genes in better opportunities and get outcomes similar to those that would have unfolded if parents or grandparents had those same improved opportunities.

(4) Clients inevitably select from the therapist's offerings whether or not that is the therapist's intent. The closer the match between the menu and client aptitudes, the greater the chance for treatment success.

(5) While there will be substantial uniformity of automatic thoughts---perhaps because we all came from the same therapsid 160 mya---there will also be substantial variability between persons. The array of automatic thoughts available to the client will vary with his or her age, reproductive standing, access to resources, seasons of the year, and significant changes in his or her niche.

(6) Therapists resemble parents: both seek opportunities to match the assets of a clients and niches. (Odd poetry: we partner with our material or human settings by finding or making them similar to us. Once more, similar, weakly-linked

---

[28]NSE and SE also overlap, respectively, with Barkley's dichotomy between goal-attracted and contingency-attracted behavior, outcomes that are driven from within and those imposed on us.

oscillators come into synchrony. A coincidence?) The obscure individual who wanted to go where the weather matched his clothes told a powerful truth.

As Popper (1992) observed, every creature seeks a better world. That world is usually characterized by the closeness of fit between the traits of their occupants and the opportunities that those occupants contrive.

"It's About Time.": Heterochrony and Remoteness

> "A few studies of children with ADHD have suggested that they may be smaller and have a younger bone age than normal children of the same chronological age." Barkley 1990, p. 127.

Males vary more than females and some of those males have ADHD whether for reasons of a deviant gene involved with neuronal release and reuptake systems or for those that come with scant maternal resources. And in the latter case, did she starve him or hand him a defective clock?

Barkley commented in regard to ADHD, "It's about time" but he's possibly correct in ways beyond what he intended (Barkley, 1994b). He referred to the tendency for some ADHD individuals to have difficulty estimating elapsed time and to have fewer memories of last weekend or plans for the one coming. They sense more than a normal six-year-old that "next Friday" is an eternity to wait and last Friday is so long ago that it never happened. There is, however, a different meaning to Barkley's phrase: shorten our time within mother and we are apt to be more impulsive, less sharing, and short-lived in ways that are correlated with our problems with remoteness in reminders, consequences, or relationships. Because of maternal fitness, poverty, or her very determined imprinted genes, she doesn't have time to finish us. The matter again becomes one of time.

Heterochrony refers to changes in developmental timing: the start, the end, and the speed of our unfolding and when links are activated or silenced between parallel developmental cascades (Gould 1977, 2003; Raff 1996; Carrington & Ambros, 2003; Kmita & Duboule, 2003; Schultz & Kay, 2003). The slowing of maternal investment, especially from an immature or ill mother, may affect one set of skills but not another and make an incomplete work of us. Less mature, more impulsive behavior can be expected in some domains but not others.

Small-world difficulties imply that remote memories, teachers, and weekends in the affected domains will be less in focus, past disasters and future goals vanish below a temporal horizon: the child experiences less inspiration or constraint from a distant teacher and he will be out of synchrony with his work group of peers who listen to her as well as to each other. There may be a very concrete if very unlikely foundation for some of these social outcomes: *the cerebellum is remote from developmentally newer frontal orbital areas and the fibers that link the two may not connect as early or reliably in ADHD children as in their peers.* (This is a recasting of Pennington's 1991 thought that that evolutionarily newer systems are more easier disrupted than older ones.)

In a far less radical vein, relative immaturity is an "ADHD fact." Mothers might object but their sons should do better if we add the following to their choices:

(1) Exclude them, as they now exclude themselves, from age-gated advancement through school. (Even if ADHD children occupy the same classroom, instructional accommodations now lower the effective grade, the nonshared environment offered to the child who also arranges his own nonshared environment. The exclusion is, again, mutual.)

(2) Introduce work groups and long term projects in late middle school or high school.

(3) Prepotent talents and skills still find opportunities in modern society. Earlier vocational or technical programs should be available for the child who can later pick up job-related formal instruction when the material is needed for vocational advancement.

(4) Maintain a richer mix of adults to students. Also, develop more use of one-gender schools.

(5) Give more time with the same teacher or a very small group of them throughout the elementary and junior high grades.

A Certain Inevitability about Mother's Work

Raff's sequence...clone, vary the clone, change timing, select a new environment, and co-opt old systems...shadows much of what we might find in ADHD, a disorder accompanied by disrupted behavioral and developmental inhibition that leaves holes in both our immediate and extended social networks. Our homework is incomplete because our personal ontogeny is likewise. The mess in our room echoes that in our minds. And poor self esteem may be not only a genetic quirk (Rowe, 1994, 2001) but also an outcome from reality: ADHD individuals really do have difficulty "fitting in" and males have these problems more often than females. Thus, our mothers and our wives train us and push aside those of will not shape up and, for that matter, nearly always have.

> "Henry, you're nearly 40. Did you outgrow your ADHD? Or does your wife manage it for you?"
>
> She looked at him and rolled her eyes.

Acknowledgments

I am grateful to Sandy Thomas, Mary Fowler and scores of other parents of ADHD children for their zeal and coherence that led to inclusion of ADHD as a qualifying educational disability in federal regulations. I also thank staff at the Barnes and Noble Store in Devon, PA, for rapid attention to my book orders and their tolerance for my sipping one cup of latté for up to 6 hours. (They eventually sold me two gallons of the stuff but one cup at a time while I wrote this manuscript. avoid a black hole: pay more but get your books from a human!) Finally, thanks to Gil Levin, Ph.D., of Behavior OnLine and Howard Bloom for their unending support.

References

Albert, Reka & Barabasi, A-L (2002) Statistical mechanics of complex networks. *Reviews of Modern Physics*. 74: 47-97.

Allport, G. (1955) *Becoming: Basic Considerations for a Psychology of Personality*. New Haven: Yale University Press.

American Psychiatric Association (1994) *Diagnostic and Statistical Manual of Mental Disorders*. (4th Ed.) Washington, D.C.

Anderson P. (1999) Computing: solving problems in finite time. *Nature*. 400: 115-116.

Axelrod, R. (1984) *The Evolution of Cooperation*. NY: Basic Books.

Axelrod, R. (1997) *The Complexity of Cooperation*. Princeton, NJ: Princeton Univ. Press.

Axelrod, R. & Hamilton, W. (1981) The evolution of cooperation. *Science*, 211, 1390-1396.

Bak, P. (1996) *How Nature Works: The Science of Self-Organized Criticality*. NY: Copernicus.

Barabasi, A-L (2002) *Linked: The New Science of Networks*. NY: Perseus.

Barkley, R. (1990) *Attention deficit Hyperactivity Disorder: A Handbook for Diagnosis and Treatment*. NY: Guilford.

Barkley, R. (1992) *ADHD: What Do We Know*. NY: Guilford Publications.

Barkley, R. (1994a) *ADHD in Adults*. NY: Guilford Publications.

Barkley, R. (1994b) It's about time. Plenary talk at the 6th Annual Meeting, Children & Adults with Attention Deficit Disorder (ChADD), New York, October 13.

Barkley, R. (1996) Attention deficit/hyperactivity disorder. In Mash, E. & Barkley, R., (Eds.) *Child Psychopathology*, Guilford, NY. p.p. 63-112.

Barkley, R. (1997) *ADHD and the Nature of Self Control*. NY: Guilford.

Barkow, J., Cosmides, L., & Tooby, J. (Eds.) (1992) *The Adapted Mind: Evolutionary Psychology and the Generation of Culture*. NY: Oxford.

Bateman, A. (1948) Intrasexual selection in *Drosophila*. *Heredity*. 2: 349-368.

Bianconi, G. & Barabasi, A-L (2000) Bose-Einstein condensation in complex networks. arXiv:cond-mat/0011224 v1 13 Nov.

Blanchard, R. (2001) Fraternal birth order and the maternal immune hypothesis of male homosexuality. *Hormones and Behavior*. 40: 105-114.

Bouchard, T., Lykken, D., McGue, M., Segal, N., & Tellegen, A. (1990) Sources of human psychological differences: The Minnesota study of twins reared apart. *Science*, 250: 223-228.

Bouchard, T. J., Lykken, D., Tellegen, A., & McGue, M. (1996) Genes, Drives, Environment, and Experience. Chapter 1 in C.P. Benbow & D. Lubinski (Eds.) *Intellectual Talent: Psychometric and Social Issues*. Baltimore: Johns Hopkins Press, pp. 5-43.

Brody, J. (2000) Life at the edge: Complicators and simplifiers in human transactions. Paper given at annual meeting, Society for Across Species Comparisons and Psychopathology, Amherst, MA, June 7.

Brody, J. (2001a) Evolutionary recasting: ADHD, mania and its variants. *Journal of Affective Disorders*. 65: 197-215.

Brody, J.F. (2001b) Sexual selection: Mind Your Mothers. Human Behavior and Evolution Society, London.

Brody, J. (2002) From Physics and Evolutionary Neuroscience to Psychotherapy: Phase Transitions and Adaptations, Diagnosis and Treatment. In G. Cory & R. Gardner (Eds.) *The Evolutionary Neuroethology of Paul MacLean: Convergences & Frontiers*, Praeger-Greenwood, pp. 231-259.

Brody, J., Bloom, H., & Turner, J. (2002) "Alternatives to the Received View of Evolution" Annual meeting, Human Behavior and Evolution Society, Rutgers, NJ. June.

Brody, J. (2003) From emergent networks to modularity and consciousness. Under review.

Brody, J. (2004) Bipolar disorder: self-interested networks, cycling, and their management. In F. Columbus (Ed.) *Progress in Bipolar Disorder Research*. Hauppage, NY: Nova Science.

Bronowski, J. (1974) Language in a biological frame. *Current Trends in Linguistics*. Reprinted in Bronowski, J. (1977) *A Sense of the Future*. Cambridge, MA: MIT Press, pp. 132-154.

Buchanan, M. (2002) *Nexus: Small Worlds and the Groundbreaking Theory of Networks*. NY: Norton.

Buss, D. (1998) The psychology of human mate selection: exploring the complexity of the strategic repertoire. In C. Crawford & D. Krebs (Eds.) *Handbook of Evolutionary Psychology*. Mahwah, NJ: Erlbaum, pp. 405-430.

Buss, D. (1999) *Evolutionary Psychology: The New Science of the Mind*. NY: Doubleday.

Buss, D. (2000) Desires in human mating. In D. LeCroy & P. Moller (Eds.) *Evolutionary Perspectives on Human Reproductive Behavior*. NY: New York Academy of Sciences, pp. 39-49.

Buss, D. (2003) *The Evolution of Desire: Strategies of Human Mating*. (2nd Ed.) New York: Basic Books.

Cagnacci, A., Renzi, A., Arangino, S., Alessandrini, C., & Volpe A. (2003) The male disadvantage and the seasonal rhythm of sex ratio at the time of conception. *Human Reproduction*. 18(4) 885-887.

Camazine, S., Deneubourg, J-L., Franks, N., Sneyd, J., Theraulaz, G., & Bonabeau, E. (2001) *Self-Organization in Biological Systems*. Princeton, NJ: Princeton Univ. Press.

Carrington, J., & Ambros, V. (2003) Role of microRNAs in plant and animal development. *Science*. 302: 336-338.

Carroll, Sean, Grenier, J., & Weatherbee, S. (2001) *From DNA to Diversity: Molecular Genetics and the Evolution of Animal Design*. Malden, MA: Blackwell.

Cavanagh, J. Van Beck, M., Muir, W., & Blackwood, D. (2002) Case-control study of neurocognitive function in euthymic patients with bipolar disorder: An association with mania. *British Journal of Psychiatry*. 180: 320-6.

Clark, L., Iversen, S., & Goodwin, G. (2002) Sustained attention deficit in bipolar disorder, *British Journal of Psychiatry*. 180:313-9.

Coen, E. (1999) *The Art of Genes: How Organisms Make Themselves* NY: Oxford.

Cohen, D. (1999) *Stranger in the Nest: Do Parents Really Shape Their Child's Personality, Intelligence, or Character*? NY: Wiley.

Cosmides L. & Tooby, J. (1992) The psychological foundations of culture. In J. Barkow, L. Cosmides, & J. Tooby (Eds.) *The Adapted Mind: Evolutionary Psychology and the Generation of Culture*. NY: Oxford, pp. 19-136.

Crawford., C. & Krebs, D. (Eds.) *Handbook of Evolutionary Psychology*. Mahwah, NJ: Erlbaum.

Daly, M., & Wilson, M. (1981) Abuse and neglect of children in evolutionary perspective. In R. Alexander & D. Tinkle (Eds.), *Natural Selection and Social Behavior*. NY: Chiron, pp. 405-416. (Cited in Buss, 1999.)

Daly, M., & Wilson, M. (1988) *Homicide*. Hawthorne, NY: Aldine. (Cited in Buss, 1999.)

Dawkins, R. (1982) An agony in five fits. In R. Dawkins (Ed.) *The Extended Phenotype*. NY: Oxford, pp. 179-194.

de Waal, F. (2001) *The Ape and the Sushi Master: Cultural Reflections of a Primatologist*. NY: Basic Books.

Divon, M., Ferber, A., Nisell., H., & Westgren, M. (2003) Male gender predisposes to prolongation of pregnancy. *Am J Obstet Gynecol*. 188(6):1665-6.

Dunn, J. & Plomin, R. (1990) *Separate Lives: Why Siblings Are So Different*. NY: Basic.

Edelman, G. (1987) *Neural Darwinism: The Theory of Neuronal Group Selection*. NY: Basic.

Edelman, G. (1992) *Bright Air, Brilliant Fire: On the Matter of the Mind*. NY: Basic.

Edelman, G. & Tononi, G. (2000) *A Universe of Consciousness: How Matter Becomes Imagination*. NY: Basic.

Fergusson, D., Horwood, L., & Beautrais, A. (1999) Is Sexual Orientation Related to Mental Health Problems and Suicidality in Young People? *Arch Gen Psychiatry*. 56: 876-880.

Ferrier, I., & Thompson, J. (2002) Cognitive impairment in bipolar affective disorder: Implication for the bipolar diathesis. *British Journal of Psychiatry*. 180: 293-5.

Fewell, J. (2003) Social insect networks. *Science*. 301: 1867-1870.

Frank, R. & Cook, P. (1995) *The Winner-Take-All Society: Why the Few at the Top Get So Much More Than the Rest of Us*. NY: Free Press.

Galton, F. (1883/1907/1911) *Inquiries into Human Faculty* (2nd Ed.) NY: Dutton. (1st Ed., 1883).

Gangestad, S. (2001) Human sexual selection: good genes, and special design. In D. LeCroy & P. Moller (Eds.) *Evolutionary Perspectives on Human Reproductive Behavior*. NY: Annals NY Acad. Sci., pp. 50-61.

Gangestad, S. & Thornhill, R. (2003) Facial masculinity and fluctuating asymmetry. *Evolution & Human Behavior*. 24: 231-241.

Gazzaniga, M. (1992) *Nature's Mind*. NY: Basic Books.

Ghiglieri, M. (1999) *The Dark Side of Man: Tracing the Origins of Male Violence*. Reading, MA: Perseus.

Gintis, H. (2000) Strong reciprocity and human sociality: game theoretic models and empirical tests. Presentation at Human Behavior and Evolution Society, Amherst, MA, 6/9/00.

Gould, S. (1977) *Ontogeny and Phylogeny*. Cambridge, MA: Harvard Belknap.

Gould, S. (2002) *The Structure of Evolutionary Theory*. Cambridge, MA: Harvard Belknap.

Granovetter, M. (1973) The strength of weak ties. *American Journal of Sociology*, 78: 1360-80.

Haig, D. (1993) Genetic conflicts in human pregnancy. *Quarterly Review of Biology*. 68, 495-532.

Haig, D. (2002) *Genomic Imprinting and Kinship*. New Brunswick, NJ: Rutgers University Press.

Harris, J. (1998) *The Nurture Assumption: Why Children Turn Out the Way They Do*. NY: Free Press.

Hawkes, K. (2004) The grandmother effect. *Nature* 428: 128-129.

Hayes B. (1997) Can't get no satisfaction. *American Scientist*, 85:108-112.

Helle, S., Lummaa, V., & Jokela, J. (2002) Sons Reduced Maternal Longevity in Preindustrial Humans. *Science*. 296:1085.

Herrell, R., Goldberg, J., True, W., Ramakrishnan, V., Lyons, M., Eisen, S., & Tsuang, M. (1999) Sexual orientation and suicidality: a co-twin control study in adult men. *Arch Gen Psychiatry*. 56: 867-874.

Hess, E. (1962) Ethology: An approach to the complete analysis of behavior. In Newcomb, T (Ed.) *New Directions in Psychology*. NY: Holt Rinehart, & Winston.

Hrdy, S. (1999) *Mother Nature: A History of Mothers, Infants, and Natural Selection*. NY: Pantheon Press.

Huxley, A. (1952) *The Devils of Loudun: A Study in the Psychology of Power, Politics, and Mystical Religion in the France of Cardinal Richelieu*. NY: Harper.

Judson, O. (2002) *Dr. Tatiana's Sex Advice to All Creation*. NY: Metropolitan.

Kauffman, S. (1993) *Origins of Order: Self-Organization and Selection in Evolution*. NY: Oxford.

Kauffman, S. (1995) *At Home in the Universe: The Search for the Laws of Self Organization and Complexity*. NY: Oxford.

Kauffman, S. (2000) *Investigations*. NY: Oxford.

Keverne, E., Fundele, R., Narasimha, M., Barton, S., & Surani, M. (1996) Genomic imprinting and the differential roles of parental genomes in brain development. *Developmental Brain Research*, 92, 91-100.

King-Hele, D. (1999) *Erasmus Darwin: A Life of Unequaled Achievement*. London, UK: Giles de la Mare.

Kirschner, M & Gerhart, J (1998) Perspective: Evolvability. *Proceedings National Academy of Science*. 95(15), 8420-8427.

Kmita, M., & Duboule, D. (2003) Organizing axes in time and space; 25 years of colinear tinkering. *Science*. **302**: 331-333.

Krebs, D. (1998) Evolution of moral behaviors. In C. Crawford & D. Krebs, *Handbook of Evolutionary Psychology*. Mahwah, NJ: Erlbaum, pp. 337-368.

Kruuk, L., Clutton-Brock, T., Albon, S., Pemberton, J. & Guinness, F. (1999) Population density affects sex ratio variation in red deer. *Nature.* 399: 459 - 461.

La Cerra, M. (1994) Evolved mate preferences in women: psychological adaptations for assessing a man's willingness to invest in offspring. Unpublished doctoral dissertation, Department of Psychology, University of California, Santa Barbara. Cited in Buss, 1999, pp. 122-123.

Lahdenpera, M, Lummaa, V., Helle, S., Tremblay, M., & Russell, A. (2004) Fitness benefits of prolonged post-reproductive lifespan in women. *Nature* 428: 178-181.

Laland, K., Odling-Smee, F., & Feldman, M. (2000) Niche construction, biological evolution and cultural change. *Behavioral and Brain Sciences* 23(1): 131-146.

Lalumière, M., Harris, G., & Rice, M. (1999) Birth order and fluctuating asymmetry: a first look. *Proceedings of the Royal Society of London*. B. Biological Sci. 266(1436): 2351-4.

Lewontin, R. (2000) *Triple helix: Gene, organism, environment.* Cambridge, MA, Harvard.

Lieberman, E., Lang, J., Cohen, A., Frigoletto, F., Acker, D., & Rao, R. (1997) The association of fetal sex with the rate of cesarean section. *Am J Obstet Gynecol.* 176(3):667-71.

Lotka, A. (1926) The frequency distribution of scientific productivity. *Journal of the Washington Academy of Sciences* 16: 317-323. Cited in Murray (2003).

Lusseau, D. (2003) The emergent properties of a dolphin social network. Biology Letters: *Proceedings of the Royal Society of London,* Series B (Suppl.).

Maguire, M., & Troisi, A. (1998) *Darwinian Psychiatry*. NY: Oxford.

Mash, E., & Dozois, D. (1996) Child psychopathology: a developmental-systems perspective. In E. Mash & R. Barkley (Eds.) *Childhood Psychopathology*. NY: Guilford, pp. 3-62.

Miller, G. (2000) *The Mating Mind: How Sexual Choice Shaped the Evolution of Human Nature.* NY: Doubleday.

Monassin, R., Zecchina, R., Kirkpatrick, S., Selman, B., & Troyansky, L. (1999) Determining computational complexity from characteristic 'phase transitions.' *Nature*, 400: 133-137.

Murray, C. (2003) *Human Accomplishment: The Pursuit of Excellence in the Arts & Sciences, 800 B.C. to 1950* NY: Harper Collins.

Odling-Smee, F., Laland, K., & Feldman, M. (2003) *Niche Construction. The Neglected Process in Evolution.* Monographs in Population Biology. Princeton, NJ: Princeton University Press.

Paul, D. (1992) Fitness: historical perspectives. In E. Keller & E. Lloyd (Eds.) *Keywords in Evolutionary Biology*. Cambridge, MA: Harvard University Press.

Pennington B. (1991) *Diagnosing Learning Disorders: A Neuropsychological Framework.* NY: Guilford.

Penton-Voak, I., Perrett, D. Castles, D., Kobayashi, T., Burt, D., Murray, L. & Minamisawa, R. (1999) Menstrual cycle alters face preference. *Nature*. 399: 741-742.

Phillips, D., Handelsman, D., Eriksson, J., Forsen, T., Osmond, C., Barker, D. (2001) Prenatal growth and subsequent marital status: longitudinal study. *British Medical Journal*. March 31. BMJ. 322: 771.

Pinker, S. (1994) *The Language Instinct: How the Mind Creates Language*. NY: Morrow.

Pinker, S. (1997) *How the Mind Works.* NY: Norton.

Pinker, S. (2002) *The Blank Slate: The Modern Denial of Human Nature.* NY: Viking.

Plomin, R. (1994) *Genetics and Experience: The Interplay between Nature and Nurture*. Thousand Oaks, CA: Sage.

Plomin, R., DeFries, J., & Loehlin, J. (1977) Genotype-environment interaction and correlation in the analysis of human behavior. *Psychological Bulletin*. 84(2), 309-322.

Plomin, R., DeFries, J., McClearn, G., & McGuffin, P. (2000) *Behavioral Genetics* (4th ed.) NY: Worth.

Popper, K. (1984/1992), *In Search of a Better World. Lectures & Essays from Thirty Years*. London: Routledge.

Poundstone, W. (1992) *Prisoner's Dilemma: John von Neumann, Game Theory, and the Puzzle of the Bomb*. NY: Anchor.

Price, J. (1967) Hypothesis: the dominance hierarchy and the evolution of mental illness. *Lancet*, 2, 243-246.

Provine, W. (1986/1989) *Sewall Wright and Evolutionary Biology*. Chicago, IL: University of Chicago Press.

Raff, R. (1996) *The Shape of Life*. Chicago, IL: University of Chicago Press.

Raff, R. & Kaufman, T. (1983) *Genes, Embryos, & Evolution*. Macmillan. Reprinted by Indiana University Press, 1991.

Ridley, M. (1993) *The Red Queen: Sex and the Evolution of Human Nature*. NY: Penguin.

Ridley, M. (1996) *The Origins of Virtue: Human Instincts and the Evolution of Cooperation*. NY: Penguin.

Robinson, R., & Jorge, R. (2002) Longitudinal course of mood disorders following traumatic brain injury. *Archives of General Psychiatry*. 59: 23-24. Reviewed by Dubovsky, S. (2002) More than a bump on the head. *Journal Watch for Psychiatry*. 8: 24.

Rowe, D. (1994) *The Limits of Family Influence: Genes, Experience, and Behavior*. NY: Guilford.

Rowe, D. (2001) Do people make environments or do environments make people? In A. Damascio, A. Harrington, J. Kagan, B. McEwen, H. Moss, & R. Shaikh (Eds.) *Unity of Knowledge: Convergence of Natural and Human Science. Annals NY Acad Sci*, 935: 62-74.

Sacks, O. (1987) *The Man Who Mistook His Wife for a Hat and Other Clinical Tales*. NY: Harper & Rowe.

Sagan, C., & Druyan, A. (1992) *Shadows of Forgotten Ancestors*. New York: Random House.

Scarr, S. & McCartney, K. (1983) How people make their own environments: A theory of genotype-->environment effects. *Child Development*. 54, 424-435.

Schiefenhoevel, W. (2002) Human birth; Cultural and evolutionary perspectives. Presentation at the Human Behavior and Evolution Society Annual Meeting, Rutgers, N.J., 6/22/2002.

Schultz, T., & Kay, S. (2003) Circadian clocks in daily and seasonal control of development. *Science*. 302: 326-328.

Singer, W. (1994) Coherence as an Organizing Principle of Cortical Functions. In O. Sporns & G. Tononi (Eds.) *Selectionism and the Brain: International Review of Neurobiology*. 37, 153-184. NY: Academic.

Sowell, T. (1987) *A Conflict of Visions: Ideological Origins of Political Struggles*. NY: Quill.

Sporns, O., (1994) Selectionist and instructionist ideas in neurobiology. In O. Sporns & G. Tononi (Eds.) *Selectionism and the Brain: International Review of Neurobiology*. 37, 4-26. NY: Academic.

Spreen, O., Risser, A., & Edgell, D. (1995) *Developmental Neuropsychology*. NY: Oxford.

Steptoe, A. (1998) (Ed.) Genius and the Mind: Studies of Creativity and Temperament. NY: Oxford.

Stevens, A., & Price, J. (2000) *Evolutionary Psychiatry: A New Beginning* (2nd Ed.). NY: Routledge.

Strogatz, S. (2003) *Sync: The Emerging Science of Spontaneous Order*. NY: Hyperion.

Suomi, S. (1997) Nonverbal communication in nonhuman primates: Implications for the emergence of culture. In Segerstrale, U. & Molnar, P. (Eds.) *Nonverbal Communication: Where Nature Meets Culture*. Mahway, NJ: Erlbaum. pp. 131-150.

Suomi, S. (1999) Attachment in rhesus monkeys. In J. Cassidy & P. Shaver (Eds.) *Handbook of Attachment: Theory, Research, and Clinical Applications*. NY: Guilford, pp. 181-197.

Suomi, S. (2000) How gene-environment interactions shape individual development trajectories in rhesus monkeys. Presentation at The Relationship System, Georgetown Family Center, April 2000.

Symons, D. (1979) *The Evolution of Human Sexuality*. NY: Oxford.

Tononi, G. (1994) Reentry and the problem of cortical integration. In O. Sporns & G. Tononi (Eds.) *Selectionism and the Brain: International Review of Neurobiology*. 37, 127-152. NY: Academic.

Trivers, R. (1972) Parental investment and sexual selection. In B. Campbell (Ed.) *Sexual Selection and the Descent of Man*. Chicago: Aldine, pp. 136-179. Reprinted in R. Trivers (Ed.) (2002) *Natural Selection and Social Theory: The Collected Papers of Robert Trivers*. Princeton, NJ: Princeton University Press, pp. 65-110.

Turner, J. (2000) *The Extended Organism: The Physiology of Animal-Built Structures*. Cambridge, MA: Harvard University Press.

Watts, D. (2002) *Six Degrees: The Science of a Connected Age*. NY: Norton.

Watts, D. (2004) *Small Worlds: The Dynamics of Networks Between Order and Randomness*. Princeton, NJ: Princeton University Press.

Watts, D. & Strogatz, S. (1998) Collective dynamics of 'small-world' networks. *Nature*. 393: 440-442.

Weiss, G., & Hechtman, L. (1993) *Hyperactive Children Grown Up* (2nd Ed). Guilford, NY.

West-Eberhard, M. (1998) Evolution in the light of developmental and cell biology, and *vice versa*. *Proceedings National Academy of Science*. 95: 8417-8419.

Whiten, A., Goodall, J., McGrew, W. Nishida, T., Reynolds, V. Sugiyama, Y, Tutin, C., Wrangham, R., & Boesch, C. (1999) Cultures in chimpanzees. *Nature*. 399: 682-685.

Wrangham, R. & Peterson, D. (1996) *Demonic Males: Apes and the Origins of Human Violence*. NY: Houghton Mifflin.

Wright, R. (2000) *NonZero: The Logic of Human Destiny*. NY: Pantheon.

Yook, S., Jeong, H., & Barabasi, A-L. Preprint. Cited in Albert & Barabasi, 2001.

Zahavi, A. & Zahavi, A. (1997) *The Handicap Principle: A Missing Piece of Darwin's Puzzle* NY: Oxford.

In: Attention Deficit Hyperactivity Disorder Research
Editor: Michelle P. Larimer, pp. 59-94
ISBN 1-59454-156-6

Chapter III

ADHD, Combined Type in Primary School Age Children: Investigations of its Association with Oppositional Defiant, Dysthymic and Anxiety Disorders

Alasdair Vance[1]
University of Melbourne
Royal Children's Hospital
Melbourne, Australia

Abstract

The association of oppositional defiant disorder with increased rates of ADHD, combined type (ADHD-CT), anxiety disorders and depressive disorders are replicated findings. However, to date, the specific associations between oppositional defiant disorder, ADHD-CT, anxiety disorders and dysthymic disorder symptoms have not been studied in primary school age children with ADHD-CT. This paper deals with these issues.

---

[1] Head Academic Child Psychiatry Department Of Paediatrics, University Of Melbourne, Royal Children's Hospital, Murdoch Childrens Research Institute, South East Building Gatehouse Street, Parkville, Melbourne VIC 3052 Australia Phone: 61 3 9345-4666 Fax: 61 3 9345-6002 email: avance@unimelb.edu.au

Introduction

Study 1 addresses this issue. Further, this chapter explores [A] the nature of and association between parent-reported child anxiety and child self-reported anxiety in (1) ADHD-CT and anxiety disorders compared to anxiety disorders alone and (2) ADHD-CT with and without dysthymic disorder in Study 2; [B] the association between neurodevelopmental measures (neurological subtle signs, parent report of motor and/or language developmental delay) and [C] psychosocial measures (parental psychopathology and family functioning) in (1) ADHD-CT with and without anxiety disorders and (2) ADHD-CT with and without dysthymic disorder in Studies 3 and 4. Data from a standard multiple regression analysis of ADHD-CT, dysthymic disorder and anxiety disorders symptoms on oppositional defiant disorder symptoms in primary school age children with ADHD-CT are presented in Study 1. Also, data from cross sectional comparison of the above groups, matched for age, gender and verbal/performance/full scale IQ and social adversity status on the above anxiety, neurodevelopmental and psychosocial measures are presented in Studies 2-4. Only ADHD-CT and dysthymic disorder symptoms make a unique contribution to oppositional defiant behaviour and only dysthymic disorder is associated with additional neurobiological dysfunction and psychosocial dysfunction in primary school age children with ADHD-CT. Parent reported anxiety in their children and child self-reported anxiety have similarities and differences that vary across ADHD-CT, anxiety and dysthymic disorders. The implications of these findings for the current construct of subtyping in ADHD-CT are discussed.

Study 1

The greater than chance association of oppositional defiant disorder with ADHD-CT, depressive disorders and anxiety disorders is a replicated finding [1]. Angold et al. [1] reported median joint odds ratios from a meta-analysis of 10.7 (95% CI = 7.7-14.8) with ADHD (primarily ADHD-CT), 6.6 (95% CI = 4.4-11.0) with depressive disorders and 3.0 (95% CI = 2.1-4.3) for anxiety disorders. Recently, Maughan et al. [2] noted previous epidemiological studies that had reported this association and confirmed it using data from their recent epidemiological study: 19.1 (95% CI = 12.5-29.3) for boys with ADHD (primarily ADHD-CT), 6.3 (95% CI = 2.1-18.7) for boys with depressive disorders and 5.4 (95% CI = 3.3-8.7) for boys with anxiety disorders.

Within the ADHD-CT literature, the greater than chance association of ADHD-CT with oppositional defiant disorder, depressive disorders and anxiety disorders has also been noted [1,3,4]. Comorbid oppositional defiant disorder rates of 14% [5] in epidemiological samples through to 30%-50% in clinical samples [3], comorbid depressive disorder rates of 15% [6] in epidemiological through to 75% in clinical samples [7,8], and comorbid anxiety disorders rates of 20%-30% in epidemiological samples [3] through to 43%-63% [9,10] in clinical samples of ADHD-CT. However, the specific associations between oppositional defiant disorder, ADHD-CT, dysthymic disorder and anxiety disorders symptoms have not been studied in primary school age children. Dysthymic disorder in children and adolescents is a mood disorder characterised by chronically depressed and/or irritable mood for more days than not, over a period of 1 or more years, with no remission longer than 2 months [11]. The clinical validity of early-onset dysthymic disorder as a diagnostic construct has been established [12]. Dysthymic disorder is important to investigate in this age group because it is more common than major depressive disorder [13], has an earlier onset of 2.3 years (8.7 versus 11.0 years) compared to major depressive disorder [13], has comorbid oppositional defiant disorder rates of 21%-83% [14], ADHD-CT rates of 24%-57.1% [14,15] and anxiety disorders of 30%-75% [14,15] in epidemiological and clinical samples, and lasts 2.5 years longer in the presence of a co-occurring externalising disorder (oppositional defiant disorder, ADHD-CT primarily) [16]. Anxiety disorders are important to investigate because they too are common in this age group, point prevalence 5.7% [17], comorbid anxiety and depressive (primarily dysthymic) disorders in children have been associated with increased severity of both anxiety and depressive disorders [18-20], comorbid ADHD-CT and anxiety disorders (parent reported) may not decrease with increasing age [21,22], and a primary school age subgroup has a lesser response to stimulant medication [23-25]. Now, anxiety is a heterogeneous construct, with many different forms [26] and hence defining which anxiety disorders will be studied is an essential initial step. From a categorical perspective, generalised anxiety disorder, separation anxiety disorder, social phobia and specific phobia are the four most common types of anxiety disorder in children [26]. Historically, they all arose from what March et al. [27] have termed 'true "neurotic" anxiety' and therefore can be considered as a group. They are readily distinguished from obsessive compulsive disorder, which has different, well described frontostriatal deficits [26] that underpin its greater-than-chance association with ADHD-CT, which also has well described, different again, frontostriatal deficits [28]. For these reasons, obsessive compulsive disorder is excluded from the anxiety disorders group(s) in this study. Remaining low prevalence anxiety disorders that are rare in primary school age children are also excluded (Panic Disorder, Agoraphobia, Post Traumatic Stress Disorder).

In this study, the association of ADHD-CT, dysthymic disorder and anxiety disorders symptoms with oppositional defiant disorder symptoms will be examined in a clinical sample of primary school age children with ADHD-CT. We hypothesise that all three symptom dimensions will be associated with oppositional defiant disorder symptoms, consistent with the replicated findings above.

Method

Subjects

One hundred and eighty-nine children aged from 6-12 years were identified in a specialised clinic for ADHD in the Western region of metropolitan Melbourne, Australia. All the children had ADHD-CT (DSM-IV criteria), defined through a semi-structured clinical interview with the child's parent(s) and by the parent and/or teacher report of the subscale scores of the core symptom domains of ADHD-CT being greater than 1.5 standard deviations above the mean for a given child's age and gender. Oppositional defiant disorder was defined through a semi-structured clinical interview with the child's parent(s). Dysthymic disorder was defined by a semi-structured clinical interview with the child's parent(s) and/or the child. Anxiety disorders diagnoses were defined from a parent and/or a child perspective using a semi-structured clinical interview. The children were all psychostimulant medication naïve and were consecutively referred for assessment because they were not responding to usual clinical psychological management approaches. The children met the inclusion criteria of living in a family home (and not in an institution) and attending normal primary schools. All had Intelligence Quotients above 70 and none had overt neurological disease, psychotic symptoms or conduct disorder. There was no refusal and parent(s) gave informed consent. Ethics committee approval was obtained for the study. The subject characteristics for this sample were as follows: Age (months) -108.90 (28.49) (range 72-151 months); Gender (M,F) - 161,28; ACRS - 22.10 (5.20); Verbal IQ - 95.39 (14.53), Performance IQ - 98.59 (14.32), Fullscale IQ - 95.96 (13.37); Social adversity scale - 7.65 (1.80) (range 4-13); oppositional defiant disorder (N%) - 142 (75); dysthymic disorder (N%) - 57 (30); anxiety disorders (N%) - 77 (41).

Measures

Anxiety Disorders Interview Schedule for Children (A-DISC) [29] is a semi-structured diagnostic interview schedule based on DSM-IV criteria with child and parent versions. It is frequently used internationally by researchers to diagnose childhood anxiety disorders and a range of other disorders, including ADHD-CT, oppositional defiant disorder /conduct disorder and depressive (including dysthymic) disorders, based on the DSM-IV criteria. It yields a categorical variable of the presence or absence of a given disorder and dimensional variables of symptoms for each diagnosis. Research findings support the clinical utility, reliability and validity of the *A-DISC*.

Abbreviated Conners' Rating Scale (ACRS) [30] is a 10-item questionnaire that outlines the core symptom domains of ADHD-CT. It is completed by parent(s) and teachers and yields a continuous variable of ADHD-CT symptoms. It has good validity and reliability and has been used extensively in the clinical research literature.

Parental Account of Childhood Symptoms (PACS) [31] is a semi-structured clinical interview developed as an instrument for the measurement of children's behaviour problems as experienced at home. It is administered by a trained interviewer. Parents are asked for detailed descriptions of what their child has done in specified situations over the previous week and over the preceding 12 month period. In all, 44 items of behaviour are enquired about in this way. Three subscales are generated as continuous variables; hyperactivity, emotional disorder and defiance. It also yields demographic data. A social adversity scale (range 3-) is formed from the summary of family income level (1-2), mother's educational level (1-2), single parent status (0-1), sibling size (0-), and broken home status (1-2). It has adequate validity and reliability and has been used extensively in published research studies.

The third edition of the *Wechsler Intelligence Scale for Children (WISC-3)* [32] was used. This provides verbal, performance and full scale scores of measured intelligence with normative data.

Procedure

The *Abbreviated Conners' Rating Scale (ACRS)* [30] parent forms were completed prior to the child's assessment. The child was initially interviewed by a registered psychologist who administered the *WISC-3* [32] to the child, while a Fellow in Child and Adolescent Psychiatry concurrently administered the *Anxiety Disorders Interview Schedule for Children (A-DISC)*- [29] parent form and the *Parental Account of Childhood Symptoms (PACS)* [31].

Statistical Analysis

The *Statistical Package for the Social Sciences (SPSS/SC)* [33] was used for all analyses in this chapter. A standard multiple regression was performed between oppositional defiant disorder symptoms as the dependent variable and ADHD-CT symptoms, dysthymic disorder symptoms and anxiety disorders symptoms as independent variables. Preliminary assumption testing was performed to ensure there were no violations of normality, linearity, outliers, multicollinearity and homoscedasticity of residuals.

Table 1 presents the correlations between variables, unstandardised and standardised regression coefficients, the semipartial correlations and the coefficient of determination, unadjusted and adjusted.

Table 1: Standard multiple regression of ADHD-CT symptoms, dysthymic disorder (DD) symptoms and anxiety disorders (ADs) symptoms on oppositional defiant disorder (ODD) symptoms in primary school age children with ADHD-CT

Variables	ODD	ADHD-CT	DD	ADs	*B*	β	sr^2
ADHD-CT	.60				0.782***	0.45	.15
DD	.55	.48			1.084***	0.35	.08
ADs	.27	.34	.44		-0.110	-0.04	

$p < .0005$ ***

a unique variability = .23

shared variability = .21

$R^2 = .45$

Adjusted $R^2 = .44$ [a]

R = .67***

B =unstandardised regression coefficient; β= standardised regression coefficient; sr^2= semipartial correlations; R^2 = coefficient of determination.

Results

ADHD-CT symptoms (15% of the variance) and dysthymic disorder symptoms (8% of the variance) made independent significant contributions to the prediction of oppositional defiant disorder symptoms. The three independent variables in combination contributed a further 21% of the variance. Altogether 44% of the variance in oppositional defiant disorder symptoms was predicted by knowing scores on these three variables. Although the correlation between anxiety disorder symptoms and oppositional defiant disorder symptoms was .27, anxiety disorders did not contribute significantly to the regression. Apparently, the relationship between anxiety disorders symptoms and oppositional defiant disorder symptoms is mediated by the relationships between ADHD-CT symptoms, dysthymic disorder symptoms and oppositional defiant disorder symptoms.

Discussion

The age, gender, ADHD-CT symptom severity, verbal/performance/fullscale IQ, social adversity level, comorbid rates of dysthymic disorder and anxiety disorders in this clinical sample of primary school age children with ADHD-CT were all consistent with the published literature [1-3]. The comorbid oppositional defiant disorder rate was higher than that of published clinical ADHD-CT samples [3] but consistent with the 30% comorbid dysthymic disorder in this ADHD-CT sample, given the known increase in oppositional defiant disorder rates with comorbid dysthymic disorder [14].

The significant independent contribution of ADHD-CT symptoms to oppositional defiant patterns of behaviour is expected [1,2], as is the lack of an independent significant contribution by anxiety disorders symptoms to oppositional defiant disorder [1,2]. In contrast, an important new finding is the significant independent contribution of dysthymic disorder symptoms to oppositional defiant patterns of behaviour in a primary school age ADHD-CT sample. This finding extends Angold et al.'s [1] reported association of conduct disorder with anxiety disorders via each disorders' link with depressive disorders by specifically demonstrating the association between oppositional defiant disorder and dysthymic disorder symptoms within a primary school age ADHD-CT sample. In addition, this finding is consistent with the known increase in severity of oppositional defiant disorder symptoms when comorbid with depressive disorders [34], but extends this association to dysthymic disorder symptoms specifically within a primary school age ADHD-CT sample. Further, the relationship between anxiety disorders symptoms and oppositional defiant disorder symptoms in this ADHD-CT group is mediated by the relationships between ADHD-CT symptoms, dysthymic disorder symptoms and oppositional defiant disorder symptoms.

Two clear implications arise from this novel finding: Firstly, dysthymic disorder is important to recognise in primary school age children with ADHD-CT. Then specific psychological and/or medication treatments can be investigated for this comorbid group. Secondly, the nature of the association between dysthymic disorder, anxiety disorders, oppositional defiant disorder and ADHD-CT needs to be systematically studied both within this developmental period and across developmental periods: for example, pre- and post-adrenarche and pre- and post-pubarche.

An important, albeit necessary methodological limitation of this study is the specific composition of the anxiety disorders group by the four most common anxiety disorders in pre-pubescent children [26] with a common historical derivation from 'true "neurotic" anxiety' [27]. This leaves unanswered the key question of whether other forms of anxiety, such as obsessive compulsive disorder and panic disorder, have a different risk inducing or resilience enhancing relationship with oppositional defiant disorder symptoms [35] in ADHD-CT within this same developmental period and across developmental periods.

The next study will address the nature of and association between parent-reported child anxiety and child self-reported anxiety in (1) ADHD-CT with and without dysthymic disorder and (2) ADHD-CT and anxiety disorders compared to anxiety disorders alone within the primary school age period.

Study 2

The parent report of anxiety in their child and the child self-report of anxiety are known to have low concordance rates [36-38]. Only approximately 50% of children with self-reported anxiety have also been reported with anxiety by their parents [39]. Further, both the child and the parent report have been noted to be important in determining comorbid anxiety associated with ADHD-CT, for significant clinical correlates, such as levels of self confidence and impairments in activities of daily living, may be associated with the child report alone [40]. Recently, March et al. [27] have noted that the parent report of their given child's anxiety disorder(s), from the Multimodal Treatment Study of children with ADHD-CT, may represent their child's 'negative affectivity and associated behavioural problems' rather than 'neurotic anxiety suffered by children with anxiety disorders alone [*sic*]'. Taken together, these findings support considering the parent report of anxiety in their child and the child self-report of anxiety, separately.

Currently, it is known that ADHD-CT is comorbid with generalised anxiety disorder, separation anxiety disorder, specific phobia and social phobia, which are also the most common anxiety disorder diagnoses reported by parents and children in pre-pubertal epidemiological samples, regardless of diagnostic category [6,17]. These findings have recently been extended by our group [21]: we found significantly higher rates of parent reported specific phobia and child self-reported separation anxiety disorder in children with ADHD-CT and anxiety disorders compared to ADHD-CT without anxiety disorders, and a significant decrease in child self-reported anxiety over 2 years in the ADHD-CT and anxiety disorders group while there was no decrease in parent reported anxiety in their children with ADHD-CT and anxiety disorders over 2 years, consistent with prior findings [8,22]. Similarly, our group has reported that generalised anxiety disorder, separation anxiety disorder, specific phobia and social phobia are also common in ADHD-CT and dysthymic disorder [41]. Further, significantly higher rates of parent reported separation anxiety disorder and social phobia in primary school age children with ADHD-CT and dysthymic disorder compared to ADHD-CT without dysthymic disorder were found.

However, to date, comparisons of the above ADHD-CT with and without anxiety disorders and ADHD-CT with and without dysthymic disorder groups with respective anxiety disorders alone and dysthymic disorders alone groups have not occurred. This study investigates these specific comparisons and explores the underlying structure of parent reported anxiety disorders in their children and child self-reported anxiety disorders in (a) ADHD-CT and anxiety disorders and anxiety disorders alone and (b) ADHD-CT and dysthymic disorder and dysthymic disorder alone.

We hypothesise that (1) the rate of parent and child reported generalised anxiety disorder, separation anxiety disorder, specific phobia and social phobia will be significantly increased in ADHD-CT and anxiety disorders, ADHD-CT and dysthymic disorder, anxiety disorders alone and dysthymic disorder alone groups compared to the ADHD-CT alone group; (2) there will be no difference between the ADHD-CT and anxiety disorders and anxiety disorders alone groups with respect to rates of parent reported specific phobia and child self-reported separation anxiety disorder; (3) there will be no difference between the ADHD-CT and dysthymic disorder and dysthymic disorder alone groups with respect to rates of parent reported separation anxiety disorder and social phobia; and (4) the same relationships will exist between parent reported anxiety disorders in their children and child self-reported anxiety disorders in (a) ADHD-CT and anxiety disorders and anxiety disorders alone and (b) ADHD-CT and dysthymic disorder and dysthymic disorder alone groups.

Method

Subjects

ADHD-CT alone, ADHD-CT and anxiety disorders and anxiety disorders alone groups

One hundred and thirteen children aged from 6-12 years were identified in specialised clinics for ADHD and anxiety disorders in the Western region of metropolitan Melbourne, Australia. 96 children had ADHD-CT (DSM-IV criteria), ADHD-CT alone (N=37) and ADHD-CT and anxiety disorders (N=59), and 17 children had anxiety disorders alone. ADHD-CT was defined through a semi-structured clinical interview with the child's parent(s) and by the parent and/or teacher report of the subscale scores of the core symptom domains of ADHD-CT being greater than 1.5 standard deviations above the mean for a given child's age and gender. Anxiety disorders were defined as generalised anxiety disorder, separation anxiety disorder, social phobia and specific phobia (DSM-IV criteria), diagnosed through a semi-structured clinical interview with the child's parent(s) and by the parent and/or child report of the total anxiety scores being greater than 1.5 standard deviations above the mean for a given child's age and gender. The children were all psychostimulant, anxiolytic and antidepressant medication naïve and were consecutively referred for assessment because they were not responding to usual clinical psychological management approaches. The children met the inclusion criteria of living in a family home (and not in an institution) and attending normal primary schools. All had Intelligence Quotients above 70 and none had overt neurological disease, endocrine disease, depressive disorders, conduct disorder or psychotic symptoms. There was no refusal and parent(s) gave informed consent. Ethics committee approval was obtained for the study.

ADHD-CT alone, ADHD-CT and dysthymic disorder and dysthymic disorder alone groups

One hundred and thirty-one children aged from 6-12 years were identified in specialised clinics for ADHD and dysthymic disorders in the Western region of metropolitan Melbourne, Australia. 95 children had ADHD-CT (DSM-IV criteria), ADHD-CT alone (N=37) and ADHD-CT and dysthymic disorder (N=58), and 36 children had dysthymic disorder alone. ADHD-CT was defined through a semi-structured clinical interview with the child's parent(s) and by the parent and/or teacher report of the subscale scores of the core symptom domains of ADHD-CT being greater than 1.5 standard deviations above the mean for a given child's age and gender. Dysthymic disorder was defined through a semi-structured clinical interview with the child's parent(s) and/or the child. Dimensional subscales of parent and child reported depression with published psychometric properties were correlated with the respective parent and child report of dysthymic disorder to confirm this diagnosis. Anxiety disorders were defined as generalised anxiety disorder, separation anxiety disorder, social phobia and specific phobia (DSM-IV criteria), diagnosed through a semi-structured clinical interview with the child's parent(s) and by the parent and/or child report of the total anxiety scores being greater than 1.5 standard deviations above the mean for a given child's age and gender. The children were all psychostimulant, anxiolytic and antidepressant medication naïve and were consecutively referred for assessment because they were not responding to usual clinical psychological management approaches. The children met the inclusion criteria of living in a family home (and not in an institution) and attending normal primary schools. All had Intelligence Quotients above 70 and none had overt neurological disease, endocrine disease, conduct disorder or psychotic symptoms. There was no refusal and parent(s) gave informed consent. Ethics committee approval was obtained for the study.

All groups were compared for age, gender, verbal/performance/fullscale IQ, social adversity and oppositional defiant disorder (see Tables 2 and 3).

Table 2: Subject characteristics ADHD-CT alone, ADHD-CT and anxiety disorders (ADs) and anxiety disorders alone groups

	1 ADHD-CT N=37	2 ADHD-CT + ADs N=59	3 ADs N=17	F	*p*
Age (months)	109.49 (27.64)	101.86 (22.05)	117.12 (21.67)	3.06	.05
Gender (M,F)	34,3	54,5	12,5	6.08#	.05
ACRS	21.60 (5.86)	21.79 (5.77)	7.06 (6.16)	42.74	**** 1=2>3
VIQ	93.41 (13.73)	96.54 (15.23)	107.00 (12.44)	2.28	.11
PIQ	97.74 (14.50)	100.71 (13.04)	97.67 (13.46)	0.56	.57
FSIQ	94.88 (12.94)	98.36 (13.49)	104.45 (8.41)	2.82	.06
SAS	7.58 (1.77)	7.77 (1.90)	6.88 (1.15)	1.53	.22
ODD (+,-)	29,8	45,14	4,13	19.42#	**** 1=2>3

VIQ/PIQ/FSIQ = verbal/performance/fullscale IQ; SAS = social adversity status; ODD = oppositional defiant disorder; # 3 x 2 χ^2 ; **** $p < .0005$

Table 3: Subject characteristics ADHD-CT alone, ADHD-CT and dysthymic disorder (DD) and dysthymic disorder alone groups

	1 ADHD-CT N=37	2 ADHD-CT + DD N=58	3 DD N=36	F	*p*
Age (months)	109.49 (27.64)	109.12 (24.15)	116.39 (21.33)	1.11	.33
Gender (M,F)	34,3	46,13	23,13	8.01#	.02 3>1##
ACRS	21.60 (5.86)	22.51 (4.53)	14.79 (7.17)	20.35	**** 1=2>3
VIQ	93.41 (13.73)	96.44 (15.19)	101.97 (14.89)	2.71	.07
PIQ	97.74 (14.50)	99.38 (14.73)	101.10 (13.05)	0.44	.65
FSIQ	94.88 (12.94)	97.67 (13.82)	100.42 (14.03)	1.40	.25
SAS	7.58 (1.77)	7.67 (1.70)	7.26 (1.50)	0.63	.54
ODD (+,-)	29,8	42,17	23,13	1.91#	.38

VIQ/PIQ/FSIQ = verbal/performance/fullscale IQ; SAS = social adversity status; ODD = oppositional defiant disorder; # 3 x 2 χ^2 ## 2 x 2 χ^2 ; **** $p < .0005$

Measures

Please note additional measures not used in Study 1 are noted here.

Child Behaviour Checklist (CBCL) [42] consists of 112 behaviour problem items, which are rated by the parent and teacher on a 3-point scale as to how well each describes the child. Parent and teacher forms are completed. An anxiety/depression subscale is generated, along with seven other behavioural subscales. All scores form continuous variables. The *CBCL* is well researched and has adequate psychometric properties.

Revised Children's Manifest Anxiety Scale (R-CMAS) [43] consists of 37 items designed to assess anxiety. The *R-CMAS* forms a total anxiety subscale, along with four other subscales. All scores form continuous variables. Good test-retest reliability and concurrent validity have been demonstrated.

Children's Depression Scale (CDS) [44] consists of 66 items designed to assess depression, including dysthymia. The *CDS* forms an affective response subscale, along with five other subscales. All scores form continuous variables. Good test-retest reliability and concurrent validity have been demonstrated.

Procedure

The *Abbreviated Conners' Rating Scale (ACRS)* [30] and *Child Behaviour Checklist (CBCL)* [42] parent forms were completed prior to the child's assessment. The child was initially interviewed by a registered psychologist who administered the *WISC-3* [32] to the child, while a Fellow in Child and Adolescent Psychiatry concurrently administered the *Anxiety Disorders Interview Schedule for Children (A-DISC)*- [29] parent form and the

Parental Account of Childhood Symptoms (PACS) [31]. At a separate session, a Fellow in Child and Adolescent Psychiatry administered the *Anxiety Disorders Interview Schedule for Children (A-DISC)*- [29] child form and the child completed the *Children's Depression Scale (CDS)* [44] and the *Revised Children's Manifest Anxiety Scale (R-CMAS)* [43].

Statistical Analysis

3 x 2 Chi-square analyses of (1) parent reported anxiety disorders in their children with ADHD-CT alone, ADHD-CT and anxiety disorders and anxiety disorders alone groups (see Table 4), (2) child self-reported anxiety disorders in ADHD-CT alone, ADHD-CT and anxiety disorders and anxiety disorders alone groups (see Table 5), (3) parent reported anxiety disorders in their children with ADHD-CT alone, ADHD-CT and dysthymic disorder and dysthymic disorder alone groups (see Table 6) and (4) child self-reported anxiety disorders in ADHD-CT alone, ADHD-CT and dysthymic disorder and dysthymic disorder alone groups (see Table 7) were initially performed. If significant, further 2 x 2 Chi-square analyses were performed to determine the source of this significance.

Hierarchical log-linear analyses were used to study the relationships between (1) parent reported anxiety disorders in their children and separately, (2) child self-reported anxiety disorders in (a) ADHD-CT and anxiety disorders and anxiety disorders alone (see Table 8 and 9) and (b) ADHD-CT and dysthymic disorder and dysthymic disorder alone (see Table 10 and 11). Anxiety disorders were only allowed in the models if two-way contingency tables provided expected frequencies in excess of 5. Individual models are described in the **Results** section.

Results

As predicted, parent reported generalised anxiety disorder, separation anxiety disorder, specific phobia and social phobia were significantly increased in the anxiety disorders alone and the ADHD-CT and anxiety disorders groups compared to the ADHD-CT alone group (see Table 4). Also, rates of obsessive compulsive disorder were high enough in the two anxiety groups for it to be analysed along with the above four most common anxiety disorders [26]. Its association was no different across the three groups. The presence of ADHD-CT did not effect the rates of these anxiety disorders except for specific phobia which was significantly lower in the ADHD-CT and anxiety disorders group compared to the anxiety disorders alone group.

Similarly, the child self-reported generalised anxiety disorder, specific phobia, social phobia and obsessive compulsive disorder were significantly increased in the anxiety disorders alone and the ADHD-CT and anxiety disorders groups compared to the ADHD-CT alone group (see Table 5). The presence of ADHD-CT did not affect the rates of these anxiety disorders. In contrast, separation anxiety disorder was significantly increased in the ADHD-CT and anxiety disorders group compared to the anxiety disorders alone group, which, in turn, was significantly increased compared to the ADHD-CT alone group.

Table 4: Parent reported anxiety disorders in their children with ADHD-CT alone, ADHD-CT and anxiety disorders (ADs) and anxiety disorders alone groups

	1 ADHD-CT N=37 N (%)	2 ADHD-CT + ADs N=59 N (%)	3 ADs N=17 N (%)	3 x 2 $\chi^2(2)$	p	2 x 2 $\chi^2(1)$
SAD	-	16 (27)	6 (35)	13.86	***	2=3>1
GAD	-	41 (70)	11 (65)	47.02	***	2=3>1
SoPh	-	13 (22)	5 (29)	6.20	*	2=3>1
SpPh	-	27 (46)	13 (77)	35.59	***	3>2>1
OCD	-	22 (38)	4 (24)	18.23	***	2=3>1
PTSD	-	5 (9)	1 (6)	#		
PD	-	3 (5)	3 (18)	#		
A	-	-	1 (6)	#		

* $p < .05$ *** $p < .005$ # insufficient expected counts in cells for analysis

SAD = separation anxiety disorder; GAD = generalized anxiety disorder; SoPh = social phobia; SpPh = specific phobia; OCD = obsessive-compulsive disorder; PTSD = post traumatic stress disorder; PD = panic disorder; A = agoraphobia.

Table 5: Child self-reported anxiety disorders in ADHD-CT alone, ADHD-CT and anxiety disorders (ADs) and anxiety disorders alone groups

	1 ADHD-CT N=37 N (%)	2 ADHD-CT + ADs N=59 N (%)	3 ADs N=17 N (%)	3 x 2 $\chi^2(2)$	p	2 x 2 $\chi^2(1)$
SAD	-	18 (31)	1 (6)	13.37	***	2>3>1
GAD	-	17 (29)	1 (6)	15.29	***	2=3>1
SoPh	-	7 (12)	1 (6)	6.59	*	2=3>1
SpPh	-	14 (24)	8 (47)	17.16	***	2=3>1
OCD	-	12 (20)	2 (11)	8.26	*	2=3>1
PTSD	-	1 (2)	-	#		
PD	-	-	-	#		
A	-	-	-	#		

* $p < .05$ *** $p < .005$ # insufficient expected counts in cells for analysis

SAD = separation anxiety disorder; GAD = generalized anxiety disorder; SoPh = social phobia; SpPh = specific phobia; OCD = obsessive-compulsive disorder; PTSD = post traumatic stress disorder; PD = panic disorder; A = agoraphobia.

Parent reported and child-self reported generalised anxiety disorder, separation anxiety disorder, specific phobia, social phobia and obsessive compulsive disorder were significantly increased in the dysthymic disorder alone and the ADHD-CT and dysthymic disorder groups compared to the ADHD-CT alone group (see Table 6 and 7). Also, rates of parent reported panic disorder were high enough in the two dysthymic disorder groups for it to be analysed along with the above five most common anxiety disorders. Its association was no different across the three groups. The presence of ADHD-CT did not affect the rates of these anxiety disorders associated with dysthymic disorder.

Table 6: Parent reported anxiety disorders in their children with ADHD-CT alone, ADHD-CT and dysthymic disorder (DD) and dysthymic disorder alone groups

	1 ADHD-CT N=37 N (%)	2 ADHD-CT + DD N=58 N (%)	3 DD N=36 N (%)	3 x 2 $\chi^2(2)$	*p*	2 x 2 $\chi^2(1)$
SAD	-	24 (41)	14 (39)	21.14	***	2=3>1
GAD	-	30 (52)	18 (50)	29.85	***	2=3>1
SoPh	-	21 (36)	12 (33)	12.06	***	2=3>1
SpPh	-	19 (33)	13 (36)	16.80	***	2=3>1
OCD	-	15 (26)	13 (36)	15.41	***	2=3>1
PTSD	-	2 (4)	4 (11)	#		
PD	-	4 (7)	6 (17)	7.27	*	2=3>1
A	-	-	2 (6)	#		

* $p < .05$ *** $p < .005$ # insufficient expected counts in cells for analysis

SAD = separation anxiety disorder; GAD = generalized anxiety disorder; SoPh = social phobia; SpPh = specific phobia; OCD = obsessive-compulsive disorder; PTSD = post traumatic stress disorder; PD = panic disorder; A = agoraphobia.

Table 7: Child self-reported anxiety disorders in ADHD-CT alone, ADHD-CT and dysthymic disorder (DD) and dysthymic disorder alone groups

	1 ADHD-CT N=37 N (%)	2 ADHD-CT + DD N=58 N (%)	3 DD N=36 N (%)	3 x 2 $\chi^2(2)$	*p*	2 x 2 $\chi^2(1)$
SAD	-	23 (40)	13 (36)	15.80	***	2=3>1
GAD	-	17 (29)	8 (22)	10.62	***	2=3>1
SoPh	-	10 (17)	8 (22)	8.25	*	2=3>1
SpPh	-	14 (24)	12 (33)	13.29	***	2=3>1
OCD	-	15 (26)	8 (22)	10.62	***	2=3>1
PTSD	-	1 (2)	2 (6)	#		
PD	-	5 (7)	4 (11)	#		
A	-	1 (2)	2 (6)	#		

* $p < .05$ *** $p < .005$ # insufficient expected counts in cells for analysis

SAD = separation anxiety disorder; GAD = generalized anxiety disorder; SoPh = social phobia; SpPh = specific phobia; OCD = obsessive-compulsive disorder; PTSD = post traumatic stress disorder; PD = panic disorder; A = agoraphobia.

A five-way frequency analysis was performed to develop a hierarchical log-linear model of parent-reported anxiety disorders in their children. Dichotamous variables analysed were SAD, GAD, SoPh, SpPh and OCD. Seventy six primary school age children with [1] ADHD-CT and anxiety and [2] anxiety alone provided data for this analysis. All two-way contingency tables provided expected frequencies in excess of five. After the model was selected, none of the 32 cells was an outlier. Stepwise selection by simple deletion of effects produced a model that included one first order effect (OCD), two of the ten possible two way associations, (SoPh by SpPh, SAD by SoPh) and one of the ten possible three-way associations (SAD by SpPh by GAD). The model had a likelihood ratio χ^2 (20) = 14.92, p = .78, indicating a good fit between observed frequencies and expected frequencies generated by the model. Table 8 records the results of tests of significance (partial likelihood ratio χ^2) and log-linear parameter estimates in raw (λ) and standardised (λ/SE) forms.

Table 8: Tests of significance (partial likelihood ratio χ^2) and log-linear parameter estimates in raw (λ) and standardised (λ/SE) forms

Effect	Partial Association χ^2	Log-linear parameter estimate (λ)	λ/SE
First order:			
SoPh	26.48**	.500	3.027
SAD	15.63**	.293	1.778
GAD	12.17**	-.397	-2.404
OCD	6.62**	.229	1.388
SpPh	0.01	-.166	-1.004
Second order:			
SoPh by SpPh	13.41**	.360	2.181
SpPh by GAD	5.11*	.311	1.884
SAD by SoPh	4.03*	.077	.466
SAD by GAD	2.71	.134	.811
SoPh by GAD	1.47	.023	.140
SAD by SpPh	0.91	-.016	-.096
SoPh by OCD	0.59	-.127	-.768
SAD by OCD	0.43	.048	.289
SpPh by OCD	0.19	-.104	-.632
GAD by OCD	0.11	.019	.114
Third order:			
SAD by SpPh by GAD	11.96**	-.274	-1.661

A three-way frequency analysis was performed to develop a hierarchical log-linear model of child self-reported anxiety disorders. Dichotamous variables analysed were SAD, GAD and SpPh. Seventy six primary school age children with [1] ADHD-CT and anxiety and [2] anxiety alone provided data for this analysis. All two-way contingency tables provided expected frequencies in excess of five. After the model was selected, none of the 8 cells was an outlier. Stepwise selection by simple deletion of effects produced a model that included two of the three possible two-way associations, (SAD by SpPh, SpPh by GAD). The model had a likelihood ratio χ^2 (2) = 1.68, p = .43, indicating a good fit between observed frequencies and expected frequencies generated by the model. Table 9 records the results of tests of significance (partial likelihood ratio χ^2) and log-linear parameter estimates in raw (λ) and standardised (λ/SE) forms.

Table 9: Tests of significance (partial likelihood ratio χ^2) and log-linear parameter estimates in raw (λ) and standardised (λ/SE) forms

Effect	Partial association χ^2	Log-linear parameter estimate (λ)	λ/SE
First order:			
SAD	24.90**	.409	2.900
SpPh	18.30**	.254	1.801
GAD	11.24**	.174	1.235
Second order:			
SAD by SpPh	8.08**	.394	2.798
SpPh by GAD	3.86*	.260	1.845
SAD by GAD	1.68	.189	1.339

A five-way frequency analysis was performed to develop a hierarchical log-linear model of parent-reported anxiety disorders in their children. Dichotamous variables analysed were SAD, GAD, SoPh, SpPh and OCD. Ninety four primary school age children with [1] ADHD-CT and dysthymic disorder and [2] dysthymic disorder alone provided data for this analysis. All two-way contingency tables provided expected frequencies in excess of five. After the model was selected, none of the 32 cells was an outlier. Stepwise selection by simple deletion of effects produced a model that included one of the ten possible two way associations, (SoPh by GAD) and three of the ten possible three-way associations (SAD by SoPh by SpPh, SoPh by SpPh by OCD, SAD by GAD by OCD). The model had a likelihood ratio χ^2 (14) = 10.18, p = .75, indicating a good fit between observed frequencies and expected frequencies generated by the model. Table 10 records the results of tests of significance (partial likelihood ratio χ^2) and log-linear parameter estimates in raw (λ) and standardised (λ/SE) forms.

Table 10: Tests of significance (partial likelihood ratio χ^2) and log-linear parameter estimates in raw (λ) and standardised (λ/SE) forms

Effect	Partial Association χ^2	Log-linear parameter estimate (λ)	λ/SE
First order:			
OCD	15.81**	.582	3.299
SpPh	9.74**	.291	1.652
SoPh	8.47**	.223	1.263
SAD	3.47	.174	0.984
GAD	0.04	.042	0.235
Second order:			
SAD by SoPh	10.50**	.355	2.013
SAD by SpPh	5.57*	.223	1.826
SoPh by GAD	3.92*	.151	.853
SAD by OCD	3.76	.131	.744
SoPh by SpPh	1.50	.223	1.263
SAD by GAD	1.15	.221	1.253
SpPh by GAD	0.82	.126	.716
SoPh by OCD	0.76	-.958	-.542
GAD by OCD	0.21	.133	.755
SpPh by OCD	0.11	.036	.206
Third order:			
SAD by GAD by OCD	4.87*	.195	1.105
SAD by SoPh by SpPh	4.59*	.126	.716
SoPh by SpPh by OCD	4.56*	-.122	-.693
SoPh by GAD by OCD	1.45	-.117	-.644
SAD by SpPh by GAD	1.21	-.080	-.435
SAD by SoPh by GAD	1.20	.039	.222
SAD by SpPh by OCD	0.86	-.096	-.545
SAD by SoPh by OCD	0.29	-.008	-.044
SpPh by GAD by OCD	0.09	.013	.075
SoPh by SpPh by GAD	0.00	-.068	-.385

A four-way frequency analysis was performed to develop a hierarchical log-linear model of child self-reported anxiety disorders. Dichotamous variables analysed were SAD, GAD, SpPh and OCD. Ninety- four primary school age children with [1] ADHD-CT and dysthymic disorder and [2] dysthymic disorder alone provided data for this analysis. All two-way contingency tables provided expected frequencies in excess of five. After the model was selected, none of the 16 cells was an outlier. Stepwise selection by simple deletion of effects produced a model that included all four of the dichotamous variables (SAD by SpPh by GAD by OCD). Table 11 records the results of tests of significance (partial likelihood ratio χ^2) and log-linear parameter estimates in raw (λ) and standardised (λ/SE) forms.

Table 11: Tests of significance (partial likelihood ratio χ^2) and log-linear parameter estimates in raw (λ) and standardised (λ/SE) forms

Effect	Partial association χ^2	Log-linear parameter estimate (λ)	λ/SE
First order:			
OCD	25.71**	.320	2.207
SpPh	19.45**	.305	2.107
GAD	17.58**	.240	1.658
SAD	5.20*	-.033	-.230
Second order:			
SAD by GAD	11.53**	.292	2.019
GAD by OCD	9.69**	.423	2.924
SpPh by OCD	7.56**	.217	1.910
SAD by SpPh	0.87	-.026	-.180
SpPh by GAD	0.65	-.078	-.536
SAD by OCD	0.55	.150	1.036
Third order:			
SAD by SpPh by OCD	1.30	.065	.451
SAD by GAD by OCD	1.17	.046	.319
SAD by SpPh by GAD	0.39	-.067	-.463
SpPh by GAD by OCD	0.37	.014	.095
Fourth order:			
SAD by SpPh by GAD by OCD		.328	2.266

Discussion

The older age of the anxiety disorders alone group compared to the ADHD-CT and anxiety disorders group approached significance, but was well within the same primary school age developmental period. Similarly, increased numbers of girls in the former group were noted but did not reach significance. Rates of oppositional defiant disorder were significantly increased in the two ADHD-CT groups compared to the anxiety disorders alone group, consistent with this known greater association [5]. The dysthymic disorder alone group had significantly increased numbers of girls compared to the ADHD-CT alone group, consistent with the known greater prevalence of girls in the former group [13]. Otherwise, the groups did not respectively differ in IQ and social adversity status.

The four most common parent reported anxiety disorders [26] were evident in the anxiety disorders groups, whether ADHD-CT was present or not. Interestingly, obsessive compulsive disorder was also present at high enough rates for it to be included in the Chi-square analyses: it had a similar association to the other anxiety disorders across the anxiety disorders with and without ADHD-CT groups. Specific phobia was particularly prevalent in the anxiety disorders alone group compared to the anxiety disorders and ADHD-CT group: this may be a sampling effect given the relatively low numbers (N=17) in the anxiety disorders alone group. The child self-reported anxiety disorders behaved in a similar way to the parent reported anxiety disorders across the groups, except for separation anxiety disorder.

Importantly, the child self-report of separation anxiety disorder was the only anxiety disorder to be significantly increased in the anxiety disorders and ADHD-CT compared to the anxiety disorders alone group. This suggests an additive or multiplicative effect between separation anxiety disorder and ADHD-CT that requires further investigation using epidemiological data with larger numbers, particularly in the anxiety disorders alone group: our calculation of the effect sizes of anxiety disorders alone: ADHD-CT alone (Cohen's d = .05) compared to ADHD-CT and anxiety disorders: anxiety disorders alone (Cohen's d = .68) compared to ADHD-CT and anxiety disorders: ADHD-CT alone (Cohen's d = .70) suggests a multiplicative effect.

The four most common parent reported and child self-reported anxiety disorders [26] were evident in the dysthymic disorder group, whether ADHD-CT was present or not. Interestingly, parent and child self-reported obsessive compulsive disorder and parent reported panic disorder were also present at high enough rates for it to be included in the Chi-square analyses: they had a similar association to the other anxiety disorders across the dysthymic disorder with and without ADHD-CT groups.

Taken together, these results suggest that parent reported anxiety in their children and child self-report of anxiety have both similarities, for example, common anxiety phenomena reported, and differences, for example, rates of specific anxiety phenomena preferentially self-reported by children in particular clinical groups [21,41]. Also, these similarities and differences vary across clinical disorders, for example, anxiety versus dysthymic disorders. The hierarchical log-linear models presented support both these assertions: parent and child reports of anxiety disorders differ in the relationships between specific anxiety disorders that were allowed entry into the models and further differ across anxiety and dysthymic disorders groups. Interestingly, parent reported obsessive compulsive disorder in the anxiety disorders alone and with ADHD-CT group was separate to the related four most common anxiety disorders [26]. This is consistent with the known aetiological differences between these two broad types of anxiety [26]. However, this difference was not evident in the dysthymic disorders alone and with the ADHD-CT group, suggesting a specific dysthymic disorder association of parent reported obsessive compulsive disorder with the related four most common anxiety disorders [26]. Importantly, child self-reported obsessive compulsive disorder was not allowed entry into the model in the anxiety disorders alone and with ADHD-CT group, unlike the dysthymic disorders alone and with ADHD-CT group. Therefore, the above parent reported difference could not be investigated in the child self-reported data.

The next study will address the association between neurobiological measures (neurodevelopmental deficits (neurological subtle signs, parent report of motor and/or language developmental delay)) and (1) ADHD-CT with and without anxiety disorders and (2) ADHD-CT with and without dysthymic disorder.

Study 3

The association between neurodevelopmental deficits (NDD) and disruptive behaviour disorders, such as ADHD-CT, is well known. Taylor et al. [31,45,46] have shown that NDD, defined by a delay in language and/or motor development and an increase in neurological 'soft signs', are associated with pervasive hyperactivity (ADHD-CT DSM-IV equivalent). Also, Piek et al. [47] examined primary school-age boys with ADHD-CT compared to a control group and determined that the ADHD-CT group had an increased parental report of motor and language delay together with increased sensorimotor incoordination. These findings are consistent with other cross-sectional and longitudinal datasets suggesting the association of increased neurological 'soft signs' and increased externalising symptoms in children [48-51].

Further, there is replicated evidence supporting the association of NDD with emotional disorders [52-54]. The important 10 year longitudinal study of Shaffer et al. [52] suggested that neurological 'soft signs' were associated with significantly more 'affective diagnoses' with 'no excess' of 'antisocial or conduct disorders'. They concluded that neurological 'soft signs' were associated with 'emotional rather than behavioural' disturbance. Subsequent longitudinal studies have reported a similar association between neurological 'soft signs' and internalising problems [53,54]. Now, NDD can be defined in a number of different ways. Therefore, Pine et al. [53] have suggested the use of standardised neurological 'soft signs' measures in this area of research. For instance, NDD can be defined by neurological subtle signs and the parent report of motor and/or language developmental delay consistent with Taylor et al.'s definition [31,45,46]. Neurological subtle signs consist of the following: choreoathetoid movements, smoothness, accuracy and mirroring of upper limb alternating movements, conjugate eye gaze, and cerebellar signs.

To date, the association between NDD and (1) ADHD-CT with and without anxiety disorders and (2) ADHD-CT with and without dysthymic disorder has not been investigated in primary school age children. We hypothesise that NDD will be increased in all the above groups and in the ADHD-CT and anxiety disorders and ADHD-CT and dysthymic disorder groups compared to the respective anxiety disorders and dysthymic disorder alone groups.

Method

Subjects

The following subject groups are defined in this chapter in Study 2 and the Subject characteristics are listed in Table 2 and 3:

ADHD-CT alone, ADHD-CT and anxiety disorders and anxiety disorders alone groups

ADHD-CT alone, ADHD-CT and dysthymic disorder and dysthymic disorder alone groups

Measures

Please note additional measures not used in Study 1 and 2 are noted here.

Scored Developmental Neurological Examination (SDNE) [55] provides a standardised assessment of current neurological subtle signs. This includes an assessment of motor coordination (choreoathetoid movements, conjugate eye gaze), complex fine-motor activities (smoothness, accuracy and mirroring of upper limb alternating movements), cerebellar signs (including dysdiadochokinesis) and parietal signs (including dysgraphesthesia and astereognosis). SDNE total score ranges from 0-80. It has demonstrated adequate validity and reliability.

Procedure

The *Abbreviated Conners' Rating Scale (ACRS)* [30] and *Child Behaviour Checklist (CBCL)* [42] parent forms were completed prior to the child's assessment. The child was initially interviewed by a registered psychologist who administered the *WISC-3* [32] to the child, while a Fellow in Child and Adolescent Psychiatry concurrently administered the *Anxiety Disorders Interview Schedule for Children (A-DISC)*- [29] parent form and the *Parental Account of Childhood Symptoms (PACS)* [31]. At a separate session, a Fellow in Child and Adolescent Psychiatry administered the *Anxiety Disorders Interview Schedule for Children (A-DISC)*- [29] child form and the *Scored Developmental Neurological Examination (SDNE)* [55] blind to the child's diagnoses, and the child completed the *Children's Depression Scale (CDS)* [44] and the *Revised Children's Manifest Anxiety Scale (R-CMAS)* [43].

Statistical Analysis

One-way analyses of variance (ANOVA) were completed to investigate the differences in total neurological subtle signs between the (1) ADHD-CT, ADHD-CT and anxiety disorders and anxiety disorders alone groups and (2) the ADHD-CT, ADHD-CT and dysthymic disorder and dysthymic disorder alone groups. One-way between-groups multivariate analyses of variance (MANOVA) were completed to investigate the differences in components of neurological subtle signs between the same respective three groups above. Five dependent variables were used: choreiform/athetoid movements, smoothness/accuracy, mirror movements, conjugate eye gaze and upper and lower limb cerebellar movements. The independent variable was membership of the respective above three groups. Preliminary assumption testing was performed to ensure there were no violations of normality, linearity, univariate and multivariate outliers, homogeneity of variance-covariance matrices and multicollinearity.

3 x 2 Chi-square analyses of parent reported motor and/or language developmental delay and (1) ADHD-CT, ADHD-CT and anxiety disorders and anxiety disorders alone groups and (2) the ADHD-CT, ADHD-CT and dysthymic disorder and dysthymic disorder alone groups were initially performed. If significant, further 2 x 2 Chi-square analyses were performed to determine the source of this significance.

Results

The ADHD-CT and ADHD-CT and anxiety disorders groups had significantly higher total neurological subtle signs than the anxiety disorders alone group, and the ADHD-CT and ADHD-CT and anxiety disorders groups did not differ from each other (see Table 12). The effect size of the difference between the ADHD-CT alone and the anxiety disorders alone groups was approximately one standard deviation (Cohen's d = .98). There was a significant difference between three groups on the combined dependent variables: Wilks' λ = .77, F (12,206) = 2.44, p = .005, partial η^2 = .12. When the results for the separate dependent variables were considered, the only differences to reach significance, using a Bonferroni corrected alpha level of .01, were smoothness/accuracy and upper and lower limb cerebellar movements. Again, the ADHD-CT and ADHD-CT and anxiety disorders groups had significantly higher levels of these particular neurological subtle signs than the anxiety disorders alone group and the ADHD-CT and ADHD-CT and anxiety disorders groups did not differ from each other. The effect sizes of the difference between the ADHD-CT alone and the anxiety disorders alone groups on smoothness/accuracy and upper and lower limb cerebellar movements were approximately 0.2 and one standard deviation, respectively (Cohen's d = .13/1.08).

Table 12: Neurological subtle signs (NSS) in ADHD-CT alone, ADHD-CT and anxiety disorders (ADs) and anxiety disorders alone groups

	1 ADHD-CT N=37 N (%)	2 ADHD-CT + ADs N=59 N (%)	3 ADs N=17 N (%)	F (2,110)	p	partial η^2
Total NSS	30.35 (15.62)	33.34 (20.07)	16.77 (12.69)	5.46	.005	1=2>3
Ch/ath	1.95 (1.30)	1.96 (1.15)	1.20 (0.80)	2.23	.11	-
SmAcc	1.69 (1.39)	1.70 (0.89)	0.80 (0.57)	4.80	.01	.08 1=2>3
Mirror	1.23 (0.69)	1.51 (0.95)	1.17 (0.72)	1.74	.18	-
Eye	0.62 (0.68)	0.92 (0.78)	0.73 (0.80)	1.91	.15	-
Cereb	1.05 (0.55)	1.22 (0.96)	0.45 (0.53)	5.58	.005	.09 1=2>3

NSS=neurological subtle signs; Ch/ath=choreiform and athetoid movements; SmAcc=smoothness/accuracy; Mirror=mirror movements; Eye=conjugate eye gaze; Cereb=upper and lower limb cerebellar movements

The ADHD-CT and dysthymic disorder group had significantly higher total neurological subtle signs than the dysthymic disorder alone group, while the ADHD-CT alone group did not differ from the ADHD-CT and dysthymic disorder and dysthymic disorder alone groups (see Table 13). The effect size of the difference between the ADHD-CT and dysthymic disorder and the dysthymic disorder alone groups was approximately 0.8 standard deviation (Cohen's d = .73). There was a significant difference between three groups on the combined dependent variables: Wilks' λ = .73, F (12,244) = 3.47, $p < .0005$, partial η^2 = .15. When the results for the separate dependent variables were considered, the only differences to reach significance, using a Bonferroni corrected alpha level of .01, were mirror movements, upper and lower limb cerebellar movements and conjugate eye gaze. Again, the ADHD-CT and dysthymic disorder group had significantly higher levels of the first two particular neurological subtle signs than the dysthymic disorder alone group while the ADHD-CT alone group did not differ from the ADHD-CT and dysthymic disorder and dysthymic disorder alone groups. The effect sizes of the difference between the ADHD-CT and dysthymic disorder and the dysthymic disorder alone groups on mirror movements and upper and lower limb cerebellar movements were approximately .1 and .5 standard deviation, respectively (Cohen's d = .09/ .62). In contrast, conjugate eye gaze was increased in the ADHD-CT and dysthymic disorder and dysthymic disorder alone groups compared to the ADHD-CT alone group. The effect size of the difference between the dysthymic disorder alone and the ADHD-CT alone groups on conjugate eye gaze was approximately .8 standard deviation (Cohen's d = .70).

Table 13: Neurological subtle signs (NSS) in ADHD-CT alone, ADHD-CT and dysthymic disorder (DD) and dysthymic disorder alone groups

	1 ADHD-CT N=37 N (%)	2 ADHD-CT + DD N=58 N (%)	3 DD N=36 N (%)	F (2,128)	*p*	partial η^2
Total NSS	30.35 (15.62)	33.35 (13.39)	24.58 (10.37)	4.81	.01	2>3
Ch/ath	1.95 (1.30)	2.25 (1.27)	1.65 (0.81)	2.53	.08	-
SmAcc	1.69 (1.39)	1.51 (0.60)	1.24 (0.91)	1.97	.14	-
Mirror	1.23 (0.69)	1.62 (1.19)	1.04 (0.74)	4.52	.01	.07 2>3
Eye	0.62 (0.68)	1.15 (0.65)	1.13 (0.77)	7.37	.001	.10 2=3>1
Cereb	1.05 (0.55)	1.22 (0.56)	0.83 (0.52)	5.77	.004	.08 2>3

NSS=neurological subtle signs; Ch/ath=choreiform and athetoid movements; SmAcc=smoothness/accuracy; Mirror=mirror movements; Eye=conjugate eye gaze; Cereb=upper and lower limb cerebellar movements

Parent report of motor delay and language delay did not differ across the ADHD-CT alone, ADHD-CT and anxiety disorders and anxiety disorders alone groups (see Table 14).

Table 14: Parent reported delay in motor and language development in their children with ADHD-CT alone, ADHD-CT and anxiety disorders (ADs) and anxiety disorders alone groups.

	1 ADHD-CT N=37 N (%)	2 ADHD-CT + ADs N=59 N (%)	3 ADs N=17 N (%)	3 x 2 $\chi^2_{(2)}$	p	2 x 2 $\chi^2_{(1)}$
Motor (+, -)	4,33	13,46	3,14	4.04	.13	-
Lang (+, -)	11,26	26,33	3,14	1.81	.40	-

Motor = parent report of motor delay; Lang = parent report of language delay.

Parent report of motor delay did not differ across the ADHD-CT alone, ADHD-CT and dysthymic disorder and dysthymic disorder alone groups (see Table 15). However, a non-significant trend was evident that was associated with the ADHD-CT and dysthymic disorder group having more parent reported motor delay than the dysthymic disorder alone group, while the ADHD-CT alone group did not differ from either group. Parent reported language delay did not differ across the above groups.

Table 15: Parent reported delay in motor and language development in their children with ADHD-CT alone, ADHD-CT and dysthymic disorder (DD) and dysthymic disorder alone groups.

	1 ADHD-CT N=37 N (%)	2 ADHD-CT + DD N=58 N (%)	3 DD N=36 N (%)	3 x 2 $\chi^2_{(2)}$	p	2 x 2 $\chi^2_{(1)}$
Motor (+, -)	4,33	14,44	3,33	5.24	.07	2>3#
Lang (+, -)	11,26	29,29	15,22	3.75	.15	-

Motor = parent report of motor delay; Lang = parent report of language delay;
# $\chi^2(1) = 3.89, p = .05$.

Discussion

ADHD-CT was associated with significantly increased neurological subtle signs whether comorbid with anxiety disorders or not. Further, there was a large effect size for increased cerebellar signs in the ADHD-CT groups compared to the anxiety disorders alone group, consistent with the current interest in cerebellar dysfunction as a central aetiological factor in ADHD-CT [56]. Although associated with a small effect size, increased smoothness/accuracy difficulties in the ADHD-CT groups compared to the anxiety disorders alone group may be an important correlate of visuospatial executive dysfunction in ADHD-CT, providing more support for the importance of aberrant frontostriatal network function in ADHD-CT [57].

Similar findings of increased neurological subtle signs and increased cerebellar signs in ADHD-CT and dysthymic disorder compared to dysthymic disorder alone were evident. However, there were important differences: Firstly, the ADHD-CT alone and dysthymic disorder alone groups did not differ on either of these measures, suggesting that dysthymic disorder alone is associated with increased neurological subtle signs, generally, and increased cerebellar signs, specifically, compared to anxiety disorders alone. This is an important new finding that further explains the prior more general findings of Shaffer et al. [52] and Pine et al. [53,54]. Secondly, in contrast to these findings, dysthymic disorder with and without ADHD-CT, was associated with significantly increased conjugate eye gaze difficulties compared to ADHD-CT alone. This is a truly remarkable finding that was not expected, given the current published literature: it has implications for the understanding of (1) equifinality and multifinality pathways between dysthymic disorder with and without ADHD-CT, (2) additional neurotransmitter networks such as $\gamma-$ amino butyric acid (GABA), aside from dopaminergic, noradrenergic and serotonergic in the pathophysiology of dysthymic disorder with and without ADHD-CT [58-60] and (3) possible synaptic gating and threshold effects that mediate and modulate regional brain neuronal networks in dysthymic disorder with and without ADHD-CT [61-64]. Of interest, the parent report of motor developmental delay was only non-significantly increased between the ADHD-CT and dysthymic disorder group compared to the dysthymic disorder alone group, which supports the need for future systematic investigation of these comorbid disorders to determine whether there is additional (either additive or multiplicative) developmental motor dysfunction.

Study 4

Primary school-age children with ADHD-CT have been associated with increased rates of parental adult ADHD, anxiety disorders, depressive disorders, antisocial personality disorder and alcohol and substance abuse disorders [65,66], negative controlling parenting [67], marital conflict and/or breakdown [23], parental distress [68] and/or psychiatric illness [69], lower socio-economic status and/or higher family adversity [70], and increased expressed emotion in the family unit, particularly increased rates of hostile criticism that is a significant predictor of long-term outcome [71]. Parental psychopathology and family functioning has been repeatedly noted to be worse in ADHD-CT and conduct disorder groups compared to ADHD-CT alone groups, suggesting that conduct disorder be controlled in any analysis of these parental and family domains of functioning [72-74].

Parental psychopathology and family functioning in dysthymic disorder in primary school age children has not been studied. Klein et al. [75] and Lizardi et al. [76] have studied an adult group with early onset dysthymic disorder, mean age of onset 10.2 years, comparing them to a normal control group. They found relatives of dysthymic probands had increased rates of mood disorders, major depressive disorder, bipolar affective disorder (bipolar 1 disorder, DSM-IV equivalent), increased recurrent major depressive disorder, relatives with increased personality disorders (of all clusters) increased rates of treatment for depressive disorder, usage of medication for depressive disorder and incapacitation due to depressive disorder compared to normal controls.

Primary school age children with anxiety disorders have been noted to not differ from healthy control children on measures of parental psychopathology [77] and family functioning [78] through to having higher rates of anxiety [79], obsessive-compulsive and depressive symptoms [78] and hostility [80] in parents, and, more troubled family relations [80], families less granting of autonomy (on an observer rated measure), and mothers of anxious children as less accepting (as rated by the child) in the families of children with anxiety disorders compared to normal control families [78].

To date, the associations between parental psychopathology and family functioning in (1) ADHD-CT with and without anxiety disorders and (2) ADHD-CT with and without dysthymic disorder have not been investigated. We hypothesise that there will be no differences between parental psychopathology and family functioning measures across the above groups.

Method

Subjects

The following subject groups are defined in this chapter in Study 2 and the Subject characteristics are listed in Table 2 and 3:

ADHD-CT alone, ADHD-CT and anxiety disorders and anxiety disorders alone groups

ADHD-CT alone, ADHD-CT and dysthymic disorder and dysthymic disorder alone groups

Measures

Please note additional measures not used in Study 1,2 and 3 are noted here.

Hopkins Symptom Checklist (HSCL) [81] comprises 58 items that measure 5 symptom dimensions: anxiety, depression, obsessive-compulsive symptoms, somatisation, and interpersonal sensitivity, using a 1-4 Likert scale. A total score provides a general measure of psychopathology. Adequate validity and reliability have been demonstrated in published research findings.

Family Assessment Device (FAD) [82] was developed from the McMaster Model of Family Functioning to measure the structural and organisational characteristics of families. It consists of 60 items that measure 6 dimensions of family functioning: problem solving, communication, affective responsiveness, affective involvement, roles and behavioural control. Each dimension forms a subscale with an additional general functioning subscale that measures the overall health/dysfunction in the family unit. Adequate validity and reliability have been demonstrated in published research findings.

Procedure

The *Abbreviated Conners' Rating Scale (ACRS)* [30] and *Child Behaviour Checklist (CBCL)* [43] parent forms were completed prior to the child's assessment. The child was initially interviewed by a registered psychologist who administered the *WISC-3* [32] to the child, while a Fellow in Child and Adolescent Psychiatry concurrently administered the *Anxiety Disorders Interview Schedule for Children (A-DISC)*- [29] parent form and the *Parental Account of Childhood Symptoms (PACS)* [31]. At a separate session, a Fellow in Child and Adolescent Psychiatry administered the *Anxiety Disorders Interview Schedule for Children (A-DISC)*- [29] child form and the child completed the *Children's Depression Scale (CDS)* [45] and the *Revised Child Manifest Anxiety Scale (R-CMAS)* [44]. Concurrently the parents completed the *Hopkins Symptom Checklist (HSCL)* [81] and the *Family Assessment Device (FAD)* [82].

Statistical Analysis

One-way analyses of variance (ANOVA) were completed to investigate the differences in total parental psychopathology and general family functioning between the (1) ADHD-CT, ADHD-CT and anxiety disorders and anxiety disorders alone groups and (2) the ADHD-CT, ADHD-CT and dysthymic disorder and dysthymic disorder alone groups. One-way between-groups multivariate analyses of variance (MANOVA) were completed to investigate the differences in components of parental psychopathology and family functioning between the same respective three groups above. Four dependent variables were used: anxiety, depression, interpersonal sensitivity and obsessive compulsive symptoms. Similarly, six dependent variables were used to investigate differences in components of family functioning between the same three groups above: problem solving, communication, roles, behavioural control, affective responsiveness and affective involvement. The independent variable was membership of the respective above three groups. Preliminary assumption testing was performed to ensure there were no violations of normality, linearity, univariate and multivariate outliers, homogeneity of variance-covariance matrices and multicollinearity.

Results

The ADHD-CT alone, ADHD-CT and anxiety disorders and anxiety disorders alone groups did not differ significantly on total parental psychopathology (see Table 16). There was no significant difference between the three groups on the combined dependent variables: Wilks' $\lambda = .90$, $F(8,184) = 1.30$, $p = .25$. However, the ADHD-CT and anxiety disorders and anxiety disorders alone groups were in the clinical range [82] for all the parental psychopathology measures while the ADHD-CT alone group was in the clinical range for the depression, interpersonal sensitivity and obsessive compulsive symptom subscales of the *HSCL*.

The ADHD-CT alone and ADHD-CT and anxiety disorders groups had significantly worse general family functioning than the anxiety disorders alone group. The effect sizes of these respective differences were approximately 1 and .8 standard deviation (Cohen's d = .96/.70). There was a significant difference between three groups on the combined dependent variables: Wilks' $\lambda = .74$, $F(12,156) = 2.16$, $p = .02$, partial $\eta^2 = .14$. When the results for the separate dependent variables were considered, the only difference to reach significance, using a Bonferroni corrected alpha level of .01, was family communication. The ADHD-CT alone group had significantly worse family communication than the anxiety disorders alone group. The effect size of this difference was approximately one standard deviation (Cohen's d = 1.16). The ADHD-CT alone and ADHD-CT and anxiety groups were in the clinical range for all the family functioning measures except the problem solving subscale of the *FAD* [83]. The anxiety disorders alone group was in the clinical range for the roles and affective involvement subscales of the *FAD* [83] only.

Table 16: Parental psychopathology and Family functioning in ADHD-CT alone, ADHD-CT and anxiety disorders (ADs) and anxiety disorders alone groups

	1 ADHD-CT N=37 N (%)	2 ADHD-CT + ADs N=59 N (%)	3 ADs N=17 N (%)	F (2,110)	*p*	partial η^2
Total PP	86.22 (19.96)	92.79 (21.96)*	90.93 (23.43)*	0.83	.44	-
anx	1.24 (0.32)	1.39 (0.40)*	1.52 (0.58)*	2.42	.09	-
dep	1.61 (0.57)*	1.71 (0.48)*	1.62 (0.51)*	0.45	.64	-
ips	1.67 (0.58)*	1.82 (0.52)*	1.68 (0.44)*	0.98	.38	-
oc	1.54 (0.36)*	1.70 (0.46)*	1.65 (0.46)*	1.27	.29	-
GF	2.26 (0.47)*	2.18 (0.46)*	1.88 (0.34)	4.02	.02	1=2>3
PS	2.17 (0.57)	2.06 (0.36)	1.99 (0.37)	0.88	.42	
C	2.37 (0.36)*	2.21 (0.40)*	1.97 (0.29)	5.54	.006	.12 1>3
R	2.55 (0.21)*	2.40 (0.25)*	2.32 (0.35)*	4.20	.02	
BC	2.24 (0.59)*	2.15 (0.57)*	1.76 (0.35)	4.17	.02	
AR	2.30 (0.52)*	2.26 (0.60)*	1.89 (0.49)	3.20	.05	
AI	2.43 (0.59)*	2.48 (0.55)*	2.44 (0.44)*	0.09	.91	

PP=parental psychopathology; anx=anxiety subscale; dep=depression subscale; ips=interpersonal sensitivity subscale; oc=obsessive compulsive subscale of the Hopkins Symptom Checklist (HSCL); GF=general functioning subscale; PS=problem solving; C=communication; R=roles; BC=behavioural control; AR=affective responsiveness; AI=affective involvement subscales of the Family Assessment Device (FAD). * clinical range

Table 17: Parental psychopathology and Family functioning in ADHD-CT alone, ADHD-CT and dysthymic disorder (DD) and dysthymic disorder alone groups

	1 ADHD-CT N=37 N (%)	2 ADHD-CT + DD N=58 N (%)	3 DD N=36 N (%)	F (2,128)	p	partial η^2
Total PP	86.22 (19.96)	105.73 (27.66)*	91.91 (22.78)*	6.55	.002	2>1=3
anx	1.24 (0.32)	1.60 (0.60)*	1.45 (0.52)*	4.46	.01	-
dep	1.61 (0.57)*	1.96 (0.55)*	1.72 (0.46)*	4.68	.01	.08 2>1
ips	1.67 (0.58)*	1.99 (0.57)*	1.74 (0.46)*	3.98	.02	-
oc	1.54 (0.36)*	1.97 (0.65)*	1.77 (0.49)*	5.70	.004	.09 2>1
GF	2.26 (0.47)*	2.14 (0.41)*	2.11 (0.48)*	0.97	.38	-
PS	2.17 (0.57)	2.07 (0.37)	2.17 (0.47)	0.49	.61	-
C	2.37 (0.36)*	2.10 (0.39)	2.13 (0.44)	3.63	.03	-
R	2.55 (0.21)*	2.40 (0.34)*	2.32 (0.37)*	3.23	.04	-
BC	2.24 (0.59)*	1.92 (0.38)*	1.85 (0.40)	5.84	.004	.14 1>2=3
AR	2.30 (0.52)*	1.95 (0.53)	2.01 (0.47)	3.76	.03	-
AI	2.43 (0.59)*	2.26 (0.45)*	2.13 (0.47)*	2.95	.06	-

PP=parental psychopathology; anx=anxiety subscale; dep=depression subscale; ips=interpersonal sensitivity subscale; oc=obsessive compulsive subscale of the Hopkins Symptom Checklist (HSCL); GF=general functioning subscale; PS=problem solving; C=communication; R=roles; BC=behavioural control; AR=affective responsiveness; AI=affective involvement subscales of the Family Assessment Device (FAD). *clinical range

The ADHD-CT and dysthymic disorder group had significantly higher total parental psychopathology than the ADHD-CT alone and the dysthymic disorder alone groups (see Table 17). The effect sizes of the differences between the ADHD-CT and dysthymic disorder and the ADHD-CT alone and dysthymic disorder alone groups were approximately 1 standard deviation and .5 standard deviation, respectively (Cohen's d = .81/.55). However, there was not a significant difference between the thrree groups on the combined dependent variables: Wilks' λ = .88, F (8,222) = 1.86, p = .07, partial η^2 = .06. Yet, both the depression and the obsessive compulsive symptoms dependent variables differed significantly between the groups with a Bonferroni corrected alpha value of .013. The ADHD-CT and dysthymic disorder group had significantly higher depression and the obsessive compulsive symptoms than the ADHD-CT alone group, respective effect sizes of approximately .5 standard deviation (Cohen's d = .65/.69). Also, the ADHD-CT and dysthymic disorder and dysthymic disorder alone groups were in the clinical range [82] for all the parental psychopathology measures from the *HSCL*, while the ADHD-CT alone group was in the clinical range for the depression, interpersonal sensitivity and obsessive compulsive symptom subscales.

The ADHD-CT alone, ADHD-CT and dysthymic disorder and dysthymic disorder alone groups did not differ on general family functioning. However, there was a significant difference between three groups on the combined dependent variables: Wilks' λ = .80, F (12,192) = 1.85, p = .04, partial η^2 = .10. When the results for the separate dependent variables were considered, the only difference to reach significance, using a Bonferroni corrected alpha level of .01, was family behavioural control. The ADHD-CT alone group had significantly worse family behavioural control than the ADHD-CT and dysthymic disorder and dysthymic disorder alone groups. The effect sizes of these differences were approximately .5 and .8 standard deviation (Cohen's d = .60/.81). The ADHD-CT alone group was in the clinical range for all the subscales of the *FAD* [83] except for the problem solving subscale, the ADHD-CT and dysthymic disorder group was in the clinical range for the general functioning, roles, behaviour control and affective involvement subscales of the *FAD* [83] as was the dysthymic disorder alone group, except for the behavioural control subscale.

Discussion

Social adversity status, a potential confounding variable noted in the literature was matched across the respective groups in this study. Another potentially confounding variable, conduct disorder, was excluded from the respective groups in this study. As predicted, parental psychopathology did not differ between the ADHD-CT alone, ADHD-CT and anxiety disorders and anxiety disorders alone groups. Also, only the ADHD-CT alone group did not have all the parental psychopathology measures in the clinical range. Interestingly, parental anxiety was not in the clinical range in this group, unlike depression, which raises the issue of parental anxiety associated with depression separate from parental anxiety alone for investigation in future studies. In contrast, family functioning was significantly worse, with a large effect size, in the ADHD-CT group, whether anxiety was present or not. In particular, family communication problems were significantly increased, with a large effect size, in the ADHD-CT alone group compared to the anxiety disorders alone group. This extends the existing literature and raises the issue of biological and environmental contributions, as main effects in themselves and as potential interaction effects, for these family communication problems in ADHD-CT. Larger epidemiological sample sizes are required.

Importantly, the ADHD-CT and dysthymic disorder group had significantly higher total parental psychopathology than either the ADHD-CT alone and dysthymic disorder alone groups. This suggests an additive or multiplicative effect between ADHD-CT and dysthymic disorder that requires further investigation using an epidemiological sample with larger numbers: our calculation of the effect sizes of dysthymic disorder alone: ADHD-CT alone (Cohen's d = .26) compared to ADHD-CT and dysthymic disorder: dysthymic disorder alone (Cohen's d = .53) compared to ADHD-CT and dysthymic disorder: ADHD-CT alone (Cohen's d = .81) suggests an additive effect. Interestingly, parental depression and obsessive compulsive symptoms were significantly increased, with a moderate effect size, in the ADHD-CT and dysthymic disorder compared to the ADHD-CT alone groups. This again extends the existing literature and supports further exploration of biological and environmental contributions, as main effects in themselves and as potential interaction effects, for these parental symptoms between these groups, and, further investigation of the association of these parental variables with the increased rates of parent and child self-reported obsessive compulsive disorder in the ADHD-CT and dysthymic disorder and dysthymic disorder alone groups is warranted.

The ADHD-CT alone group had significantly higher levels of behavioural control difficulties, with a moderate-large effect size, compared to the dysthymic disorder with and without ADHD-CT groups, although the dysthymic disorder and ADHD-CT group was in the clinical range for behavioural control difficulties and all three groups were in the clinical range for general family functioning, role definition and affective involvement difficulties. This again extends the existing literature and supports further exploration of biological and environmental contributions, as main effects in themselves, and as potential interaction effects, for these family functioning symptoms between these groups.

Integration and Implications of these Findings

Studies one to four present data that enhance our understanding of dysthymic disorder, anxiety disorders and ADHD-CT, both alone and in combination. The implications for the concept of subtyping in ADHD-CT are considered below.

Dysthymic disorder is *quite distinct* from anxiety disorders: (1) Dysthymic disorder rather than anxiety disorders makes an independent contribution to oppositional defiant patterns of behaviour in primary school age children with ADHD-CT whereas anxiety disorders do not. (2) Dysthymic disorder is significantly associated with anxiety disorders, parent and child reports of these child anxiety disorders are similar, in that the same anxiety phenomena are reported by parent(s) and children, and different as relationships between specific anxiety disorders differ between the parent and child reports in the dysthymic disorder group. However, the relationships between parent and child reports of anxiety disorders differ again in the anxiety disorders group compared to the dysthymic disorder group. For example, parent reported obsessive compulsive disorder in dysthymic disorder is not separate from the four most common anxiety disorders [26], as it is in the anxiety disorders group. (3) Dysthymic disorder is associated with increased neurological subtle signs and is specifically associated with significantly increased conjugate eye gaze difficulties, whether ADHD-CT is present or not. (4) Dysthymic disorder and ADHD-CT is associated with significantly increased parental psychopathology compared to ADHD-CT alone and dysthymic disorder alone groups. This may be an additive effect.

Taken together, these data emphasise the importance of distinguishing comorbid dysthymic disorder from comorbid anxiety disorders in ADHD-CT. These data do not support the construct of a distinct subtype [83], but rather a co-occurrence with additional neurodevelopmental and psychosocial vulnerabilities that arise from either disorder and specific interactional effects. Since 1982 [83], the question of an anxiety subtype of ADHD-CT has been raised. These data do not support any additional neurodevelopmental or psychosocial vulnerabilities arising from the co-occurrence of anxiety disorders with ADHD-CT. In contrast, additional neurodevelopmental vulnerability and an interactional (may be additive) psychosocial vulnerability is evident with dysthymic disorder co-occurring with ADHD-CT. However, an intriguing interactional (may be multiplicative) effect between child self-reported separation anxiety disorder and ADHD-CT is evident in the absence of dysthymic disorder.

All these additional and interactional (additive or multiplicative) vulnerabilities between co-occurring disorders warrant further investigation to explore (1) biological and/or environmental associations as main effects or interactional effects within equifinality and multifinality developmental psychopathology models [84], (2) their developmental phase specific or independent association through longitudinal study designs, particularly pre-through to post-puberty, (3) their primary or secondary nature through different developmental phases and (4) their risk factor and/or resilience factor status at different developmental phases: given the complex interplay of multi-levelled human adaptation to core pathological processes, a given risk factor for a given group of individuals at one developmental stage may be a resilience factor for that same group of individuals at another developmental stage [85].

References

[1] Angold A, Costello J, Erkanli A. Comorbidity. *J Child Psychol Psychiatry*. 1999; 40: 57-97.

[2] Maughan B, Rowe R, Messer J, Goodman R, Meltzer H. Conduct disorder and oppositional defiant disorder in a national sample: developmental epidemiology. *J Child Psychol Psychiatry*. 2004; 45: 609-621.

[3] Biederman J, Newcorn J, Sprich S. Comorbidity of attention deficit hyperactivity disorder with conduct, depressive, anxiety, and other disorders. *Am J Psychiatry*.1991; 148: 564-577.

[4] Lahey BB, McBurnett K, Loeber R. Are ADHD and ODD developmental precursors to conduct disorder? In: Lewis M, Sameroff A, eds. *Handbook of Developmental Psychopathology*. Volume 2. New York: Plenum, 2000.

[5] Angold A, Costello EJ. Towards establishing an empirical basis for the diagnosis of oppositional defiant disorder. *J Am Acad Child Adolesc Psychiatry*. 1996; 35: 1205-1212.

[6] Anderson JC, Williams S, McGee R, Silva PA. DSM-III disorders in preadolescent children: prevalence in a large sample from the general population. *Arch Gen Psychiatry*.1987; 44: 69-76.

[7] Jensen JB, Burke N, Garfinkel BD. Depression and symptoms of attention deficit disorder with hyperactivity. *J Am Acad Child Adolesc Psychiatry*. 1988; 27:742-747.

[8] Woolston JL, Rosenthal SL, Riddle M. Childhood co-morbidity of anxiety/affective disorder and behavior disorders. *J Am Acad Child Adolesc Psychiatry*. 1989; 28:707-713.

[9] Lahey BB, Schaughency EA, Hynd GW, Carlson CL, Nieves N. Attention deficit disorder with and without hyperactivity: comparison of behavioural characteristics of clinic-referred children. *J Am Acad Child Adolesc Psychiatry*. 1987; 26:718-723.

[10] Vance AL, Luk ES, Costin J, Tonge BJ, Pantelis C. Attention deficit hyperactivity disorder: anxiety phenomena in children treated with psychostimulant medication for 6 months or more. *Aust N Z J Psychiatry*. 1999; 33:399-406.

[11] American Psychiatric Association. *Diagnostic and Statistical Manual of Mental Disorders, fourth edition*. Washington, DC: American Psychiatric Association, 1994.

[12] Klein DN, Taylor EB, Dickstein S, Harding D. The early-late onset distinction in DSM-III-R Dysthymia. *J Affect Disord*. 1988; 14:25-33.

[13] Kovacs M. The course of childhood onset depressive disorders. *Psychiatric Annals*. 1996; 26: 326-330.

[14] Angold A, Costello EJ. Depressive comorbidity in children and adolescents: empirical, theoretical and methodological issues. *Am J Psychiatry*. 1993; 150: 1779-1791.

[15] Kovacs M, Akiskal HS, Gatsonis C, Parrone PL. Childhood-onset dysthymic disorder. Clinical features and prospective naturalistic outcome. *Arch Gen Psychiatry*. 1994; 51:365-374.

[16] Kovacs M, Obrosky DS, Gatsonis C, Richards C. First-episode major depressive and dysthymic disorder in childhood: clinical and sociodemographic factors in recovery. *J Am Acad Child Adolesc Psychiatry*.1997; 36:777-784.

[17] Costello EJ, Angold A, Burns BJ. The great smoky mountain study of youth: goals, design, methods and prevalence of DSM-III-R disorders. *Arch Gen Psychiatry*. 1996; 53: 1129-1136.

[18] Mitchell J, McCauley E, Burke PM, Moss SJ. Phenomenology of depression in children and adolescents. *J Am Acad Child Adolesc Psychiatry*. 1988; 27:12-20.

[19] Strauss CC, Last CG, Hersen M, Kazdin AE. Association between anxiety and depression in children and adolescents with anxiety disorder. *J Abn Child Psychol*. 1988; 16:57-68.

[20] Bernstein GA. Comorbidity and severity of anxiety and depressive disorders in a clinic sample. *J Am Acad Child Adolesc Psychiatry*. 1991; 30:43-50.

[21] Vance A, Costin J, Barnett R, Luk E, Maruff P, Tonge B. Characteristics of parent- and child-reported anxiety in psychostimulant medication naive, clinically referred children with attention deficit hyperactivity disorder, combined type (ADHD-CT). *Aust N Z J Psychiatry*. 2002; 36:234-239.

[22] Kashani JH, Orvaschel H. A community study of anxiety in children and adolescents. *Am J Psychiatry*.1990; 147: 313-318.

[23] Taylor E, Schachar R, Thorley G, Wieselberg HM, Everitt B, Rutter M. Which boys respond to stimulant medication? A controlled trial of methylphenidate in boys with disruptive behaviour. *Psychol Med*. 1987; 17: 121-143.

[24] Buitelaar Jan K, Van-der-Gaag RJ, Swaab-Barneveld H, Kuiper M. The prediction of clinical response to methylphenidate in children with attention deficit hyperactivity disorder. *J Am Acad Child Adolesc Psychiatry.*1995; 34: 1025-1032.

[25] Tannock R, Ickowicz A, Schachar R. Differential effects of methylphenidate on working memory in ADHD children with and without comorbid anxiety. *J Am Acad Child Adolesc Psychiatry* 1995; 34: 886-896.

[26] Silverman WK, Treffers PDA, eds. *Anxiety Disorders in children and adolescents.* Cambridge: Cambridge University Press, 2001.

[27] March JS, Swanson JM, Arnold LE, Hoza B, Conners CK, Hinshaw SP, Hechtman L, Kraemer HC, Greenhill LL, Abikoff HB, Elliot GE, Jensen PS, Newcorn JH, Vitlello B, Severe J, Wells KC, Pelham WE. Anxiety as a Predictor and Outcome Variable in the Multimodal Treatment Study of Children with ADHD (MTA). *J Abn Child Psychol.* 2000; 28: 527-541.

[28] Barkley RA. Behavioural inhibition, sustained attention, and executive functions: Constructing a unified theory of ADHD. *Psychol Bulletin.*1997; 121: 65-94.

[29] Silverman WK, Albano AM. *Anxiety Disorders Interview Schedule for DSM-IV.* Texas: Graywind, 1996.

[30] Conners CK. Parent Symptom Questionnaire. *Psychopharm Bull.*1985; 21: 816-822.

[31] Taylor E, Schachar R, Thorley G, Wieselberg M. Conduct disorder and hyperactivity: I, Separation of hyperactivity and antisocial conduct in British child psychiatric patients. *B J Psychiatry.*1986; 149: 760-767.

[32] Wechsler D. *Wechsler Intelligence Scale for Children (3rd Ed.).* Texas: The Psychological Co-operation, 1991.

[33] Nie NH, Hadlai Hull C, Jenkins JG, Steinbrenner K, Bent DH. *Statistical package for the social sciences.* New York: McGraw Hill, 1970.

[34] Loeber R, Burke JD, Lahey BB, Winters A, Zera M. Oppositional defiant and conduct disorders: a review. *J Am Acad Child Adolesc Psychiatry.*2000; 39: 1468-1484.

[35] Kerr M, Tremblay RE, Pagani L, Vitaro F. Boy's behavioural inhibition and the risk of later delinquency. *Arch Gen Psychiatry.*1997; 54: 809-816.

[36] Bird HR, Gould MS, Staghezza B. Aggregating data from multiple informants in child psychiatry epidemiological research. *J Am Acad Child Adolesc Psychiatry.* 1992; 31: 78-85.

[37] Ialongo N, Edelsohn G, Wertharner-Larsson L, Crockett L, Kellam S. The significance of self-reported anxious symptoms in first grade children. *J Abn Child Psychol.* 1994; 22: 441-455.

[38] Jensen PS, Rubio-Stipec M, Canino G, Bird HR, Dulcan MK, Schwab-Stone ME, Lahey BB. Parent and Child Contributions to Diagnosis of Mental Disorder: Are Both Informants Always Necessary? *J Am Acad Child Adolesc Psychiatry.*1999; 38: 1569-1579.

[39] Tannock R. Attention Deficit disorders and Anxiety disorders. In: Brown TE, ed. *Subtypes of Attention Deficit Disorders in Children, Adolescents and Adults.* New York: American Psychiatric Press, 1994.

[40] Pliszka SR. Comorbidity of Attention Deficit Hyperactivity Disorder and Overanxious Disorder. *J Am Acad Child Adolesc Psychiatry.* 1992; 31: 197-203.

[41] Vance ALA, Harris K, Boots M, Talbot J, Costin J, Karamitsios M, Maruff P. (2003) Attention Deficit Hyperactivity Disorder, combined type (ADHD-CT) with and without dysthymic disorder: characteristics of parent and child reported anxiety. *Aust N Z J Psychiatry.*2003; 37: 563-569.

[42] Achenbach TM, Edelbrock CS. *Manual for the Child Behaviour Checklist and Behaviour Profile.* University of Vermont: Burlington, 1983.

[43] Reynolds CR, Richmond BO. *Revised Children's Manifest Anxiety Scale: Manual.* Los Angeles, CA: Western Psychological Services, 1985.

[44] Lang M, Tisher M. *Children's Depression Scale.* Melbourne: ACER, 1983.

[45] Taylor E, Everitt B, Schachar R, Thorley G, Rutter M, Wieselberg M. Conduct disorder and hyperactivity: 11, A cluster analytic approach to the identification of a behavioural syndrome. *Br J Psychiatry.* 1986; 149:768-777.

[46] Taylor E, Sandberg S, Thorley G, Giles S. *The epidemiology of childhood hyperactivity. Institute of Psychiatry Maudsley monograph.* London: Oxford University Press, 1991.

[47] Piek JP, Pitcher TM, Hay DA. Motor Coordination and Kinaesthesis in Boys with Attention Deficit Hyperactivity Disorder. *Dev Med Child Neurol.* 1999; 41:159-165.

[48] Kadesjo B, Gillberg C. Developmental Coordination Disorder in Swedish 7-year old children. *J Am Acad Child Adolesc Psychiatry.* 1999; 38:820-828.

[49] Neeper R, Greenwood RS. On the psychiatric importance of neurological soft signs. In: Lahey B, Kazdin AE, eds. *Advances in Clinical Child Psychology.* New York: Plenum, 1987.

[50] Tupper D, ed. *Soft Neurological Signs.* New York: Grune and Stratton, 1987.

[51] Raine A, Brennan P, Mednick B, Mednick SA. High rates of violence, crime, academic problems, and behavioural problems in males with both early neuromotor deficits and unstable family environments. *Arch Gen Psychiatry.* 1996; 53:544-549.

[52] Shaffer D, Schonfeld I, O'Connor P et al. Neurological soft signs: their relationship to psychiatric disorder and intelligence in childhood and adolescence. *Arch Gen Psychiatry* 1985; 42:342-351.

[53] Pine DS, Shaffer D, Shonfeld IS. Persistent emotional disorders in children with neurological soft signs. *J Am Acad Child Adolesc Psychiatry.* 1993; 32:1229-1236.

[54] Pine DS, Wasserman GA, Fried JE, Parides M, Shaffer D. Neurological soft signs: one-year stability and relationship to psychiatric symptoms in boys. *J Am Acad Child Adolesc Psychiatry.* 1997; 36:1579-1586.

[55] Sandberg ST, Rutter M, Taylor E. Hyperkinetic disorders in clinic attenders. *Dev Med Child Neurol.* 1978; 20:279-299.

[56] Castellanos FX, Tannock R. Neuroscience of ADHD: the search for endophenotypes. *Nat Rev Neuroscience.* 2002; 3: 617-628.

[57] Castellanos FX, Sharp WS, Gottesman RF, Greenstein DK, Giedd JN, Rapoport JL. Anatomic brain abnormalities in monozygotic twins discordant for attention deficit hyperactivity disorder. *Am J Psychiatry.* 2003;160:1693-6.

[58] Viggiano D, Grammatikopoulos G, Sadile AG. Evidence for a hyperfunctioning mesolimbic system-animal model of ADHD. *Beh Br Research.*2002; 130: 181-189.

[59] MacMaster FP, Carrey N, Sparkes S, Kusumaker V. Proton spectroscopy in medication free pediatric ADHD. *Biol Psychiatry.*2003; 53: 184-187.

[60] Cairney S, Maruff P, Vance A, Barnett R, Luk E, Currie J. Abnormalities using task context to voluntarily inhibit saccades in children with attention deficit hyperactivity disorder. *Exp Br Research.*2001; 141: 507-518.

[61] French SJ, Totterdell S. Individual nucleus accumbens-projection neurons receive both basolateral amygdala and ventral subicular afferents in rats. *Neuroscience.*2003; 119: 19-31.

[62] Grace AA. Gating of information flow within the limbic system and the pathophysiology of schizophrenia. *Br Res Reviews.* 2000; 31: 330-341.

[63] Grace AA. Psychostimulant actions on dopamine and limbic system function: relevance to the pathophysiology and treatment of ADHD. In: Solanto MV, Arnsten AFT, Castellanos FX, eds. *Stimulant drugs and ADHD: Basic and clinical neuroscience.* Oxford: Oxford University Press, 2001: 134-157.

[64] Arnsten AFT. Catecholamine modulation of prefrontal cortical function. *Trends Cog Sciences.* 1998; 2: 436-446.

[65] Biederman J, Faraone SV, Keenan K, Steingard R, Tsuang MT. Familial Association Between Attention Deficit Disorder and Anxiety Disorders. *Am J Psychiatry.*1991;148: 251-256.

[66] Biederman J, Faraone SV, Keenan K, Tsuang MT. Evidence of Familial Association Between Attention Deficit Hyperactivity Disorder and Major Affective Disorders. *Arch Gen Psychiatry.*1991; 48: 633-642.

[67] Befera MS, Barkley RA. Hyperactive and normal girls and boys: mother child interaction, parent psychiatric studies and child psychopathology. *J Child Psychol Psychiatry.*1985; 26: 439-452.

[68] Zarin DA, Suarez AP, Pincus HA, Kupersanin E, Zito JM. Clinical and treatment characteristics of children with Attention deficit/Hyperactivity Disorder in psychiatric practice. *J Am Acad Child Adolesc Psychiatry.*1998; 37: 1262-1270.

[69] McGee R, Williams S, Silva PA. Background characteristics of aggressive, hyperactive and aggressive-hyperactive boys. *J Am Acad Child Adolesc Psychiatry.*1984; 23: 280-284.

[70] August GJ, Stewart MA. Is there a syndrome of pure hyperactivity? *B J Psychiatry.* 1982; 140: 305-311.

[71] Rutter M, Maughan B, Meyer J, Pickles A, Sillberg J, Simonoff E, Taylor E. Heterogeneity of antisocial behaviour: causes, continuities, and consequences. *Neb Symp Motivation.* 1997; 44: 45-118.

[72] Lahey BB. Piacentini JC. McBurnett K. Stone P. Hartdagen S. Hynd G. Psychopathology in the parents of children with conduct disorder and hyperactivity. *J Am Acad Child Adolesc Psychiatry.*1988; 27:163-70.

[73] Schachar R, Wachsmuth R. Family Dysfunction and Psychosocial Adversity: Comparison of Attention Deficit Disorder, Conduct Disorder, Normal and Clinical Controls. *Can J Beh Science.* 1991; 23: 332-348.

[74] Barkley RA, Fischer M, Edelbrock C, Smallish L. The Adolescent Outcome of Hyperactive Children Diagnosed by Research Criteria – III. Mother-Child Interactions,

Family Conflicts and Maternal Psychopathology. *J Child Psychol Psychiatry.* 1991; 32: 233-255.

[75] Klein D, Riso L, Donaldson SK, Schwartz JE, Anderson RL, Ouimette PC, Lizardi H, Aronson T. Family Study of Early-Onset Dysthymia: Mood and Personality Disorders in Relatives of Outpatients With Dysthymia and Episodic Major Depression and Normal Controls. *Arch Gen Psychiatry.* 1995; 52: 487-496.

[76] Lizardi H, Klein D. Parental Psychopathology and Reports of the Childhood Home Environment in Adults with Early-Onset Dysthymic Disorder. *J Nerv Ment Disease.* 2000; 188: 63-70.

[77] Siqueland L, Kendall PC, Steinberg L. Anxiety in Children: Perceived Family Environments and Observed Family Interaction. *J Child Psychol Psychiatry.*1996; 25: 225-237.

[78] Messer SC, Beidel DC. Psychosocial Correlates of Childhood Anxiety Disorders. *J Am Acad Child Adolesc Psychiatry.* 1994; 33: 975-983.

[79] Last CG, Hersen M, Kazdin A, Francis G, Grubb H. Psychiatric Illness in the Mothers of Anxious Children. *Am J Psychiatry.* 1987; 144: 1580-1583.

[80] Kashani JH, Vaidya AF, Soltys SM, Dandoy AC, Katz LM, Reid JC. Correlates of Anxiety in Psychiatrically Hospitalised Children and Their Parents. *Am J Psychiatry.* 1990; 147:3:319-323.

[81] Derogatis LR, Lipman RS, Rickels K, Uhlenhuth EH, Covi L. The Hopkins Symptom Checklist (HSCL): a self-report symptom inventory. *Beh Science.* 1974; 19: 1-15.

[82] Epstein NB, Baldwin LM, Bishop DS. The McMaster Family Assessment Device. *J Mar Fam Therapy.*1983; 9: 171-180.

[83] Jensen, PS, Martin, D, Cantwell, DP. Comorbidity in ADHD: Implications for Research, Practice, and DSM-V. *J Am Acad Child Adolesc Psychiatry.*1997; 36: 1065-1079.

[84] Cicchetti D. Reflections on the past and future of developmental psychopathology. In: Green J, Yule W eds. *Research and innovation on the road to modern child psychiatry: Volume 1: Festschrift for Professor Sir Michael Rutter.* Glasgow: Gaskell and the Association of child psychology and psychiatry, 2001: 37-53.

[85] Vance ALA. Attention Deficit Hyperactivity Disorder: towards an innovative developmental model. *Aust N Z J Psychiatry.* 2002; 36: 485-487.

In: Attention Deficit Hyperactivity Disorder Research
Editor: Michelle P. Larimer, pp. 95-110 ISBN 1-59454-156-6

Chapter IV

Laterality and Perceptual Bias in ADHD

Jill M. Norvilitis[1] ***and Howard M. Reid***
State University of New York College at Buffalo

Abstract

Research indicates that children with ADHD suffer from frontal striatal and right hemisphere dysfunction. As would be expected, children with ADHD have been found to be deficient on measures of executive functioning and are more likely to exhibit nonrighthandedness. We have recently found that ADHD is associated with anomalous lateralization across domain (Reid & Norvilitis, 2000). Relatedly, data suggest that a significant proportion of children with ADHD pay less attention to objects and events presented to their left than to their right visual fields (Malone, Couitis, Kershner, & Logan, 1994; Sandson, Bachna, & Morin, 2000; Voeller & Heilman, 1988). To further examine this association, we recently utilized three measures of visual neglect to ascertain the extent to which children with and without ADHD (N = 36) exhibit perceptual biases. As predicted, the ADHD participants showed an attention deficit for the left visual field on the line bisection test. Significant differences were not found with either the letter cancellation task or the Bells Test. The results, therefore, provide some support for the hypothesis that children with ADHD exhibit a perceptual bias. The results also indicate that caution should be noted in considering the extent to which these biases occur. Finally, this chapter discusses implications for further research and how lateralization/perceptual bias findings may, potentially, affect treatment of the neuropsychological deficits associated with ADHD.

ADHD is found in between 3 and 5% of school-age children (Daley, Griffin, & Onwuegbuzie, 1997; Ross & Ross, 1982; Shaffer et al, 1996) and is one of the most frequent causes for referral to child guidance centers (Barkley, 1990). Symptoms are most severe between the ages of three and six (Mash & Johnston, 1982) and lessen considerably during

[1] Correspondence: Jill M. Norvilitis, Ph.D.; Associate Professor of Psychology; SUNY College at Buffalo; 1300 Elmwood Avenue; Buffalo, NY 14222. Electronic mail may be sent to norviljm@buffalostate.edu.

adolescence (e.g. Barkley, 1990). Nevertheless, Weiss, Hechtman, Milroy and Perlman (1985) estimate that up to 30% of these children will fail to complete high school and few will continue for advanced education. Unfortunately, recent studies indicate that ADHD characteristics often continue into adulthood (Goldstein, 1996; Murphy & Barkley, 1996).

Individuals diagnosed with ADHD exhibit a constellation of symptoms, including deficiencies in sustained attention, as well as for what are known as executive functions, such as the ability to follow directions, control impulses and plan efficiently (Kibby, Cohen & Hynd, 2002). As just noted, individuals with this diagnosis are more likely to receive poor grades and to drop out of school (Hinshaw, 1992). In addition, they have been found to exhibit a higher incidence of drug abuse and are more likely to develop an antisocial personality (Mannuzza, Klein, Bessler & Malloy, 1993). However, the characteristic that has most commonly been associated with ADHD is being male. An increased frequency of males in studies of ADHD has been reported since at least 1902 (Still, cited in Barkley, 1990). Depending upon the sample's characteristics, modern estimates of the male to female ratio vary from 4:1 to as high as 9:1 (American Psychiatric Association, 1994), although the ratio is somewhat lower for the inattentive subtype (Weiler, Bellinger, Marmor, Rancier, & Waber, 1999).

A variety of etiological factors have been proposed to account for ADHD. For instance, it has been noted that ADHD symptoms run in families. Cantwell (1972) found an approximately four-fold increase in ADHD symptoms in parents of children diagnosed with ADHD as with control parents. Further, a number of studies have reported higher concordance rates for MZ than for DZ twins (Gilger, Pennington, & DeFries, 1995; Gillis, Gilger, Pennington, & DeFries, 1992; Goodman & Stevenson, 1989). These findings suggest that a genetic mechanism may be involved and a number have been hypothesized. Among these have been Fragile X Syndrome (Marshall, 1989) and the XYY chromosome configuration in males (Hier, 1980). Neither is currently viewed to provide an adequate explanation for ADHD. Further, La Hoste et al (1996) examined the DRD4 gene, which encodes the D4 (dopamine) receptor. This receptor is involved in impulsiveness and excitability as well as other factors that have been associated with ADHD. As anticipated, they determined that children with ADHD exhibited a higher incidence of D4 gene polymorphism than controls. However, there was substantial overlap between the two groups and a subsequent attempt to replicate the finding was not successful (Castellanos et al., 1998).

In addition, a variety of environmental factors have been proposed to account for ADHD's prevalence. These include lead poisoning as well as dietary variables including food additives and reactions to sugar (See Hynd, Hern, Voeller, & Marshall, 1991 for a review). However, subsequent research has failed to support the view that most children with ADHD are particularly sensitive to any aspect of their diet, such as food additives or sugar. Studies have shown, though, that children with ADHD who are also allergic to food additives are helped by the removal of these additives (See Bradley & Golden, 2001 for a review). What has been consistently supported is that an enhanced incidence of learning and behavioral problems is associated with prenatal and perinatal events that affect nervous system functioning (Hynd et al., 1991). For example, a substantial literature links maternal smoking with an increased incidence of ADHD in their children. Thus, Milberger, Biederman,

Faraone, Chen, and Jones (1996) reported an almost three-fold increase in the rate of ADHD among boys of mothers who smoked a pack of cigarettes a day during their pregnancy compared to control children.

Although older research failed to locate structural differences in the brains of children with and without ADHD (e.g. Shaywitz, Shaywitz, Byrne, Cohen, & Rothman, 1983), it has long been thought that ADHD is related to frontal striatal dysfunction (e.g., Benson, 1991; Giedd, Castellanos, Casey, & Kozuch, 1994; Vaidya, Austin, & Kirkorian, 1998). Children with ADHD perform poorly on tasks traditionally purported to assess frontal lobe deficits in basic and higher mental control, such as the Wisconsin Card Sorting Task (WCST), the Stroop Test, and the Tower of Hanoi (See Aman, Roberts, & Pennington, 1998 for a review). However, results become less predictable if adolescents or adults, rather than younger children, serve as participants. Thus, Gansler et al (1998) did not obtain a significant difference between performance on the WCST for a group of adults with ADHD compared with controls. When the ADHD group was divided into inattentive and hyperactive groups and each was compared to the controls, though, a significant difference was obtained. Specifically, the ADHD participants who had exhibited hyperactivity during childhood, but not those who were inattentive, were found to make more perseveration errors on the WCST than the control subjects.

Newer technology has begun to identify the long-hypothesized structural differences in the frontal region (Hynd, Semrud-Clikeman, Lorys, Novey & Eliopulos, 1990). For instance, Lou, Hendrickson, and Bruhn (1984) examined cerebral blood flow in eight children diagnosed with ADHD. All eight children were found to exhibit below normal blood flow bilaterally in the frontal lobes. Subsequent studies have replicated this finding (Lou, 1996; Lou, Hendrickson, Bruhn, Borner, & Nielson, 1989). Support for the view that ADHD is associated with frontal dysfunction also comes from the work of Giedd et al. (1994), which employed magnetic resonance imaging to assess the midsagital cross-sectional areas of seven regions of the corpus callosum of 18 boys with ADHD and 18 matched controls. As expected, the areas of two anterior regions of the corpus callosum were found to be significantly smaller in the children with ADHD. The authors concluded that their findings supported the hypothesis that ADHD is correlated with abnormal frontal lobe development.

ADHD has also begun to be identified with right-hemisphere dysfunction. In an early study by Voeller (1986), children with right hemisphere lesion or dysfunction were found to have a high probability of meeting the diagnostic requirements of attention deficit disorder or hyperactivity. These subjects were found to be deficient in perceiving the emotional states of others, as well as in demonstrating interpersonal skills, deficits that have been repeatedly identified in children with ADHD (e.g. Norvilitis, Casey, Brooklier, & Bonello, 2000). In a subsequent study, Casey et al (1997) correlated the outcomes of three response inhibition tasks with the magnetic resonance images of children with ADHD as well as age-matched controls. They concluded that both the right prefrontal cortex and the basal ganglia appeared to be implicated in the response inhibition deficits exhibited by children with ADHD. Neuropsychological tests also indicate the presence of right-hemisphere dysfunction. For example, Snow (1990) reported that children with ADHD perform more poorly on a mental rotation measure, a task sensitive to right-hemisphere disturbance.

The presence of a lateralized physiological correlate with ADHD symptoms might also lead one to anticipate differences in behavioral lateralization between children with and without ADHD. This expectation has been confirmed by a number of studies which have found a higher than expected rate of non-righthandedness (ambidexterity or left-handedness) in the ADHD population (e.g., Shaw & Brown, 1990; 1991; Yamamoto & Hatta, 1982). Surprisingly, little interest has been devoted to the issue of whether ADHD is specifically linked with handedness or, alternatively, is associated with anomalous laterality across domain. In fact, we are aware of only one study that has explored the relationship between ADHD and other measures of laterality. In this study, Biederman, et al (1994) failed to find any evidence of unusual or anomalous lateralization beyond handedness in children based upon parental report of ADHD symptoms.

We recently re-examined this issue utilizing clinically assessed children with ADHD (Study One) and college students identified on the basis of responses to the Wender Utah Rating Scale (WURS) (Study Two) (Reid & Norvilitis, 2000). In the first study, parental reports of greater attentional symptoms in children were only related to non-righthandedness, but teacher reports were related to anomalous laterality of foot, ear, and eye, as well as hand. This suggests that the previously reported association between ADHD and non-righthandedness may not be unique, but instead indicative of a more general condition of anomalous lateralization. This possibility was examined in Study Two, in which 234 undergraduates were assessed. In a replication of Study One, enhanced WURS scores were associated with anomalous lateralization beyond handedness. In this case, ADHD characteristics were associated with a shift away from a right bias for hand, foot, and ear, but not eye. Factor analysis of the extensive Steenhuis and Bryden (1989) handedness questionnaire was then undertaken to determine whether all aspects of handedness, or only a subset, are associated with ADHD. The factor analysis indicated that the retrospective reports of ADHD characteristics were associated with only two of the three dimensions. Though limitations such as the gender composition of the groups in Study One temper the conclusions, the results of both studies support previous findings that ADHD is associated with anomalous laterality, but also indicate that non-righthandedness is not an adequate characterization of this relationship. This interpretation is supported by the results of a recent study that has reported the lack of a right ear advantage in subjects with ADHD (Combs, 2002).

Another indication of differences in hemispheric lateralization would be visuospatial attention. Though not universally found (Ben-Artsy, Glicksohn, Soroker, Margalit & Myslobodsky, 1996; Klimkeit, Mattingly, Sheppard, Lee, & Bradshaw, 2003), an association between ADHD and a reduction in attention to the left visual hemispace is currently widely accepted (e.g., Carter, Krener, Chaderjian, Northcutt & Wolfe, 1995; Heilman, Voeller, & Nadeau, 1991). Specifically, Rothlind, Posner, and Schaughency (1991) examined this by tracking the eye movements of children with and without ADHD in response to a target. Although children without ADHD responded more quickly in the leftward direction, children with ADHD did not show this expected asymmetry. Epstein, Conners, Erhardt, March, and Swanson (1997) similarly examined reaction time in the left and right visual field among adults with and without ADHD, as did McDonald, Bennett, Chambers, and Castiello (1999) in a study with children. In both studies, the participants with ADHD showed a delayed response to targets in the left visual field. In one of the studies to not report a strong perceptual bias, Klimkeit et al. (2003) examined perceptual asymmetries in two different tasks, one requiring children to attend to both sides of a face and another that required children to identify which of two gray rectangles appeared to be darker. They failed to find the expected bias on the faces task, but did find it with the rectangles measure. It is possible that the emotional nature of the faces task was strong enough to overcome any asymmetry that the children might have shown. Thus, even among studies not reporting strong evidence of bias, the implications are unclear.

Many studies examining left visuospatial inattention have employed letter cancellation tasks (e.g., Malone, Couitis, Kershner, & Logan, 1994; Sandson, Bachna, & Morin, 2000; Voeller & Heilman, 1988). Thus, Voeller and Heilman (1988) noted that 7 right-handed boys with ADD made significantly more errors on the left side of the task than did the 5 right-handed controls. More recently, Sandson and colleagues (2000) extended this finding to adults. Specifically, 58 adults meeting the DSM-IV criteria for ADHD were found to make significantly more omission errors on the left side compared with the 29 matched controls.

A number of studies have reported that methylphenidate will counteract the right visual field bias exhibited by subjects with ADHD. For instance, an early study by Malone, Kersher and Siegel (1988) utilized tachistoscopic presentation of word pairs under medication and placebo conditions. They found that methylphenidate counteracted the right visual field advantage of children with attention deficit disorder. This outcome was replicated in a more recent study by Malone and colleagues (1994) that also compared children with ADHD while on placebo versus methylphenidate and noted that the left visual field neglect was counteracted by the stimulant medication. Finally, Nigg, Swanson and Hinshaw (1996) conducted a dose-response study of methylphenidate and found that it equalized visual field responses for the ADHD group.

We recently completed a study that was designed to clarify the extent to which children with ADHD exhibit a consistent perceptual bias away from information presented in the left visual field. Though many studies have noted such a shift in focus of attention, we are unaware of a study which has directly compared the performance of a group of children with ADHD on a series of tests designed to detect perceptual biases, as has been recommended by prior research (Voeller, 1991).

Method

Participants

Data were analyzed from 36 children between the ages of 7 and 13, ADHD $M = 10.37$, $SD = 1.67$, comparison $M = 10.19$, $SD = 1.51$; $t\ (31) = .29$, $p = .77$. Of these, 10 had previously been diagnosed with ADHD. There were 5 males in the ADHD group and 16 males in the comparison group ($X^2 = .40$, $p = .53$). In the ADHD group, all children were Caucasian. In the comparison group, 25 were Caucasian and 1 was African-American ($X^2 = .40$, $p = .53$). Eight of the ADHD group were taking stimulant medication, but none of the comparison group were taking any psychotropic medication ($X^2 = 26.74$, $p < .001$).

Measures and Procedure

Families were recruited through newspaper advertisements in local newspapers. Parents gave written consent and the children gave written assent. A battery of tests was then administered to each participant, with children and parents in adjacent rooms. Although all children with ADHD were diagnosed prior to the study, parents completed the Conners' Parent Rating Scale (Conners, 1995a) and teachers completed the Conners' Teacher Rating Scale (Conners, 1995b) to confirm diagnostic status. Because of its strong correlation with overall IQ, children also completed the Peabody Picture Vocabulary Test-Third Edition (PPVT-III, Dunn & Dunn, 1997) to assure that the groups had comparable verbal receptive language.

Of particular interest for the examination of visual neglect in children with ADHD were the line bisection task, a letter cancellation task, and the Bells Test. The line bisection task is a commonly used test for perceptual bias. For this task, the individual is asked to mark the midsection of all lines on a sheet of paper (the lines are of different lengths and point in varying directions). For each line a bias from the midpoint was calculated, with a positive sign indicating a left bias and a negative sign indicating a right bias. Data for the analysis consisted of the total of each subject's biases on each half of the page. It was expected that children with ADHD would be biased away from the left half of space. Thus, when lines are on the left side it was predicted that he or she would bisect them toward the right, as if the line did not extend all the way to the left (Banich, 1997).

Similarly, cancellation tasks can be utilized to test for perceptual bias. In such a task, an individual is presented with an array of letters, for instance, and is asked to cross out a specific letter, such as 'A', every time it is found. In the current study, there were 90 letters in each quadrant, 15 of which were the letter A. Data consisted of the number of the letter A's crossed out in each quadrant in a total of one minute. It was expected that individuals with ADHD would cancel far fewer targets on the left half of the page than on the right (Voeller, 1991).

Finally, the Bells Test (Gauthier, Dehaut, & Joanette, 1989) allows for an assessment of scanning patterns. In this task, a child is asked to cross out all pictures of bells that appear on the sheet, in the midst of representations of many other objects. The individual administering the test follows along with his or her own copy, marking the order in which the bells are located. As a result, the order in which objects are noticed by the child can be recorded. The test sheet was divided into seven equal vertical sections and the number of bells crossed out in each section was examined.

Results

ADHD Status

As expected, children with ADHD received significantly higher scores on the Conners' measures. Using the Conners' ADHD Index, children with ADHD received a mean score of 73.40 (*SD* = 12.04), while the comparison group received a mean score of 51.04, *SD* = 10.94,

t (31) = 5.24, $p < .001$. Three children were home schooled. Of the remaining 33, 27 teachers responded. Again using the Conners' ADHD Index, children with ADHD received a mean score of 71.71 (*SD* = 13.71), while the comparison group received a mean score of 49.95, *SD* = 8.36, t (25) = 5.00, $p < .001$.

Verbal Receptive Language

There was no difference between groups on the PPVT-III; ADHD *M* = 96.90, *SD* = 10.90, Comparison *M* = 104.35, *SD* = 13.64; t (31) = 1.52, p = .14; and both groups performed in the average range of functioning.

Hemispatial Neglect

The predicted association of ADHD and hemispatial neglect was partially supported by the results. Although analyses for the letter cancellation task and the Bells Test were not significant, differences were noted in the line bisection task. Specifically, the line bisection data were analyzed with a 2 X 2 (Diagnosis X Side of Page) analysis of variance. The interaction was significant, F (1, 34) = 8.087, $p < .01$. This was primarily due to the bisection of lines within the left visual field being significantly different between those subjects with ADHD, who neglected the left side of the lines, and the control subjects, who were biased away from the right side of the lines, t (34) = 2.758, $p < .01$. Additionally, there was a main effect for the control subjects in that neglect of the right half of lines occurred when the lines were displayed on the left half of the sheet but not when displayed on the right half, t (25) = -2.077, $p < .05$. A similar main effect did not exist for those individuals with ADHD. However, the numerical difference between marginal means for the children diagnosed with ADHD (neglected the left side of lines when located in the left visual field and, to a lesser extent, the right side of lines in the right visual field) was greater than for the control subjects. It is suggested, therefore, that this difference might have been found to be significant had the number of ADHD participants tested been greater.

In addition, the bisection of lines in the top half of the visual field versus the bottom half was investigated, as well as those within a central circle as compared to those lines existing outside the circle. However, neither of these analyses was statistically significant.

Discussion

Thus, even with a small sample, the reviewed study's findings provide some support for the view that subjects with ADHD exhibit a perceptual bias away from the left region of stimuli in the left visual field. Further, that all three measures did not indicate the presence of a perceptual bias is not surprising. Maeshima et al. (2001), for instance, found only modest correlations among the line bisection scores and scores on other measures of unilateral spatial neglect in right hemisphere stroke patients. This is likely due to the differing nature of the tasks: cancellation tasks involve motor exploration and line bisection involves a perceptual judgment (Bailey, Riddoch, & Crome, 2000). Further, Ferber and Karnath (2001) argue that cancellation tests are much more sensitive to neglect than line bisection tasks. Thus, letter cancellation tasks have frequently been employed in studies that have found evidence of a lateralized perceptual bias in children with ADHD. The lack of a significant finding with this measure is, accordingly, something of a surprise. Finally, this report supports recent evidence that suggests that normal children also exhibit evidence of a developmental perceptual bias in the left visual field, but in the opposite direction than that found with ADHD subjects (Cairo Valcarcel et al., 2002). According to Cairo Valcarcel and colleagues, brain maturation eliminates this bias at about age 13 or 14.

Because the research just reviewed was a pilot study, the sample size was limited and there were not enough participants to divide the ADHD group into subtypes. Thus, one future goal is to examine how perceptual neglect varies among the three ADHD subtypes. Prior research has noted differences between those with ADHD primarily inattentive type or combined type and those with ADHD primarily hyperactive type. Specifically, Garcia-Sanchez, Estevez-Gonzalez, Suarez-Romero, and Junque (1997) reported that, although both those with and without hyperactivity performed worse on measures of right hemisphere functioning, the deficits were more pronounced in those without hyperactivity. These results are consistent with other research that has found greater behavioral difficulties in children with hyperactivity, but greater cognitive deficits in those without hyperactivity (Carlson, Shin, & Booth, 1999; McBurnett, Pfiffner, & Frick, 2001). Therefore, we expect to find that neglect, like other right hemisphere deficits, is more pronounced in children with inattentive or combined-type hyperactivity.

We are also in the early stages of a study examining a potential new treatment for ADHD. More specifically, this therapeutic intervention is designed to counteract the perceptual neglect of children with ADHD. Current therapy heavily emphasizes medication, which has been found in the Multimodal Treatment Study (MTA) to be more effective at reducing symptoms of ADHD than behavioral interventions alone (Jensen et al., 2001). It is no surprise, then, that prescription of psychostimulants increased 2.9 fold between 1990 and 1995 (Robison, Sclar, Skaer, & Galin, 1999). This emphasis upon a medical solution to ADHD has a number of well-publicized drawbacks, including the obvious concern associated with the long-term use of any drug. Notably, despite the general effectiveness of medication, approximately one-quarter of children do not benefit from stimulants (Wicks-Nelson & Israel, 2000). Among those who are least likely to benefit are older children, those with anxiety, and those with less severe forms of the disorder (Gray & Kagan, 2000). Further, while stimulant medication undoubtedly calms the recipient, the efficacy of this therapy on improving academic performance has not been well established (Rapport, Denney, DuPaul, & Gardner, 1994). Among studies that find that academic functioning is helped by medication, it appears that low doses are best for academics, though higher doses may be necessary to change behavior (Evans et al., 2001). Still another concern is that children on medication and their parents are more likely to attribute successes to the medication and failures to themselves (Johnston & Leung, 2001; Treuting & Hinshaw, 2001).

Unfortunately, there is not currently a non-medication alternative therapy that is practical for all children with ADHD. Although behavioral treatments have been found to be effective, they are labor intensive because children with ADHD require strong, continuous reinforcement (Wicks-Nelson & Israel, 2000) and the conditioned behaviors often fail to generalize to other settings. Further, they are less effective than medication, according to the recent MTA, although when combined with medication efficacy improves (Jensen et al., 2001).

Given that children with ADHD have perceptual deficits similar to those with hemispheric neglect due to right hemispheric lesions, it seems plausible that techniques used in rehabilitation of neglect might prove useful for ADHD. Several categories of rehabilitation have emerged for sensory neglect. For example, one involves training patients to attend to the cues on the left side. Most of the research in this area has been behaviorally oriented and requires patients to learn to turn their heads or move their hands, etc. (Manly, 2002). This method has shown some success, but is quite labor intensive. Other labor intensive approaches include such techniques as limb activation in which neglect is reduced when patients are forced to use their left hands to perform tasks (Manly, 2002).

Another method involves forcing patients to attend to the neglected information by blocking or altering non-neglected stimuli. Initial research on this possibility simply covered the right eye with a patch (Butter & Kirsch, 1992). Although this technique did not fully limit sensory input from the right, the authors still reported some success. However, others have not reported positive outcomes. In fact, Barrett, Crucian, Beversdorf, and Heilman (2001) described a case in which monocular patching actually worsened attentional neglect. Recently, however, two studies (Arai, Ohi, Sasaki, Nobuto & Tanaka, 1997; Beis, Andre, Baumgarten & Challier, 1999) have refined this technique and reported that right, half-field eye patches accelerated the recovery of patients with left visual field neglect resulting from a right cerebral vascular lesion. That is, instead of simply covering the right eye and assuming that the uncovered left eye would lead to an enhanced emphasis upon the left visual field, patients were fitted with glasses that block the right visual field from both eyes. This forced both eyes to attend to the left visual field rather than the right.

We hypothesize that a similar eye patching treatment may be effective for children with ADHD, either by itself or in combination with other well-established techniques. Although this is a novel approach, prior research has indicated that children with ADHD are overattending to left hemisphere (right visual field) stimulation, leading them to process information in a faulty manner (Becker, Doane, & Wexler, 1993). Becker and colleagues (1993) go on to suggest that these deficits lead to many of the difficulties associated with ADHD: heightened focus on continuous positive reinforcement, high levels of comorbid psychopathology, and a possible explanation for the high rates of learning disorders. McDonald and colleagues (1999) further suggest that the right hemisphere deficits in orienting and focusing attention may be related to the failure of children with ADHD to stop ongoing responses. That is, they may engage in a particular behavioral response set and be unable to learn from instruction and their own mistakes. Becker and colleagues believe that cognitive remediation, rather than traditional approaches, may be effective for children with right hemisphere deficits.

In our research we are utilizing the half-field eye patch technique as a treatment of the perceptual bias associated with ADHD. Specifically, as in the Arai et al (1997) and Beis et al (1999) studies with brain injured patients, those ADHD participants exhibiting neglect are being fitted with glasses which prevent input from the right visual field. Thus the ADHD participants are forced to attend more strongly to information in the left visual field, and are simultaneously being spared sensory extinction that might occur as a result of right side stimulation. Following exposure to this intervention, we would expect that their left side neglect would be reduced and we would hope for a positive effect on ADHD symptomatology, academic achievement, social interactions, cognitive deficits associated with ADHD (e.g., a continuous performance test) and emotion appraisal. If successful, this will be followed with a more refined technique. Specifically, we currently employ glasses in which the right visual field of each eye is completely blocked by an opaque region of each lens, while the left visual field and the region directly ahead are unaffected. We anticipate that in the future we will employ more sophisticated glasses in which the degree of attenuation of the input from the right visual field will gradually become greater the farther the stimulus is from the midline. Thus, instead of the subject having glasses in which the left side of each lens is clear while the right is opaque, in the future we anticipate employing lenses in which there will be a gradual increase in the level of attenuation of visual input as one goes farther into the right visual field. Further, the rate at which this attenuation occurs will be matched to the individual subject's level of visual neglect: the more strongly the bias to the right side, the more rapid the attenuation of this input will be. This approach is clearly still in the preliminary stages of testing. However, given both the prior research on right-hemisphere dysfunction in children with ADHD and our recent studies on hemispheric neglect, we anticipate positive results.

In conclusion, the search for interventions to counter ADHD's effects began as soon as the disorder was identified early in the 20th century. The recent trend that emphasizes biological interventions has many supporters, but, as was reviewed, also raises serious concerns. Furthermore, the use of medications has not proven to be effective for all users. Unfortunately, alternative therapies have either not been found to be effective, are labor intensive, or both. The urgency to identify new treatments has been increased by the recent findings which indicate that a substantial proportion of ADHD symptoms continue into adulthood. Thus, what was once thought of as a childhood disorder that would be outgrown is now realized to be a more chronic, perhaps lifelong, condition. Fortunately, a clearer understanding of the physiological correlates of ADHD is also being obtained. Frontal cortical involvement is now strongly supported by the research and the role of lateralized brain processes is being appreciated. These advances potentially will lead to new interventions for the treatment of ADHD. Most notably, children for whom current medications are less effective or for whom behavioral interventions prove too time consuming for parents and teachers to implement may benefit the most from future research in this area.

References

American Psychiatric Association (1994). *Diagnostic and statistical manual of mental disorders* (4th ed.). Washington, D. C.: Author.

Aman, C. J., Roberts, R. J., & Pennington, B. F. (1998). A neuropsychological examination of the underlying deficit in attention deficit hyperactivity disorder: Frontal lobe versus right parietal lobe theories. *Developmental Psychology*, 34, 956-969.

Arai, T., Ohi, H., Sasaki, H., Nobuto, H., & Tanaka, K. (1997). Hemispatial sunglasses: Effect on unilateral spatial neglect. *Archives of Physical Medicine and Rehabilitation*, 78, 230-232.

Bailey, M. J., Riddoch, M. J., & Crome, P. (2000). Evaluation of a test battery for hemineglect in elderly stroke patients for use by therapists in clinical practice. *NeuroRehabilitation*, 14, 139-150.

Banich, M. T. (1997). *Neuropsychology: The neural bases of mental function*. Boston: Houghton Mifflin Company.

Barkley, R. A. (1990). Attention deficit disorders: History, definition, and diagnosis. In M. Lewis & S. M. Miller (eds.) *Handbook of Developmental Psychopathology*. New York: Plenum Press.

Barrett, A. M., Crucian, G. P., Beversdorf, D. Q., & Heilman, K. M. (2001). Monocular patching may worsen sensory-attentional neglect: A case report. *Archives of Physical Medicine and Rehabilitation*, 82, 516- 518.

Becker, D. F., Doane, J. A., & Wexler, B. E. (1993). Effects of emotion on perceptual asymmetry in adolescent inpatients with attention deficit hyperactivity disorder. *Journal of the American Academy of Child and Adolescent Psychiatry*, 32, 318-321.

Beis, J. M., Andre, J. M., Baumgarten, A., & Challier, B. (1999). Eye patching in unilateral spatial neglect: Efficacy of two methods. *Archives of Physical Medicine and Rehabilitation*, 80, 71-76.

Ben-Artsy, A., Glicksohn, J., Soroker, N., Margalit, M. & Myslobodsky, M., (1996). An assessment of hemineglect in children with attention deficit hyperactivity disorder. *Developmental Neuropsychology*, 12(3), 271-281.

Benson, D. F. (1991). The role of frontal dysfunction in attention deficit hyperactivity disorder. *Journal of Child Neurology*, 6, S9- S12.

Biederman, J., Lapey, K. A., Milberger, S., Faraone, S. V., Reed, E. D., & Seidman, L. J. (1994). Motor preference, major depression, and psychosocial dysfunction among children with attention deficit hyperactivity disorder. *Journal of Psychiatric Research*, 28, 171-184.

Bradley, J. D. D., & Golden, C. J. (2001). Biological contributions to the presentation and understanding of attention deficit/hyperactivity disorder: A review. *Clinical Psychology Review*, 21, 907-929.

Butter, C., & Kirsch, N. (1992). Combined and separate effects of eye patching and visual stimulation on unilateral neglect following stroke. *Archives of Physical Medicine and Rehabilitation*, 73, 1133-1139.

Cairo Valcarcel, E., Ijalba, E., Obler, L. K., Lozano, R. G., Llanes, R. M., Collazos, C. D., & Herrera, C. B. (2002). Bias in visual attention behavior in a normal school-aged population. *Brain & Cognition*, 48, 291-296.

Cantwell, D. (1972). Psychiatric illness in the families of hyperactive children. *Archives of General Psychiatry,* 27, 414-417.

Carlson C. L., Shin, M., & Booth, J. (1999). The case for DSM-IV subtypes in ADHD. *Mental Retardation and Developmental Disabilities Research Reviews*, 5 (3), 199-206.

Carter, C. S., Krener, P., Chaderjian, M., Northcutt, C. & Wolfe, V. (1995). Asymmetrical visual-spatial attentional performance in ADHD: Evidence for a right hemisphere deficit. *Biological Psychiatry*, 37, 789-797.

Casey, B. J., Castellanos, F. X., Giedd, J. N., Marsh, W. L., Hamburger, S. D., Schubert, A. B., Vauss, Y. C., Vaituzis, A. C., Dickstein, D. P., Sarfatti, S. E., & Rapoport J. L. (1997). Implication of right frontostriatal circuitry in response inhibition and attention deficit/hyperactivity disorder. *Journal of Child and Adolescent Psychiatry*, 36, 374-383.

Castellanos, F. X., Lau, E., Tayebi, N., Lee, P., Long, R. E., & Giedd, J. N. (1998). Lack of an association between a dopamine-4 receptor polymorphism and attention/deficit hyperactivity disorder: Genetic and brain morphometric analyses. *Molecular Psychiatry*, 3, 431-434.

Combs, J. T. (2002). Lack of right ear advantage in patients with attention deficit/hyperactivity disorder. *Clinical Pediatrics,* 41, 231-234.

Conners, C. K. (1995a). *Conners' Parent Rating Scale Revised—Long Version*. North Tonawanda, NY: Multi-Health Systems, Inc.

Conners, C. K. (1995b). *Conners' Teacher Rating Scale Revised—Long Version*. North Tonawanda, NY: Multi-Health Systems, Inc.

Daley, C. E., Griffin, H., & Onwuegbuzie, A. J. (1997). Prevalence and identification of attention deficit hyperactivity disorder in a mid-southern state. *Research in the Schools*, 4 (2), 49-56.

Dunn, L. M. & Dunn, L. M. (1997). *Peabody Picture Vocabulary Test* (3rd ed.). Circle Pines, MN: American Guidance Service, Inc.

Epstein, J. N., Conners, C. K., Erhardt, D., & March, J. S. (1997). Asymmetrical hemispheric control of visual-spatial attention in adults with attention deficit hyperactivity disorder. *Neuropsychology*, 11, 467-473.

Evans, S. W., Pelham, W. E., Smith, B. H., Bukstein, O., Gnagy, E. M., Greiner, A. R., Altenderfer, L., & Baron-Myak, C. (2001). Dose-response effects of methylphenidate on ecologically valid measures of academic performance and classroom behavior in adolescents with ADHD. *Experimental and Clinical Psychopharmacology*, 9, 163-175.

Ferber, S., & Karnath, H. O. (2001). How to assess spatial neglect—Line bisection or cancellation tasks? *Journal of Clinical and Experimental Neuropsychology*, 23, 599-607.

Gansler, D. A., Fucetola, R., Krengel, M., Stetson, S., Zimering, R., & Makary, C. (1998). Are there cognitive subtypes in adult attention deficit/hyperactivity disorder? *The Journal of Nervous and Mental Disease*, 186, 776-781.

Garcia-Sanchez, C., Estevez-Gonzalez, A., Suarez-Romero, E., & Junque, C. (1997). Right hemisphere dysfunction in subjects with attention deficit disorder and without hyperactivity. *Journal of Child Neurology*, 12, 107-115.

Gauthier, L., Dehaut, F., & Joanette, Y. (1989). The Bells Test: A quantitative and qualitative test for visual neglect. *International Journal of Clinical Neuropsychology*, 11, 49-54.

Giedd, J. N., Castellanos, F. X., Casey, B. J., & Kozuch, P. (1994). Quantitative morphology of the corpus callosum in attention deficit hyperactivity disorder. *American Journal of Psychiatry, 151,* 665-669.

Gilger, J. W., Pennington, B. F., & DeFries, J. C. (1992). A twin study of the etiology of comorbidity: Attention deficit hyperactivity disorder and dyslexia. *Journal of the American Academy of Child and Adolescent Psychiatry*, 31, 343-348.

Gillis, J. J., Gilger, J. W., Pennington, B. F., & DeFries, J. C. (1992). Attention deficit disorder in reading-disabled twins: Evidence for a genetic etiology. *Journal of Abnormal Child Psychology*, 20, 303-315.

Goldstein, S. (1996, November). Attention deficit hyperactivity disorder in adults: What we know, think we know, and need to know. *Paper presented at the 16th Annual National Academy of Neuropsychology*, New Orleans, LA.

Goodman, R., & Stevenson, J. (1989). A twin study of hyperactivity-II. The aetiological role of genes, family relationships, and perinatal adversity. *Journal of Child Psychology and Psychiatry,* 30, 691-709.

Gray, J. R., & Kagan, J. (2000). The challenge of predicting which children with attention deficit-hyperactivity disorder will respond positively to methylphenidate. *Journal of Applied Developmental Psychology,* 21, 471-489.

Heilman, K. M., Voeller, K. K. S., & Nadeau, S. E. (1991). A possible pathophysiologic substrate of attention deficit hyperactivity disorder. *Journal of Child Neurology*, 6, S76-S81.

Hier, D. (1980). Learning disorders and sex chromosome aberrations. *Journal of Mental Deficiency Research,* 24, 17-26.

Hinshaw, S. P. (1992). Externalizing behavior problems and academic underachievement in childhood and adolescence: Causal relationships and underlying mechanisms. *Psychological Bulletin*, 111, 127-155.

Hynd, G. W., Hern, K. L., Voeller, K. K., & Marshall, R. M. (1991). Neurobiological basis of attention deficit hyperactivity disorder (ADHD). *School Psychology Review*, 20, 174-186.

Hynd, G. W., Semrud-Clikeman, M., Lorys, A., Novey, E. S., & Eliopulos, D. (1990). Brain morphology in developmental dyslexia and attention deficit hyperactivity. *Archives of Neurology,* 47, 919-926.

Jensen, P. S., Hinshaw, S. P., Swanson, J. M., Greenhill, L. L., Conners, C. K., Arnold, L. E., Abikoff, H. B., Elliott, G., Hechtman, L., Hoza, B., March, J. S., Newcorn, J. H., Severe, J. B., Vitiello, B., Wells, K., & Wigal, T. (2001). Findings from the NIMH Multimodal Treatment Study of ADHD (MTA): Implications and application for primary care providers. *Journal of Developmental and Behavioral Pediatrics*, 22, 60-73.

Johnston, C., & Leung, D. W. (2001). Effects of medication, behavioral, and combined treatments on parents' and children's attributions for the behavior of children with attention deficit hyperactivity disorder. *Journal of Consulting and Clinical Psychology*, 69, 67-76.

Kibby, M. Y., Cohen, M. J., & Hynd, G. W. (2002). Clock face drawing in children with attention deficit/hyperactivity disorder. *Archives of Clinical Neuropsychology*, 17, 531-546.

Klimkeit, E. I., Mattingley, J. B., Sheppard, D. M., Lee, P., & Bradshaw, J. L. (2003). Perceptual asymmetries in normal children and children with attention deficit/hyperactivity disorder. *Brain & Cognition*, 52, 205-215.

La Hoste, G. J., Swanson, J. M., Wigal, S. B., Glabe, C., Wigal, T., King, N., & Kennedy, J. L. (1996). Dopamine D4 receptor gene polymorphism is associated with attention deficit hyperactivity disorder. *Molecular Psychiatry*, 1, 121-124.

Lou, H. C. (1996). Etiology and pathogenesis of attention deficit hyperactivity disorder (ADHD): Significance of prematurity and perinatal hypoxic-haemodynamic encephalopathy. *Acta Paediatrica*, 85, 1266-1271.

Lou, H. C., Hendrickson, L., & Bruhn, P. (1984). Focal cerebral hypoperfusion in children with dysphasia and/or attention deficit disorder. *Archives of Neurology*, 41, 825-829.

Lou, H. C., Hendrickson, L., Bruhn, P., Borner, H., & Nielsen, J. B. (1989). Striatal dysfunction in attention deficit disorder and hyperkinetic disorder. *Archives of Neurology*, 46, 48-52.

Maeshima, S., Truman, G., Smith, D. S., Dohi, N., Shigeno, K., Itakura, T., & Komai, N. (2001). Factor analysis of the components of 12 standard test batteries for unilateral spatial neglect reveals that they contain a number of discrete and important clinical variables. *Brain Injury*, 15, 125-137.

Malone, M. A., Couitis, J., Kershner, J. R., & Logan, W. J. (1994). Right hemisphere dysfunction and methylphenidate effects in children with attention deficit/hyperactivity disorder. *Journal of Child and Adolescent Psychopharmacology*, 4, 245-253.

Malone, M. A., Kershner, J. R., & Siegel, L. (1988). The effects of methylphenidate on levels of processing and laterality in children with attention deficit disorder. *Journal of Abnormal Child Psychology*, 16, 379-395.

Manly, T. (2002). Cognitive rehabilitation for unilateral neglect: Review. *Neuropsychological Rehabilitation,* 12, 289-310.

Mannuzza, S., Klein, R. G., Bessler, A., & Malloy, P. (1993). Adult outcome of hyperactive boys: Educational achievement, occupational rank, and psychiatric status. *Archives of General Psychiatry*, 50, 565-576.

Marshall, P. (1989). Attention deficit disorder and allergy: A neurochemical model of the relation between the illnesses. *Psychological Bulletin*, 106, 434-446.

Mash, E. J., & Johnston, C. (1982). Comparison of the mother-child interactions of younger and older hyperactive and normal children. *Child Development*, 53, 1371-1381.

McBurnett, K., Pfiffner, L. J., & Frick, P. (2001). Symptom properties as a function of ADHD type: An argument for continued study of sluggish cognitive tempo. *Journal of Abnormal Child Psychology,* 29, 207-213.

McDonald, S., Bennett, K. M. B., Chambers, H., & Castiello, U. (1999). Covert orienting and focusing of attention in children with attention deficit hyperactivity disorder. *Neuropsychologia*, 37, 345-356.

Milberger, S., Biederman, J., Faraone, S. V., Chen, L., & Jones, J. (1996). Is maternal smoking a risk factor for attention deficit hyperactivity disorder in children? *American Journal of Psychiatry,* 153, 1138-1142.

Murphy, K., & Barkley, R. A. (1996). Attention deficit / hyperactivity disorder adults: Comorbidities and adaptive impairments. *Comprehensive Psychiatry*, 37, 393-401.

Nigg, J. T., Swanson, J. M., & Hinshaw, S. P. (1997) Covert spatial attention in boys with attention deficit hyperactivity disorder: Lateral effects, methylphenidate response and results for parents. *Neuropsychologia*, 35, 165-176.

Norvilitis, J. M., Casey, R. J., Brooklier, K. M., & Bonello, P. J. (2000). Emotion appraisal in children with attention deficit-hyperactivity disorder and their parents. *Journal of Attention Disorders,* 4, 15-26.

Rapport, M. D., Denney, C., DuPaul, G. J., & Gardner, M. J. (1994). Attention deficit disorder and methylphenidate: Normalization rates, clinical effectiveness, and response prediction in 76 children. *Journal of the American Academy of Child and Adolescent Psychiatry*, 33, 882-893.

Reid, H. M. & Norvilitis, J. M. (2000). Evidence for anomalous lateralization across domain in ADHD children as well as adults identified with the Wender Utah Rating Scale. *Journal of Psychiatric Research*, 34, 311-316.

Robison, L. M., Sclar, D. A., Skaer, T. L., & Galin, R. S. (1999). National trends in the prevalence of attention deficit/hyperactivity disorder and the prescribing of methylphenidate among school-age children: 1990-1995. *Clinical Pediatrics*, 38, 209-218.

Ross, D. M., & Ross, S. A. (1982). *Hyperactivity: Current issues, research, and theory* (2nd ed.). New York: John Wiley & Sons.

Rothlind, J. C., Posner, M. I., & Schaughency, E. A. (1991). Lateralized control of eye movements in attention deficit hyperactivity disorder. *Journal of Cognitive Neuroscience*, 3, 377-381.

Sandson, T. A., Bachna, K. J., & Morin, M. D. (2000). Right hemisphere dysfunction in ADHD: Visual hemispatial inattention and clinical subtype. *Journal of Learning Disabilities,* 33, 83-90.

Shaffer, D., Fisher, P., Dulcan, M. K., Davies, M., Piacentini, J., Schwab-Stone, M. E., Lahey, B., Bourdin, K., Jensen, P. S., Bird, H. R., Canino, G., & Regier, D. A. (1996). The NIMH Diagnostic Interview Schedule for Children version 2.3 (DISC-2.3): Description, acceptability, prevalence rates, and performance in the MECA study. *Journal of the American Academy of Child and Adolescent Psychiatry*, 35, 865-877.

Shaw, G. A., & Brown, G. (1990). Laterality and creativity concomitants of attention problems. *Developmental Neuropsychology*, 6, 39-56.

Shaw, G. A., & Brown, G. (1991). Laterality, implicit memory and attention disorder. *Educational Studies*, 17, 15-23.

Shaywitz, B. A., Shaywitz, S. E., Byrne, T., Cohen, D. J., & Rothman, S. (1983). Attention deficit disorder: Quantitative analysis of CT. *Neurology*, 33, 1500-1503.

Snow, J. H. (1990). Investigation of a mental rotation task with school-age children. *Journal of Psychoeducational Assessment*, 8, 538-549.

Steenhuis, R. E., & Bryden, M. P. (1989). Different dimensions of hand preference that relate to skilled and unskilled activities. *Cortex,* 25, 289-304.

Treuting, J. J., & Hinshaw, S. P. (2001). Depression and self-esteem in boys with attention deficit/hyperactivity disorder: Associations with comorbid aggression and explanatory attributional mechanisms. *Journal of Abnormal Child Psychology*, 29, 23-39.

Vaidya, C. J., Austin, G., & Kirkorian, G. (1998). Selective effects of methylphenidate in attention deficit hyperactivity disorder: A functional magnetic resonance study. *Proceedings of the National Academy of Sciences in the United States of America*, 95, 11494-11498.

Voeller, K. K. S. (1986). Right-hemisphere deficit syndrome in children. *American Journal of Psychiatry,* 143, 1004-1009.

Voeller, K. K. S. (1991). What can neurological models of attention, intention, and arousal tell us about attention deficit hyperactivity disorder. *Journal of Neuropsychiatry*, 3, 209-216.

Voeller, K. K. S., & Heilman, K. M. (1988). Attention deficit disorder in children: A neglect syndrome? *Neurology,* 38, 806-808.

Weiler, M. D., Bellinger, D., Marmor, J., Rancier, S., Waber, D. (1999). Mother and teacher reports of ADHD symptoms: DSM-IV questionnaire data. *Journal of American Academy of Child and Adolescent Psychiatry*, 38, 1139-1147.

Weiss, G., Hechtman, L., Milroy, T., & Perlman, T. (1985). Psychiatric status of hyperactives as adults: A controlled prospective 15-year follow-up of 63 hyperactive children. *Journal of the American Academy of Child Psychiatry,* 24, 211-220.

Wicks-Nelson, R. & Israel A. C. (2000). *Behavior disorders of childhood* (4th ed.). Upper Saddle River, N.J.: Prentice-Hall.

Yamamoto, M., & Hatta, T. (1982). Handedness and imbalance lateralization on the Tapping Test in MBD children. *International Journal of Neuroscience*, 17, 215-218.

In: Attention Deficit Hyperactivity Disorder Research
Editor: Michelle P. Larimer, pp. 111-137
ISBN 1-59454-156-6

Chapter V

Story Comprehension in Children with ADHD: Research Findings and Treatment Implications

Richard Milich[1], Elizabeth P. Lorch and Kristen S. Berthiaume
University of Kentucky
Lexington, KY 40506

Abstract

Children with attention deficit hyperactivity disorder (ADHD) are at risk for significant academic difficulties. Although academic problems are well documented for these children, there is little information about specific ways in which children with ADHD may differ from comparison children in their comprehension of and memory for complex, interconnected information such as that represented in stories. This chapter explores such issues, addressing three major goals:

1) Theories of the development of story comprehension are reviewed, to establish a framework for guiding research in this area among children with ADHD. Notable theories include story grammar theory and the network model of story comprehension. These theories stress the importance of character goals and connections among story events in building a coherent representation of a story.
2) A series of studies, employing several different methodologies, is reviewed that document the nature of the difficulties in story comprehension experienced by children with ADHD. One of the major methodologies reviewed concerns children's comprehension of televised stories because this approach permits systematic investigation of the impact of variations in visual attention on story comprehension. The results of these studies indicate that children with ADHD have more difficulty than their nonreferred peers in making connections among events when their visual attention is disrupted and they are thereby unable to sustain cognitive engagement with the televised material. In addition, all the methodologies converge on the

[1] Corresponding author: Richard Milich, email: milich@uky.edu; fax = 859-323-1979; phone = 859-257-4396

conclusion that these children have difficulty utilizing causal relations and the goal structure of a story to create a coherent representation.

3) The treatment implications of the research findings are discussed, and future directions for research are offered. The traditional interventions recommended for children with ADHD, such as stimulant medication and behavior modification, focus on increasing children's on-task behavior but may not address deficits in processing complex information represented in story comprehension. In contrast, treatment interventions are discussed that target the specific deficits exhibited by children with ADHD.

Attention deficit hyperactivity disorder (ADHD) is often identified as the most prevalent childhood behavior disorder (APA, 1994). In addition, it may well be the most widely investigated childhood disorder, with literally thousands of studies examining the etiology, symptom patterns, treatment, and long-term outcomes of this disorder. Despite this wealth of information, there are still many important questions that remain to be answered. One of the most intriguing concerns how the specific symptoms associated with ADHD may contribute to the well-documented academic difficulties experienced by these children. The goals of this chapter are to review a series of studies that attempt to address this question, and then to offer both research and treatment recommendations that arise from the results of these studies.

ADHD is considered to affect between 5% and 10% of school-age children, which translates into an average of one child per classroom. The primary symptoms of the disorder are developmentally inappropriate levels of inattention, overactivity, and impulsivity (APA, 1994). Translated into everyday behaviors, this means that these children are more often off task and complete less school work than their classmates, they are more likely to be fidgety or actually out of their seats during class time, and they engage in disruptive behaviors such as calling out in class or cutting in line. These disruptive, age-inappropriate behaviors result in significant impairment in many aspects of these children's daily functioning. For example, these children are often actively rejected by their peers, even after relatively brief interactions with a new peer (Diener & Milich, 1997). Children with ADHD have similar aversive interactions with the adults in their lives, especially parents and teachers.

Although the symptoms of ADHD adversely impact most areas of a child's functioning, perhaps the domain that is most impaired is academic functioning. No matter which outcome measure is examined, children with ADHD perform more poorly than their classmates. For example, these children are more likely to fail subjects, to be held back, and to drop out of school. Associated with these academic difficulties are problems during adulthood, including being less likely to enter or complete college, having lower than expected occupational status, and having more frequent changes in occupation. Additionally, when children with ADHD grow up, they are at risk for substance use/abuse, psychiatric disorders including depression and personality disorders, and traffic violations and car accidents (Barkley, 1998).

It is easy to document that children with ADHD have significant academic impairment. It is less clear how the symptoms associated with ADHD contribute to these academic difficulties. Certainly there are a number of potential 'suspects.' Children with ADHD are at increased risk for having a comorbid learning disability, with comorbidity estimates ranging anywhere from 20% to 70% (Barkley, 1997). Research has attempted to disentangle which aspects of the academic impairment may be due to ADHD versus LD (see Douglas, 1999;

Pennington, Groisser, & Welsh, 1993; Purvis & Tannock, 1997). For example, Pennington et al. found that ADHD alone was associated with deficits in executive functioning, LD alone was associated with phonological deficits, and the functioning of children with comorbid ADHD/LD was more similar to that of the LD alone group. In a similar vein, Purvis and Tannock found that children with ADHD had difficulty utilizing the causal connections among story events in guiding their recall of the story, whereas the performance of children with LD was similar to that of the comparison children. These findings suggest that there are clear differences between groups of children with ADHD versus LD, and that the academic difficulties of the former cannot be explained entirely by their comorbid LD status.

In accounting for the academic difficulties of children with ADHD, focus must be given to the role of their attentional problems. Certainly if children are off task at high rates, this will adversely impact their productivity, which in turn will impair their academic performance. Academic productivity is an important indicator of school performance and decreased levels of productivity will certainly impair performance. However, by itself this decreased productivity tells us little about how problems in sustaining attention may directly affect the children's learning, especially when considering higher order cognitive processing. Higher order cognitive processing involves skills such as applying, analyzing, synthesizing, and evaluating information, and is required for many academic tasks, such as understanding texts and lectures.

Perhaps the major reason for the dearth of information on how the attentional problems of children with ADHD may contribute to their academic difficulties is that the traditional methods of assessing these attentional difficulties do not offer ready linkages to higher order cognitive processing. Historically, children with ADHD have been found to have problems sustaining attention over time, and these problems have been documented using either laboratory measures or observations of in-class behavior. For example, a traditional laboratory measure employed would be a vigilance task such as a continuous performance test (CPT). Research has clearly indicated that children with ADHD do poorly on such tasks, committing more errors of omission over time (Hooks, Milich, & Lorch, 1994). However, the nature of this task does not lend itself to examining higher order cognitive processing. Typically, the task requires the children to attend to a computer screen while individual letters are displayed sequentially. The children's task is to press a computer key when a certain pattern of letters appears, and inhibit responding to all other letters. Such a task may be appropriate for measuring problems in sustaining attention but it makes no higher order cognitive processing demands on the children.

A second common procedure for documenting attentional problems among children with ADHD is to observe their rates of on-task behavior in the classroom. Studies employing this methodology reliably document decreased rates of attending among children with ADHD, and these rates can be linked to decreased productivity. However, the global nature of these observations do not allow for more fine-grained analyses of the link between attention and higher order cognitive processing.

Thus, the studies examining the nature of the attention deficit have provided valuable information about the initial stages of information processing by children with ADHD (Sergeant & van der Meere, 1990). This research, however, sheds light on only one component of the total information processing capabilities of these children, and leaves many important issues unaddressed. For example, there is little information about specific ways in which children with ADHD may differ from comparison children in their comprehension of and memory for complex, interconnected information such as that represented in stories. As Low and Durkin (1998, p. 202) argue, story comprehension abilities are regarded as "... fundamental organizational processes which underpin representational development, the construction of knowledge bases and problem-solving strategies."

As this brief review would suggest, better understanding of the basis of the academic problems of children with ADHD requires two major elements. First, a strong theoretical foundation is needed that can guide research examining higher order cognitive processing. Second, a methodology is needed that can link specifically the attentional problems experienced by children with ADHD to their higher order cognitive processing difficulties, thereby further clarifying the etiology of and potential treatment for the academic problems documented among these children. In the next two sections each of these two elements is discussed.

Theories of Story Comprehension

The study of children's story comprehension provides a unique opportunity to evaluate their understanding of complex events (van den Broek, Bauer, & Bourg, 1997). Effective story comprehension is a significant component of school performance in the early school years, and requires a number of cognitive skills. As such, story comprehension is a powerful gauge of cognitive processing and cognitive development. By investigating story comprehension, we gain insight into many aspects of children's cognitive functioning. These include the strategic allocation of attention, the selection, encoding and interpretation of important information, the use of story structure features to guide comprehension, the retrieval of relevant background information, the generation of inferences that allow an interpretation of the presented information, the monitoring of comprehension, and the use of retrieval skills (Lorch & Sanchez, 1997). Thus, story comprehension provides a microcosm for investigating virtually all aspects of comprehension in general. In turn, an examination of the major theoretical ideas guiding research on the development of story comprehension is a necessary first step in understanding the story comprehension abilities of children with ADHD.

In the story comprehension literature, many theories emphasize the importance of causal relations among story events (Ackerman, Silver, & Glickman, 1990; Graesser & Clark, 1985; Trabasso & Nickels, 1992). That is, in order to achieve a coherent understanding of a story, individuals must determine the *causes* of a given event and the *effects* of that event on subsequent events. A *network model* has been proposed to represent different kinds of story events, the types of *causal relations* among events, and the overall *structure* of causal relations (Trabasso & van den Broek, 1985; Trabasso, van den Broek, & Suh, 1989; van den Broek, 1990).

According to this network model, one property of events in a story concerns the number of *causal connections* that an event has to other events in the story. If an event is connected to many other events in a story through antecedents and/or consequences, it has many causal connections and plays an important role in maintaining the coherence of the story. Research has demonstrated that even young children's story comprehension is influenced by causal connections. Children as young as 4 years of age recall events with many causal connections more often than events with few causal connections (van den Broek, Lorch, & Thurlow, 1996). In addition, as children develop, they become better able both to identify causal relations in a story and to use them to guide recall (Ackerman, Paine, & Silver, 1991; van den Broek, 1989).

A second feature of the network model is a focus on the *goals* arising from certain story events that in turn motivate other actions and outcomes (Mandler & Johnson, 1977; Stein & Glenn, 1979). The goals of a character in a story may be stated explicitly, or they may need to be inferred from other events that suggest the character's motivations. A given goal may motivate a number of subsequent action sequences. Thus, understanding the character's goals is an important influence on overall story comprehension. Young children show considerable difficulty in using goal information to enhance their story comprehension. This is true regardless of whether the task involves memory demands (i.e., recalling a story) or minimizes such demands (i.e., narrating a story from a sequence of pictures). With increasing age, goals take on added importance, to the point where they become a dominant feature in older children's story representations (Goldman & Varnhagen, 1986; Trabasso & Nickels, 1992; Trabasso, Secco, & van den Broek, 1984; van den Broek et al., 1996).

A third feature of the network model concerns the *organizational structure* of causal relations in a story. Story events can be grouped into episodes, each of which centers around a goal (Johnson & Mandler, 1980). In many stories, entire episodes are hierarchically organized and causally dependent on each other, with one episode enabling successful completion of another. As children develop, they first achieve the ability to grasp causal relations *within* episodes, and later become able to comprehend the causal relations *between* these groups of events (Goldman & Varnhagen, 1986; van den Broek, 1989; 1997).

As this brief review indicates, the network model identifies crucial components in story comprehension, and specifies relations among them (see Table 1 in van den Broek et al., 1996, for a concrete example of the network model applied to a story). Recent research has demonstrated that this model provides a coherent framework for understanding developmental trends in children's story comprehension. As such, this model can provide a useful theoretical basis for investigating story comprehension among children with ADHD. However, in order to understand how the attentional problems exhibited by children with ADHD may affect their story comprehension, a methodology is needed that can link their attentional problems to their higher order cognitive processing difficulties. Fortunately, the television viewing methodology fulfills this criterion.

Television Viewing Methodology

The television viewing methodology involves presenting to a child two programs, once in the presence of toys and once without any toys available. The presence of toys is included to simulate what routinely occurs in the home while children are watching television. This manipulation also allows for the assessment of how children allocate attention to the programs versus the toys. In order to measure children's attention, they are videotaped while the program is presented, and the videotapes are coded for moment-to-moment visual attention. After the program is over comprehension is assessed through free and cued recall.

The television viewing methodology has a number of positive features, especially when studying the attention and comprehension of children with ADHD (Lorch & Sanches, 1997). The average school age child watches 20 hours or more of television per week (Anderson, Lorch, Field, Collins, & Nathan, 1986), and recent research suggests that children with ADHD watch even more than that of their nonreferred peers (Acevedo, Lorch, & Milich, 2004). Thus, this procedure reflects children's everyday experiences. In addition, children have been shown to be active, strategic viewers of television from an early age (Anderson, Lorch, Field, & Sanders, 1981; Huston & Wright, 1983; Lorch, Anderson, & Levin, 1979), demonstrating that television programming can actively engage children's attention. Television studies also allow for systematic examination of the relation between visual attention and comprehension (Field & Anderson, 1985; Lorch et al., 1979; Pezdek & Hartman, 1983), as well as factors that mediate this relation (Alwitt, Anderson, Lorch, & Levin, 1980; Calvert, Huston, Watkins, & Wright, 1982). Finally, structural properties defined in research on recall of written stories also predict children's recall of televised stories (van den Broek et al., 1996). Therefore, the study of children's attention to and comprehension of television provides a rich context for gaining information about children's higher order cognitive processing.

As noted earlier, the television viewing methodology is especially appropriate for understanding the attention and comprehension difficulties of children with ADHD. The manipulation of the presence of toys allows for a determination of the allocation of attention, an important issue when studying children noted to have problems sustaining attention. This also allows for examination of the impact of salient distractors on children's attention and comprehension, an issue of great importance among children with ADHD. Further, this methodology is especially appropriate when studying story comprehension of preliterate children or children with significant reading problems, as is often the case in ADHD. This methodology can present strong narrative text without making any demands on the children's reading ability. Thus, important questions about higher order cognitive processing, as reflected in story comprehension, can be addressed.

In what follows we review studies that have applied the network model in building an understanding of these children's story comprehension abilities and difficulties. First, a series of studies is reviewed that employed the television viewing methodology to examine how variations in attention contribute to difficulties children with ADHD have in understanding causal relations among story events. Second, studies employing other methodological approaches to investigate different features of the network model are reviewed. For example, some of these studies employed an online story narration procedure to understand children's use of goal structure in constructing a story representation. Still others have focused on how children's recall can be predicted from the causal structure of the story. The review of these studies will reveal difficulties encountered by children with ADHD in story comprehension that are consistent across the different methodologies. These identified difficulties in turn lead to treatment recommendations for improving the academic performance of children with ADHD.

Television Viewing Studies among Children with ADHD

Landau, Lorch, and Milich (1992) examined the television viewing and comprehension of 19 boys with ADHD and 20 comparison boys, ranging in age from 6 to 12 years. The children viewed two different 14-minute segments from the PBS program "3-2-1 Contact," once in the presence of toys and once in their absence. At the end of each viewing session, the children were asked a series of questions about the programs they had seen. The children were videotaped while viewing the programs so that a measure of the children's visual attention to the television could be obtained. The results revealed a significant group x viewing condition interaction for percent visual attention to the television. There was no difference between the two groups in attention to television when toys were absent, with both groups attending at very high rates (i.e., above 90%). However, in the presence of toys the visual attention of both groups decreased significantly, but the decrease for the boys with ADHD was significantly greater than that of the comparison boys.

In terms of comprehension, although there was a trend toward poorer overall recall for the boys with ADHD, the presence or absence of toys did not differentially affect the comprehension of the two groups. Thus, despite the lower visual attention of children with ADHD when toys were present, their recall of discrete, factual information was no more adversely affected by the presence of toys than that of comparison children. Such a finding might suggest that the children with ADHD are actually strategic viewers of television, since they could decrease their attention without adversely affecting their comprehension. However, a more complex picture of the impact of visual attention on the comprehension of children with ADHD emerged as we incorporated the network model to guide our future studies. Specifically, the findings from Landau et al. (1992) seem to apply to comprehension of factual information, but not necessarily to comprehension of how events in a story are causally related.

The procedures of Landau et al. (1992) were replicated and extended in Study 1 of Lorch et al. (2000). Specifically, 40 boys with ADHD and 52 nonreferred boys, ages 7 to 12, viewed two television programs, once in the presence of toys and once in their absence. However, the programs employed differed somewhat from the Landau et al. (1992) study. First, the length of the programs was increased to 23 minutes, which is more typical of regular programming. Second, two different types of programs were employed, the "3-2-1 Contact" segments from Landau et al. and a more traditional situation comedy, "Growing Pains."

The results concerning visual attention replicated those from Landau et al. (1992), in that there was no group difference in the absence of toys but in the presence of toys the visual attention of the boys with ADHD decreased significantly more than that of the comparison boys. However, a somewhat different pattern of results emerged for the comprehension measures. Once again, in the toys-absent condition there was no group difference, but the recall of the comparison boys was greater than that of the boys with ADHD in the toys-present condition. Because this latter finding was somewhat different from what was found in Landau et al., exploratory analyses were undertaken to reconcile this difference. Specifically, it was noted that the inclusion of the situation comedy, with its strong narrative structure, led to the inclusion of questions that went beyond asking mere factual information and instead examined comprehension of causal connections between story events. When the factual (i.e., 'what') and causal relations (i.e., 'why') questions were reanalyzed separately, the reason for the discrepant findings became clear. Specifically, similar to Landau et al., there were no group differences in the recall of factual information, regardless of viewing condition. However, in terms of causal relations, there was no group difference in the toys-absent condition, but the comparison boys performed better on these questions than the boys with ADHD in the toys-present condition.

The analyses involving the causal relations questions offer an intriguing explanation for the discrepant findings between Landau et al. (1992) and Study 1 of Lorch et al. (2000). Study 2 was designed to directly test this hypothesis by only including programming with a strong narrative structure and explicitly generating questions designed to test both factual information and causal relations. The participants in this study included 44 boys with ADHD and 59 nonreferred boys, ranging in age from 7 to 12. The boys viewed two different episodes of 'Growing Pains,' once in the presence of toys and once in their absence. At the end of each program the boys were asked cued recall questions tapping both factual information and causal relations.

The results concerning percent visual attention replicated those from Landau et al. (1992) and Study 1 of Lorch et al. (2000)—no group differences in the toys-absent condition, the boys with ADHD showing a steeper decline in the toys-present condition. In terms of number of discrete looks at the television, however, there were no group differences in either viewing condition. In terms of recall, there were no group differences for factual information, regardless of viewing condition. This replicates the findings from Landau et al. and Study 1. In terms of causal relations questions, the results were consistent with the explanation offered in Study 1. Specifically, there was no group difference in the toys-absent condition, but the nonreferred boys answered significantly more of these questions than the boys with ADHD in the toys-present condition.

Taken together, the results of Landau et al. (1992) and the two studies of Lorch et al. (2000) lead to some consistent conclusions about the attention and comprehension of boys with ADHD. First, results for visual attention are entirely consistent across the three studies. Both groups of boys sustained high levels of visual attention to television in the absence of toys, whereas the presence of toys reduced visual attention of boys with ADHD to a greater degree than for comparison boys. Second, also consistent across the three studies, the groups did not differ significantly in cued recall of discrete, factual information, regardless of the presence of toys during viewing. Third, differences in story comprehension of boys with ADHD and comparison boys emerged when tasks tapped the understanding of specific causal relations between story events, but only in the presence of toys. This third point indicates that boys with ADHD do not necessarily have a generalized deficit in understanding causal relations. Instead, their ability to understand how story events are connected is more easily disrupted by distractors than is that of the nonreferred boys. This raises the question of how the attentional problems of children with ADHD may impair their understanding of causal relations, an issue addressed in a subsequent study.

Look Lengths and Cognitive Engagement

Why might children with ADHD maintain their understanding of factual events but not causal relations when the presence of toys reduces their visual attention? To answer this question we need to look more closely at differences in the patterns of attention between the comparison children and children with ADHD. One possibility is that children with ADHD shift visual attention more frequently, thus disrupting the continuity of their story processing. However, studies consistently have failed to find group differences in the number of looks at the television in the toys present condition (Landau et al., 1992; Lorch et al., 2000). A second possibility is that children with ADHD engage in shorter looks at the television during the toys-present condition, thus impeding their construction of a coherent story representation. Indeed, these same studies consistently found that the average length of looks at the television is significantly shorter for children with ADHD than for comparison children. The question thus becomes how the group differences in look lengths might account for the problems children with ADHD have in understanding causal relations. One viable explanation stems from evidence that long looks at the television reflect greater cognitive engagement (Anderson, Choi, & Lorch, 1987).

A link between look length and cognitive engagement is suggested by studies of a phenomenon known as attentional inertia. Attentional inertia is defined as an increasing probability of a look continuing, the longer the look already has been in progress (Anderson, Alwitt, Lorch, & Levin, 1979). That is, a look at the television is most likely to be terminated early in the look (within the first 3 seconds), with an increasing probability of the look being maintained until around 15 seconds, when the probability begins to level off (Anderson & Lorch, 1983). Research also suggests that long looks are indicative of increased cognitive engagement and deeper processing.

Perhaps the most direct evidence indicating that length of look is related to cognitive engagement comes from a study by Burns and Anderson (1993). Employing adult participants, the investigators demonstrated that recognition memory was the highest for parts of television segments occurring during the later parts of long looks (looks $\geq$ 15 s). Conversely, recognition memory declined the longer a look away from the television continued. Building on the notion that long looks represent increased cognitive engagement, Hawkins, Tapper, Bruce, and Pingree (1995) hypothesized that such engagement may reflect both the processing demands of a televised story and the degree to which the viewer actively integrates story events as the program continues. In a study of adult participants, Hawkins et al. found that the longer a look was in progress, the longer it continued beyond a content boundary. Further, this effect was stronger the more the information prior to the content boundary needed to be linked to information following the content boundary. Hawkins et al. concluded that these long looks were not merely an automatic process but that their continuation across boundaries also was due to deeper processing of thematically connected material.

Two studies with child participants also offer support for the hypothesized relations between look length and cognitive engagement. In a study of 3 to 5 year olds, Anderson et al. (1987) found that during long looks at a *Sesame Street* program children were both less likely and slower to turn toward a distractor, indicating more involvement with the program during these long looks. Similarly, Lorch and Castle (1997) found that 5-year-old children were slower to respond to a secondary auditory probe the longer a look at a *Sesame Street* program was in progress. However, this was not true for segments of the program edited to be low in comprehensibility. Lorch and Castle concluded that if children were able to comprehend content, deeper processing occurred as longer looks were maintained.

Thus, several studies suggest a relation between long looks and cognitive engagement in both children and adults. No studies, however, had compared differences in look length and story recall between children with ADHD and their nonreferred counterparts. Previous studies using a television viewing paradigm found that if toys are present, children with ADHD do not suffer in their recall of factual information from the story, but show a decrement in their performance on questions testing causal relations (Lorch et al., 2000). One possible explanation for the difficulties children with ADHD have in answering causal relations questions when their attention is divided is that these children spend less time engaged in long looks at the television. If long looks are indicative of increased cognitive engagement, these children would be less engaged with the material and thereby less likely to make connections among events.

Lorch et al. (2004) was designed specifically to address the question of whether time spent in look looks, but not short looks, accounts for the differences between children with ADHD and comparison children in performance on causal relations questions when toys are present during viewing. The sample for the study consisted of 134 boys and girls ranging in age from 7 to 11. Of the total sample, 70 of the children had been diagnosed with ADHD, whereas 64 children were free of any behavior or learning problems. The procedures replicated those of earlier studies, with the children viewing two episodes of the situation comedy, *Growing Pains*, once in the presence of toys and once in their absence. On the basis of causal network analyses and importance ratings of the program scripts, 30 cued recall questions were generated for each episode—10 questions tapping factual information and 20 questions tapping causal relations.

Before analyses could be undertaken testing the cognitive engagement hypothesis, it was necessary to determine whether the results for visual attention and recall replicated those from Landau et al. (1992) and the two studies of Lorch et al. (2000). In terms of percent visual attention, the results were quite consistent with those from the earlier studies. There were no group differences in the toys-absent condition, but children with ADHD showed a greater decrease in visual attention than the comparison children in the toys-present condition. There were no group differences in terms of number of looks the children made to the television, but in the toys-present condition the comparison children spent more time in long looks (i.e., $\geq$ 15 seconds) than did the children with ADHD.

In terms of recall, the results once again replicated those from the earlier studies. Specifically, there were no group differences for recall of factual information regardless of viewing condition. In terms of the causal relations questions, there was no group difference in the toys-absent condition but the comparison children answered significantly more questions than the children with ADHD in the toys-present condition. In fact, the comparison children showed no decrement in recall of causal relations in the toys-present condition, despite their significant drop in overall visual attention.

Having replicated the pattern of results for performance on causal relations questions from Lorch et al. (2000), the next set of analyses focused on the primary purpose of the Lorch et al. (2004) study, which was to test the hypothesis that differences in cognitive engagement accounted for group differences in recall of causal relations in the toys-present condition. This set of analyses included three different analytic strategies that focused on how patterns of attention in the toys-present condition relate to recall. The first analyses tested whether time spent in long looks, but not time spent in short (i.e., < 15 s) looks, significantly mediated group differences in recall of causal relations. The second set of analyses compared the groups in their distributions of long looks, short looks, and looks away during presentation of information necessary to answer causal relations questions. The third set of analyses compared the groups' performance on the causal relations questions for long looks, short looks, and looks away during the relevant information.

The results of these three analytic strategies converged to offer compelling support for the hypothesis that greater cognitive engagement enables the comparison children to form a more coherent representation of the relations among story events, thereby accounting for group differences when toys are present. First, time spent in long looks, but not time spent in short looks, significantly mediated group differences in recall of causal relations. Second, comparison children were found to be engaged in long looks during information relevant to causal relations questions for significantly more questions than were children with ADHD. In contrast, children with ADHD were found to be looking away during information relevant to causal relations questions for significantly more questions than were comparison children. Third, children with ADHD and the comparison children performed comparably on causal relations questions when both groups of children were looking away during presentation of information needed to answer the questions. In contrast, the comparison group significantly outperformed the children with ADHD on these questions when the children were engaged in short looks during presentation of the relevant information. Finally, and most importantly, the two groups did not differ significantly when the participants were engaged in long looks during the information necessary to answer the causal relations questions.

Taken together, the findings from Lorch et al. (2004) are consistent with the literature on attentional inertia and provide further support for the interpretation that long looks lead to deeper cognitive processing (Burns & Anderson, 1993; Hawkins et al., 1995). Of greater significance, these findings constitute the first evidence that the amount of time spent in deeper cognitive processing during long looks helps explain the differential patterns of recall in children with ADHD and comparison children reported here and by Lorch et al. (2000). That is, the similar performance on causal relations questions by the two groups of children when toys are absent can be explained by the fact that in this condition both groups engage primarily in long looks. In contrast, the deficiency in the recall of causal relations shown by children with ADHD in the toys-present condition is attributable to the fact that they spend significantly less time engaged in long looks than comparison children. The most compelling support for this interpretation is that when toys are present, children with ADHD do process information more deeply during long looks, as shown by their impressive performance on causal relations questions testing information presented while they are engaged in long looks.

What is it about long looks that leads to deeper processing? A possible explanation is that comparison children's greater time in long looks means that these children engage in deeper processing of more story content, in turn enabling construction of more coherent story representations. Comparison children can then use these more coherent representations to guide further processing and thereby make causal connections, even during short looks. In contrast, children with ADHD had difficulty making such connections during short looks. There are several possible mechanisms for how extended time in long looks could enhance comprehension of causal relation information presented during short looks. First, by developing a more coherent story representation, comparison children may more systematically monitor their ongoing understanding of the story than do children with ADHD, which enables the comparison children to use short looks to fill in missing information. Second, more coherent story representations among comparison children may provide a structure for connecting incoming information, even that obtained during short looks. Finally, more coherent story representations may allow comparison children to make inferences about the connections among events during cued recall testing, even if short looks did not allow for deeper processing at the time of viewing.

The results of Lorch et al. (2004) suggest that variations in cognitive engagement may account for the problems that children with ADHD have with causal relations questions. However, cognitive engagement is an internal construct that cannot be measured directly. In that study, the degree of cognitive engagement was inferred from time spent in long looks. There are other ways to operationalize cognitive engagement and a better understanding of this construct can be gained from combining methodologies in a converging operations approach. For example, one method for measuring moment-to-moment variations in cognitive engagement is the secondary task procedure (Britton, Westbrook, & Holdredge, 1978). In this procedure, children's reaction times to a secondary probe (e.g., an auditory tone) are measured while they are watching a television program. The assumption underlying this procedure is that slower reaction times reflect greater cognitive engagement with the televised material. Research with nonreferred children has indicated that levels of cognitive engagement, as measured by the secondary task procedure, vary with the comprehensibility of the material and the centrality of story content (Lorch & Castle, 1997; Meadowcroft & Reeves, 1989).

Whirley, Lorch, Lemberger, and Milich (2003) was designed to employ the secondary task methodology to investigate patterns of cognitive engagement among children with ADHD, and how these patterns may differ depending on whether the information was either central or incidental to the story plot. Specifically, we examined whether boys with ADHD became more cognitively engaged (i.e., their reaction times slowed down) as a sequence of central information continued, and less engaged (i.e., faster reaction times) as a sequence of incidental information progressed, as theory and research suggests (Lorch & Castle, 1997; Meadowcroft & Reeves, 1989).

Participants were 22 boys with ADHD and 36 nonreferred boys, ranging in age from 9 to 11. The boys viewed one episode of the situation comedy, *Growing Pains*, for which sequences of high (i.e., central) and low (incidental) importance had been identified. For each central or incidental sequence, auditory probes were placed at the beginning (i.e., 2 s), middle (7 s) or end (12 s and $\geq$ 24 s) in order to measure changes in cognitive engagement as the sequence progressed. The boys were instructed to view the television program but to respond as quickly as possible whenever they heard one of the auditory probes. At the end of the program the boys were asked a series of questions about the show, tapping information of either high or low importance.

The results revealed that overall the boys with ADHD responded significantly slower than the nonreferred boys, a common finding in reaction time studies. More importantly, the patterns of reaction times across the central sequences differed between the two groups of boys. Specifically, the nonreferred boys showed the typical pattern of slower reaction times (i.e., increased cognitive engagement) the longer into a central sequence the probes appeared. In contrast, the boys with ADHD actually showed faster reaction times from the beginning to the middle of the central sequences, suggesting decreased cognitive engagement as the central sequences progressed. It was only at the final probes that the reaction times of the boys with ADHD showed the expected increase.

In terms of cued recall performance, there was a significant main effect of group, with the comparison boys answering more questions correctly. However, group did not interact with question importance. Analyses also compared the relation between reaction times and cued recall performance for the two groups. For questions testing both central and incidental story information, there was a significant main effect, such that reaction times were slower for questions that were answered correctly. This is consistent with the hypothesis that slower reaction times are associated with deeper cognitive processing. However, these patterns were comparable for the two groups of boys.

Although the methodologies of Lorch et al. (2004) and Whirley et al. (2003) operationalized cognitive engagement somewhat differently, the results of the two studies are consistent in documenting that children with ADHD have difficulty sustaining cognitive engagement over extended periods of time. In the case of Lorch et al., this conclusion held only in the presence of appealing distractors. In the Whirley et al. study, the difficulty sustaining cognitive engagement was true even in the absence of such distractors. Further, Lorch et al. did not observe a group difference in the recall of factual information whereas Whirley et al. found such a difference. These discrepancies in the results of the two studies may be reconciled by considering differences in how toys and secondary probes may have functioned as distractors. In the Lorch et al. study, attention to the distractors (i.e., toys) was under the voluntary control of the children. That is, children determined when and for how long they directed their attention away from and back to the television. In contrast, in Whirley et al. the children could not anticipate when the probes were presented, and they were placed to coincide with information needed to answer the cued recall questions. Although not planned as such, the probes in the Whirley et al. study may have been especially distracting to the children with ADHD, thereby disrupting both the ability of these children to sustain cognitive engagement and to answer the factual recall questions.

Another possible explanation for the differences in the results of Lorch et al. (2004) and Whirley et al. (2003) concerns how cognitive engagement was operationalized in the two studies. In Lorch et al., cognitive engagement is inferred from long looks. However, look length is influenced not only by level of cognitive engagement but can reflect other factors (e.g., salient program features that may hold the child's attention but not require deep levels of engagement). As such, look length measures cognitive engagement at a relatively gross level. In contrast, reaction times to secondary probes, as used in Whirley et al., provide a more immediate, moment-to-moment index of cognitive engagement. Therefore, it may be a more sensitive measure of cognitive engagement in its ability to detect more subtle variations in engagement. This contrast is evident in that group differences in engagement were detected in Whirley et al., even though the children in both groups predominantly engaged in long looks.

Studies Using other Story Comprehension Methodologies

To this point, this review has focused on studies employing television programs as the stimuli from which comprehension is assessed. As noted earlier, such an approach has many benefits. These include the ability to link attention to comprehension, the appealing nature of the stimuli so that the children will be actively engaged, and the fact that these stimuli allow for the assessment of story comprehension in populations (such as ADHD) where reading is a documented problem. However, as with any single experimental methodology, there are limitations with the television viewing approach. First, as noted earlier, television programs have high appeal to children and, as such, may not reflect the more mundane nature of classroom lectures and textbooks. The best evidence for this statement is the very high rate of visual attention (> 90%) exhibited by children with ADHD in the toys-absent condition (e.g., Lorch et al., 2000; Lorch et al., 2004). We know of no classroom observation study of (unmedicated) children with ADHD that reveals rates of on-task behavior anywhere approaching such high levels of attention. As such, the ecological validity of the television viewing methodology may be somewhat limited, although the lessons learned from these studies can still inform us about the cognitive processing difficulties of children with ADHD.

Second, the studies reviewed so far all have used cued recall performance as their measure of comprehension. Specifically, recall is assessed after the program is over and comprehension is inferred from recall. Thus, if children with ADHD exhibit deficits in comprehension in these studies, any of a number of cognitive processes may account for these deficits. For example, the problems in recall could reflect difficulties in encoding the initial information, difficulties in working memory, difficulties in the story representations created, and/or difficulties in retrieving the relevant information. The studies reviewed so far cannot specifically address these different possibilities.

The following studies begin to address each of the two limitations noted for the television viewing studies. First, we review two studies in which the stories to be recalled are presented on audio tapes. Such an approach more closely approximates what may occur in a typical classroom lecture. The second of these two studies also addresses the question of whether studying can improve the overall story recall of children with ADHD. Then we review two studies that use an online story telling procedure to address more directly the building of story representations by children with ADHD. Such a methodology relies less on memory and instead informs us how children with ADHD employ important story grammar categories, such as the protagonist's goals, to guide their story representation.

Recall of Auditory Stories among Children with ADHD

Lorch et al. (1999) examined the role of causal relations, as well as importance, in predicting the recall of children with ADHD and their nonreferred classmates. The sample of children consisted of 71 children with ADHD and 64 comparison children, ranging in age from 7 to 11. The children listened to audiotape presentations of two relatively brief (e.g., 4 min) folk tales, used previously by Brown and Smiley (1977) and Tannock, Purvis, and Schachar (1993). After hearing each story, the children were asked to retell the stories. Importance ratings and causal network analyses of the folk tales were available, and regression analyses were used to predict recall of each story unit from the number of causal connections and importance of each story unit for the two groups of children.

Consistent with the story comprehension literature (van den Broek et al., 1996), as the number of causal connections and importance increased, recall increased for both groups. However, each story structure variable interacted significantly with group status. Specifically, the relation of each variable to recall was stronger for comparison children than for children with ADHD. Further examination revealed that the number of causal connections was the only predictor variable to make a unique contribution to the interaction. Thus, although the children with ADHD showed sensitivity to the causal structure of the stories, the results indicated that they benefited less from the story structure properties than did the comparison children. That is, as the number of causal connections to a story event increased, the increase in recall was steeper for comparison children than for children with ADHD. This group difference may reflect greater sensitivity among the nonreferred children in identifying causal relations, in effectively encoding them, and/or in using causal relations to guide retrieval of story information.

Lorch et al. (2004) was designed to replicate and extend the findings of Lorch et al. (1999). The study had three major goals. First, the study examined group differences in the extent to which number of causal connections predicts story recall. The second major purpose was to investigate group differences in changes in story recall as a function of studying and story structure. Specifically, we examined the relation between time spent studying specific information and the recall of that information, as well as group differences in the relation between story structure and information gained or retained as a result of studying. Finally, we compared the study behavior of children with ADHD and nonreferred children in terms of time spent studying, variations in their use of different study strategies, and allocation of study time to specific story ideas.

The sample for this study consisted of 36 children with ADHD and 43 nonreferred children, ranging in age from 7 to 11. The children were asked to listen to one of the two folk tale stories used in Lorch et al. (1999), and then were asked to recall the story immediately after hearing it. After completing the first recall, children were given a written version of the story they had just heard, with each page of the story containing one story event. Children were given pencils, highlighters, and paper and were instructed that they could do anything they wished to study the story so that they could remember it better. Children were given up to ten minutes to study, and were stopped at this time if they had not yet finished studying. When children finished studying, a second recall was recorded. Prior to giving this recall, children were reminded to tell the whole story, including everything that they recalled the first time.

The results revealed that the number of causal connections predicted recall, such that the more causal connections an event had, the more often it was recalled. Further, the number of causal connections interacted significantly with diagnostic group in predicting recall. Consistent with Lorch et al. (1999), the difference in the proportion of items recalled for the two groups increased as the number of causal connections increased, such that children with ADHD benefited less than comparison children in their recalls as the number of causal connections increased.

The next set of analyses concerned the impact of studying on recall. There was a main effect for study time, such that children spent more time studying the items they later recalled. We next examined group differences in the relation between number of causal connections and information gained or retained as a result of studying. It is important to note that for story events that were not recalled in the immediate recall prior to studying, post-study recall scores represent events *gained*; for story events that were recalled prior to studying, post-study recall scores represent events *retained*. The following results are presented separately for information gained and information retained.

No systematic difference in *gain* occurred for children with IQs below the median, such that the proportion of items gained was small for both diagnostic groups of children with lower IQs. In contrast, significant differences did appear between the two diagnostic groups with higher IQs, such that differences in *gain* became greater between the higher IQ diagnostic groups as the number of causal connections increased. At low numbers of causal connections (i.e., 1 to 4 connections), there was no significant difference between diagnostic groups, but across the two highest numbers of causal connections (i.e., 5 and 6 connections) the comparison children gained considerably more than children with ADHD. Thus, studying appears to be more effective for the higher IQ comparison children in helping them add the information that is the most important for a coherent understanding of the story.

In terms of information *retained*, no group differences were observed for children with IQs below the median, and both groups retained less than their higher IQ counterparts. For children with IQs above the median, both diagnostic groups retained most of the information at the highest levels of causal connections. The superiority of the comparison group occurred only for recall of units with four causal connections.

The third purpose of the study was to examine group differences in study strategies and behavior. There were no significant main effects of group status for any of the variables examined, including time spent studying, the distribution of study time across story events, and the specific study strategies employed (e.g., rereading, highlighting). The lack of group differences in study behaviors was somewhat unexpected, especially given the differential impact of studying on the recall of the two groups.

To integrate the studies reviewed to this point, it is important to note that there are several ways in which the methodology of the Lorch et al. (1999) and Lorch et al. (2004) studies differs from that employed in the television viewing studies. First, in the audiotape recall studies, the story is presented in a single modality, most likely resulting in a presentation that is less engaging than professionally produced television programs that communicate audiovisually and utilize appealing formal features (e.g., sound effects, rapid action sequences). Second, only in the television viewing studies is attention systematically manipulated and measured. Third, comprehension is assessed differently in the two types of studies, with cued recall employed in the television viewing studies and free recall in the audiotape recall studies. As such, testing demands in the audiotape recall studies are considerably greater, in that children must retrieve information without cues and supply their own organizational structure for retelling the story.

Despite these potentially important methodological differences in the two types of studies, the results point to similar conclusions regarding story comprehension difficulties of children with ADHD. Most notably, these children have more difficulty than their nonreferred peers in representing and utilizing the causal relations that underlie the structure of a story. In the television viewing studies, this was only true when toys were present. However, this methodology presents stories in an appealing format and supplies children with considerable structure in the cued recall testing. Both of these factors are absent in the audiotape recall studies, which may explain why the children with ADHD are less effective than comparison children in benefiting from the causal structure of a story, even in the absence of distractors or after studying the story. It is important to note that the methodology of the audiotape recall studies more closely approximates classroom presentations, suggesting that children with ADHD will have difficulty in making connections among events and in using connections to guide recall of information, even in the absence of salient distractors.

Online Story Narrations among Children with ADHD

Many studies of children's story comprehension use recall to assess comprehension. However, asking a child to listen to or watch a story and then later questioning him or her about the story not only explores knowledge of causal connections and goal plans, but also tests the child's memory. Thus, although memory deficits are hypothesized to be an integral aspect of ADHD (Barkley, 1997), researchers have attempted to tease out the effects of memory on comprehension by using an online narrative approach.

Online narration involves asking a child to tell a story from a series of pictures. The pictures are not accompanied by words, and the child must generate the story. This task reduces memory demands because an element of the story is available to the child at all times. However, in order to narrate the story coherently, the child needs to understand the importance of a goal plan in resolving the dilemma in the story (Trabasso, Stein, Rodkin, Munger, & Baughn, 1992). The child also needs to grasp the importance of causal connections to establish why one event follows another and make connections between events occurring at different times in the story. A narration missing these elements is indicative of deficits in story comprehension.

Several research groups have specifically examined the online story comprehension of children with ADHD. Milch-Reich, Campbell, Pelham, Connelly, and Geva (1999) investigated story narration among school-aged children with ADHD and nonreferred children. They asked children to narrate a series of seven pictures and then examined the organizational structure of the narratives. Specifically, Milch-Reich et al. (1999) looked at the ability of the children to integrate events within and between the pictures in the narration. They also analyzed two types of links between the pictures: concrete and inferential/causal. Concrete links lacked an explanation of why events occurred, whereas inferential/causal links made explicit the causal connections between events.

Analyses of the children's narratives revealed a pattern similar to studies using recall. In general, younger children produced shorter narratives (Milch-Reich et al., 1999; Zentall, 1988). Older nonreferred children and older children with ADHD included the same number of ideas in their narratives, but the type of ideas differed. Consistent with the pattern shown by younger children, older children with ADHD produced narratives that contained discrete ideas and few causal connections, evidence of a lack of understanding of the importance of causal structure. Children with ADHD also made more errors in their narrations than nonreferred children. Milch-Reich et al. (1999) attributed this to impulsivity interfering with the organizational processes of these children.

The Milch-Reich et al. (1999) study demonstrated that children with ADHD and non-referred children differ in their ability to organize a story and in their understanding of causal connections. However, the story used in this study only contained seven pictures. In order to truly capture differences in the cohesion and organization of on-line narrations, a longer story is needed. Story-grammar theory provides an explicit technique for examining understanding of causal connections and goal-based categories, which are important in the cohesion and organization of a story.

To this end, Renz et al. (2003) used both a longer story and the story grammar coding categories in order to explore differences in narrations between 9- to11-year-old children with ADHD and their nonreferred peers. The story used by Renz et al. (2003), *Frog Where Are You?* by Mercer Mayer (1969), contains 24 pictures and includes an hierarchical goal structure. The story begins with a frog escaping from its owner, a little boy. After the boy establishes his overall goal of finding the frog and bringing it back home, the story progresses with a number of unsuccessful attempts to meet the goal, creating subgoals. Ultimately, the boy does find the frog, and to his surprise, the frog's family. The boy is then allowed to take a baby frog home, thus resolving his overall goal of bringing a frog back home.

In their study, Renz et al. (2003) coded the children's narratives using the story grammar categories. The establishment of the overall goal, the subsequent subgoal attempts and outcomes, and the resolution to the overall goal were the most important story grammar categories coded. The subgoal attempts were classified into unlinked attempts (i.e., not explicitly related to finding the frog), linked attempts (i.e., specifying the overall goal of finding the frog), and specific linked attempts (i.e., when the boy searched specific locations for the frog). Linked attempts suggest an understanding of both goal structure and causal connections because the child restates the boy's goal of searching to recover the frog, which was established at the beginning of the story.

Renz et al. (2003) found that nonreferred children included the resolution of the overall goal significantly more often than children with ADHD, suggesting that nonreferred children ages 9 to11 are better able to maintain a goal plan throughout the narration of a story. Children with ADHD also used fewer specific linked attempts than did nonreferred children. This suggests that children with ADHD have a less developed understanding of goal plans and their narratives lack cohesion and organization compared to their nonreferred peers.

Finally, children with ADHD made more errors in their narrations than did nonreferred children. Specifically, children with ADHD repeated themselves more often, suggesting problems with working memory. They also used more ambiguous references within their sentences.

Although the Renz et al. (2003) study is important to understanding the organization of narratives of children with ADHD, the age range of children within the study may not have captured major developmental changes in story comprehension. According to Trabasso et al. (1992), the most important ages for the development of the understanding of causal structure and goal plan are between three and nine. Thus, in a subsequent study (Flory et al., 2004), the methodology of Renz et al. (2003) was replicated using 7- to 9-year-old children with and without ADHD. In addition, the Flory et al. study went beyond prior comprehension studies and examined how the core deficits of ADHD (e.g., inattention, executive functioning deficits, working memory) may account for the problems these children have with online story comprehension and narration.

The sample for the Flory et al. (2004) study consisted of 49 children with ADHD and 67 nonreferred children, ranging in age from 7 to 9. The children narrated one of two wordless picture books, both authored by Mercer Mayer. One book was *Frog Where Are You?* (Mayer, 1969), the one employed by both Renz et al. (2003) and Trabasso et al. (1992). The second story, *A Boy, A Dog, and A Frog* (Mayer, 1967), is the prequel to *Frog Where Are You?* and also contains a series of 24 pictures. The children's story narrations were coded according to the story grammar categories employed in Renz et al. (2003).

In addition to the story narration procedure, three tasks measuring the core deficits of ADHD were collected. The three tasks were the Tower of London-Drexel (TOL^{DX}; Culbertson & Zillmer, 2000), which supplied measures of planning and executive functioning; the Stop-Signal Task (Schachar & Logan, 1990), which supplied measures of inattention and problems in inhibitory control; and Digits Forward and Backward from the *WISC-III*, measures of memory and working memory, respectively.

The results revealed that the two groups of children did not differ in the lengths of stories they narrated. However, there were group differences on several of the story grammar categories related to the causal structure of the stories, and on all three error categories. Specifically, nonreferred children were significantly more likely to mention the initiating event than were the children with ADHD. The former were also more likely to include Goal-Attempt-Outcome (GAO) sequences in their narratives, and to state the completion of the overall goal. The children with ADHD made significantly more errors in each of the three categories—within clause, whole clause, and repetition errors.

Consistent with the research literature, the children with ADHD did more poorly on most of the measures of core deficits, including those of planning, memory and working memory, inattention and disinhibition. Mediation analyses revealed that all of these core deficits accounted to some degree account for the problems children with ADHD have in narrating a coherent, goal-based story. However, further analyses revealed that the standard deviation of the reaction times on go-trials of the stop-signal task, a measure of the ability to sustain attention, consistently was the most influential mediator. This measure was a significant mediator for all seven categories and it always accounted for the largest percent reduction of all of the mediators.

The results of the Renz et al. (2003) and Flory et al. (2004) online story narration studies both revealed problems that children with ADHD have in narrating a coherent, goal-based story. Just as earlier we noted that the studies using the audiotape recall and television viewing methodologies revealed common bases for the deficits among children with ADHD, so too the results of the online narration studies can be linked to these explanations. The earlier explanations focused on deficiencies in how children with ADHD used the causal relations that structure a story in guiding their recall, or structuring a coherent representation that can be used to answer causal relations questions. In contrast to the focus on individual causal relations in these methodologies, the online methodology emphasizes the protagonist's overall goal, which serves as the linchpin of a causal structure. To create a coherent story representation, children need to recognize events that motivate the overall goal, actions and outcomes that result from the goal, and subgoals that may follow from actions and outcomes. The results of Renz et al. and Flory et al. reveal that such goal-based story events are the very areas in which children with ADHD are deficient in their story narrations. Further, as the results of the online studies reveal, these deficiencies are evident even when memory and attentional demands are reduced. Thus, regardless of the methodology used, children with ADHD demonstrate deficiencies in employing causal structure in guiding comprehension and recall.

Treatment Implications

The results of these studies offer important implications for improving the academic performance of children with ADHD. Currently, the empirically-validated treatments recommended for children with ADHD are stimulant medication and behavior modification. Such treatments tend to focus on and have proven effective in decreasing the children's disruptiveness and increasing their on-task behavior and the quantity of academic work completed. In contrast, results of the studies on story comprehension demonstrate that such interventions may prove insufficient in helping children with ADHD understand and construct coherent representations of information presented in lectures or texts. Instead, appropriate interventions will need to target ways to assist these children in seeing connections among events so that they use these connections to build a complete and articulated understanding of the presented material.

Given that children with ADHD show less sensitivity to the causal structure of stories and are less able to use it to guide their understanding and recall, academic interventions should place greater emphasis on the causal relations among story events. Day-to-day-instruction of elementary school-aged children often primarily focuses on helping children gain factual information from a lecture or story but this method of instruction ignores the importance of how story events or ideas in a lecture are related to one another. Emphasizing causal relations among events or ideas may help sensitize children with ADHD to structures that organize stories and lectures and thus assist them in building more effective representations for guiding recall. One way to accomplish this is for teachers to systematically ask students why certain events occurred as the information is being presented. These ongoing causal relations questions should help students to appreciate the underlying coherence of story events, rather than as a series of discrete facts. The research is clear that the more children can make connections among events, the greater their recall of a story (van den Broek, 1997).

One aspect of stories that has special importance in understanding the causal relations among events consists of the protagonist's major goals and the subgoals that may result from a protagonist's thwarted attempts to achieve these goals. Research has shown that comprehending how these goals and subgoals drive characters' actions and story outcomes are critical in developing a coherent narrative representation (Trabasso & Stein, 1997). Children with ADHD have been shown to have difficulty maintaining focus on the protagonist's goals as they build a story representation (Flory et al., 2004; Renz et al., 2003). To rectify this deficiency, teachers could help children to relate ongoing events to what the protagonist is trying to achieve, and how the protagonist must alter his/her behavior in response to outcomes that result from initial attempts.

Another approach to emphasizing causal relations is to provide students with the opportunity to practice predicting upcoming story events and explain those predictions in terms of prior events. From any given event, causal relations may connect backward to explain past occurrences or lead forward to produce future events. Research has shown that among more skilled comprehenders, forward connections are a better predictor of overall story recall than backward connections (van den Broek et al., 1996). Thus, in helping children to grasp causal relations, it is important that teachers emphasize not only the reasons for a current event, but also the ways in which the current event sets the stage for future events.

Finally, children with ADHD appear to need help discriminating information of greater and lesser importance. For example, teachers could present information from a story and ask the children to indicate whether this information is important to developing the plot of the story, and then ask them to explain the thinking behind their judgments. The goal of such an intervention is to enable the students to build an explicit understanding of determinants of what makes events important to a plot. This type of explicit understanding should help children in guiding their recall of information.

Unfortunately, a search of the treatment literature for children with ADHD fails to mention any interventions that focus on having these children utilize causal relations to enhance their ability to represent information coherently. Findings from the story comprehension studies indicate that these types of interventions may have potential for improving the story comprehension and thus the academic performance of children with ADHD. As indicated in the next section, these suggested interventions need to be tested in future research.

Future Directions

As this review has indicated, children with ADHD exhibit reliable deficiencies in their story comprehension skills, across a variety of research methodologies. Specifically, the problems these children experience include using the causal relations that structure a story in guiding their recall and structuring a coherent representation that can be used to answer causal relations questions. In addition, children with ADHD have difficulty employing the protagonist's overall goal, and goal-based events, to create coherent story representations. Although these studies have given us important leads in understanding the story comprehension difficulties experienced by children with ADHD, there still remain other aspects of story comprehension that need to be explored. For example, studies can examine these children's inferencing ability. This is especially germane for furthering our understanding of these children's deficits because causal relations among story events often are not explicitly stated, and the reader must infer connections among the events. Given the previously documented difficulties children with ADHD have in making connections among events, a potential contributing factor may be problems in drawing the appropriate inferences. In a similar vein, studies can explore comprehension monitoring among children with ADHD. Comprehension monitoring is defined as both the ability to detect gaps in one's understanding of a story, as well as the skills to fill in the gaps to create a coherent story (Wagoner, 1983). To the extent that children with ADHD have difficulty in drawing appropriate inferences and monitoring their comprehension, these children will have increased difficulty as they progress to more demanding materials and story comprehension tasks.

A second area of future research concerns the generalizability of the laboratory studies reported here to the actual classroom environment. For example, the television viewing studies reliably documented that salient distractors impaired the ability of children with ADHD to understand causal relations. However, these studies all involved the children sitting alone in a room with toys available while they viewed a television program. However, in the real-world classroom environment, the children are rarely alone, rarely allowed to play with toys, and rarely viewing television programs. Thus, it is difficult to know how the present results generalize to actual classroom behavior. It may well be that the performance of children with ADHD is even more impaired in the classroom, because there are many more distractors and the presentation format is often not as engaging as are television programs. Studies can be undertaken to examine the ability of children with ADHD to comprehend classroom lectures and expository text, to determine whether similar or even more pronounced difficulties are evident.

A third line of future research investigations concerns attempts to intervene to rectify the story comprehension difficulties experienced by children with ADHD. An obvious starting point concerns the impact of stimulant medication on story comprehension abilities. This is the most widely used treatment for ADHD, and such treatment has shown significant efficacy in decreasing disruptive behavior and increasing on-task behavior. However, very few studies have been undertaken examining the impact of stimulant medication on the higher order processing abilities of children with ADHD. One of the few studies addressing this issue is a study examining the effects of stimulant medication on story retelling among children with ADHD (Francis, Fine, & Tannock, 2001). The results revealed that the number of story events included in retellings and performance on factual and inferential cued recall questions showed no medication effects, although on medication children were more likely to report story characters' internal responses and attempts. Similar studies can be undertaken examining the impact of stimulant medication on other aspects of story comprehension among children with ADHD.

As noted earlier, there are reasons to believe that treatment with stimulant medication may not be sufficient to ameliorate the story comprehension difficulties of children with ADHD. First, such deficits showed up on tasks, such as the online narrations, that placed limited demands on attention and working memory, areas that tend to be positively impacted by stimulant medication. Second, the Francis et al. (2001) study only found limited improvements in story comprehension due to stimulant medication, findings that are consistent with other studies examining medication's effects on higher order cognitive processing (Murphy, Pelham, & Lang, 1992). Thus, interventions that more directly target the specific story comprehension deficits exhibited by children with ADHD may be necessary. For example, the educational literature reveals gains in comprehension abilities among children identified as poor comprehenders following training in areas such as comprehension monitoring (McGee & Johnson, 2003) and inference making (Hansen, 1981). To date, no study could be located examining the impact of such training on the story comprehension abilities of children with ADHD. The systematic study of interventions targeting the story comprehension deficits of children with ADHD may significantly advance our ability to address the academic difficulties experienced by these children.

In this chapter we have reviewed a series of studies examining the story comprehension abilities of children with ADHD. We have attempted to make the point that this is an important but neglected research area in understanding the academic difficulties of children with ADHD. In reviewing the television viewing studies, we have shown how story comprehension research can complement and build upon the literature examining the core deficits of ADHD, such as problems in sustaining attention. We believe that this line of investigation can offer valuable insights into both the bases for academic difficulties among children with ADHD and the interventions necessary to address these difficulties.

Author Notes

This research was supported by National Institute of Mental Health grant MH47386 to the second author. Requests for reprints should be addressed to: Richard Milich, Department of Psychology, University of Kentucky, Lexington, KY 40506-0044. Electronic mail can be sent to milich@uky.edu.

References

Acevedo, D., Lorch, E. P., & Milich, R., (2004). TV or not TV: The media habits of children with ADHD. Unpublished manuscript.

Ackerman, B. P., Paine, J., & Silver, D. (1991). Building a story representation: The effects of early concepts on later causal inferences by children. *Developmental Psychology, 27*, 370-380.

Ackerman, B. P., Silver, D., & Glickman, I. (1990). Concept availability in the causal inferences by children and adults. *Child Development, 61*, 230-246.

Alwitt, L. F., Anderson, D. R., Lorch, E. P., & Levin, S. R. (1980). Preschool children's visual attention to television. *Human Communication Research, 7*, 52-67.

American Psychiatric Association. (1994). *Diagnostic and statistical manual of mental disorders* (Fourth edition). Washington, DC: Author.

Anderson, D., Alwitt, L., Lorch, E., & Levin, S. (1979). Watching children watch television. In G. Hale & M. Lewis (Eds.), *Attention and cognitive development* (pp. 331-361). NY: Plenum Press.

Anderson, D. R., Choi, H. P., & Lorch, E. P. (1987). Attentional inertia reduces distractibility in young children's television viewing. *Child Development, 58,* 798-806.

Anderson, D. R. & Lorch, E. P. (1983). Looking at television: Action or reaction? In J. Bryant & D. R. Anderson (Eds.), *Children's understanding of television: Research on attention and comprehension* (pp. 1-33). New York: Academic Press.

Anderson, D. R., Lorch, E. P. Field, D. E., Collins, P. & Nathan, J. (1986). Television viewing at home: Age trends in visual attention and time with TV. *Child Development, 57*, 1024-1033.

Anderson, D. R., Lorch, E. P., Field, D. E., & Sanders, J. (1981). The effects of TV program comprehensibility on preschool children's visual attention to television. *Child Development, 52*, 151-157.

Barkley, R. A. (1997). Behavioral inhibition, sustained attention, and executive functions: Constructing a unifying theory of ADHD. *Psychological Bulletin, 121,* 65-94.

Barkley, R.A. (1998). *Attention deficit hyperactivity disorder: A handbook for diagnosis and treatment* (2nd ed.). New York: Guilford.

Britton, B. K., Westbrook, R. D., & Holdredge, T. S. (1978). Reading and cognitive capacity usage: Effects of text difficulty. *Journal of Experimental Psychology: Human Learning and Memory, 4*, 582-591.

Brown, A. L. & Smiley, S. S. (1977). Rating the importance of structural units of prose passages: A problem of metacognitive development. *Child Development, 48*, 1-8.

Burns, J. J. & Anderson, D. R. (1993). Attentional inertia and recognition memory in adult television viewing. *Communication Research, 20,* 777-799.

Calvert, S., Huston, A. Watkins, B., & Wright, J. (1982). The effects of selective attention to television forms on children's comprehension of content. *Child Development, 53*, 601-610.

Culbertson, W. C. & Zillmer, E. A. (2000). *Tower of London^{DX}*. Multi-Health Systems Inc: North Tonawanda, NY.

Diener, M. B. & Milich, R. (1997). The effects of positive feedback on the social interactions of boys with ADHD: A test of the self-protective hypothesis. *Journal of Clinical Child Psychology, 26*, 256-265.

Douglas, V. I. (1999). Cognitive control processes in attention deficit/hyperactivity disorder. In H. C. Quay and A. E. Hogan (Eds.), *Handbook of disruptive behavior disorders* (pp. 105-138). NY: Kluwer Academic.

Field, D. E. & Anderson, D. R. (1985). Instruction and modality effects on children's television attention and comprehension. *Journal of Educational Psychology, 77*, 91-100.

Flory, K., Hayden, A. N., Milich, R., Lorch, E. P., Strange, C., & Welsh, R. (2004). Online story comprehension among children with ADHD: Which core deficits are involved? Unpublished manuscript.

Francis, S., Fine, J., & Tannock, R. (2001). Methylphenidate selectively improves storyretelling in children with attention deficit hyperactivity disorder. *Journal of Child and Adolescent Psychopharmacology, 11*, 3, 217-228.

Graesser, A. C. & Clark, L. F. (1985). *Structures and procedures of implicit knowledge.* Norwood, NJ: Ablex.

Goldman, S. R. & Varnhagen, C.K. (1986). Memory for embedded and sequential story structures. *Journal of Memory and Learning, 25,* 401-418.

Hansen, J. (1981). The effectcs of inference training and practice on young children's reading comprehension. *Reading Research Quarterly, 3*, 391-417.

Hawkins, R.P., Tapper, J., Bruce, L., and Pingree, S. (1995) Strategic and nonstrategic explanations for attentional inertia. *Communication Research, 22*, 188-206.

Hooks, K., Milich, R., & Lorch, E. P. (1994). Sustained and selective attention in boys with attention deficit hyperactivity disorder. *Journal of Clinical Child Psychology, 23*, 69-77.

Huston, A. & Wright, J. (1983). Children's processing of television: The informative functions of formal features. In J. Bryant & D. Anderson (Eds.), *Children's understanding of television: Research on attention and comprehension* (pp. 35-68). New York: Academic Press.

Landau, S., Lorch, E. P., & Milich, R. (1992). Visual attention to and comprehension of television in attention deficit hyperactivity disordered and normal boys. *Child Development, 63,* 928-937.

Lorch, E. P., Anderson, D. R., & Levin, S. R. (1979). The relationship of visual attention to children's comprehension of television. *Child Development, 50*, 722-727.

Lorch, E. P. & Castle, V. J. (1997). Preschool children's attention to television: Visual attention and probe response times. *Journal of Experimental Child Psychology, 66,* 111-127.

Lorch, E. P., Diener, M. B., Sanchez, R. P., Milich, R., van den Broek, P., & Welsh, R. (1999). The effects of story structure on the recall of stories in children with attention deficit hyperactivity disorder. *Journal of Educational Psychology, 92*, 273-283.

Lorch, E. P., Eastham, D., Milich, R., & Lemberger, C. C. (2004). Difficulties in comprehending causal relations among children with ADHD: The role of cognitive engagement. *Journal of Abnormal Psychology*.

Lorch, E. P., Milich, R., & Sanchez, R. P. (1998). Story comprehension in children with ADHD. *Clinical Child and Family Psychology Review, 1,* 163-178.

Lorch, E. P., Milich, R., Sanchez, R. P., van den Broek, P., Baer, S., Hooks, K., Hartung, C., & Welsh, R. (2000). Comprehension of televised stories in attention deficit hyperactivity disordered and nonreferred boys. *Journal of Abnormal Psychology, 109,* 321-330.

Lorch, E. P., O'Neil, K., Berthiaume, K. S., Milich, R., Eastham, D., & Brooks, T. (2004). Study time and story recall by children with ADHD and nonreferred children. *Journal of Clinical Child and Adolescent Psychology,* 33, 506-515.

Lorch, E. P., & Sanchez, R. P. (1997). Children's memory for televised events. In P.W. van den Broek, P. J. Bauer, & T. Bourg, (Eds.), *Developmental spans in event comprehension and representation: Bridging fictional and actual events.* (pp. 271-294). Mahwah, NJ: Lawrence Erlbaum Associates.

Low, J. & Durkin, K. (1998). Structure and causal connections in children's online television narratives: What develops? *Cognitive Development, 13,* 201-225.

McGee, A., & Johnson, T.H. (1978-1979). The development and evaluation of a self-questioning study technique. *Reading Research Quarterly, 14*, 605-623.

Mandler, J.M., & Johnson, N.S. (1977). Remembrance of things parsed: story structure and recall. *Cognitive Psychology, 9*, 111-151.

Mayer, M. (1967). *A boy, a dog, and a frog.* New York: Dial.

Mayer, M. (1969). *Frog, where are you?* New York: Dial.

Meadowcroft, J. M., & Reeves, B. (1989). Influence of story schema development on children's attention to television. *Communication Research, 16,* 352-374.

Milch-Reich, S., Campbell, S. B., Pelham, W. E., Connelly, L. M., & Geva, D. (1999). Developmental and individual differences in children's online representations of dynamic social events. *Child Development, 70*, 2, 413-431.

Murphy, D.A., Pelham, W.E., & Lang, A.R. (1992). Aggression in boys with attention deficit-hyperactivity disorder: Methylphenidate effects on naturally observed aggression, response to provocation, and social information processing. *Journal of Abnormal Child Psychology, 20*, 451-466.

Pennington, B. F., Groisser, D., & Welsh, M. C. (1993). Contrasting cognitive deficits in attention deficit hyperactivity disorder versus reading disability. *Developmental Psychology, 29*, 511-523.

Pezdek, K., & Hartman, E. F. (1983). Children's television viewing: Attention and comprehension of auditory versus visual information. *Child Development, 54*, 1015-1023.

Purvis, K. L., & Tannock, R. (1997). Language abilities in children with attention deficit hyperactivity disorder, reading disabilities, and normal controls. *Journal of Abnormal Child Psychology, 25,* 133-144.

Renz, K., Lorch, E. P., Milich, R., Lemberger, C., Bodner, A., & Welsh, R. (2003). On-line story representation in boys with attention deficit hyperactivity disorder. *Journal of Abnormal Child Psychology, 31,* 93-104.

Sanchez, R. P., Lorch, E. P., & Milich, R. (1999). Comprehension of televised stories by preschool children with ADHD. *Journal of Clinical Child Psychology, 28*, 376-385.

Schachar, R. & Logan, G. D. (1990). Impulsivity and inhibitory control in normal development and childhood psychopathology. *Developmental Psychology, 26,* 710-720.

Sergeant, J. & van der Meere, J. J. (1990). Convergence of approaches in localizing the hyperactivity deficit. In B. B. Lahey & A. E. Kazdin (Eds.), *Advances in clinical child psychology* (Vol. 13, pp. 207-245). New York: Plenum.

Stein, N. L. & Glenn, C. G. (1979). An analysis of story comprehension in elementary school children. In R. Freedble (Ed.), *Multidisciplinary Approaches to Discourse Comprehension*. Hillsdale, N.J.: Lawrence Erlbaun Associates.

Tannock, R., Purvis, K. L., & Schachar, R. J. (1993). Narrative abilities in children with attention deficit hyperactivity disorder and normal peers. *Journal of Abnormal Child Psychology, 21,* 103-117.

Trabasso, T. & Nickels, M. (1992). The development of goal plans of action in the narration of a picture story. *Discourse Processes, 15*, 249-275.

Trabasso, T., Secco, T., & van den Broek, P. W. (1984). Causal cohesion and story coherence. In H. Mandler, N. L. Stein, & T. Trabasso (Eds.), *Learning and comprehension of text* (pp. 83-111). Hillsdale, NJ: Erlbaum.

Trabasso, T., Stein, N. L., Rodkin, P. C., Munger, G. P., & Baughn, C. (1992). Knowledge of goals and plans in the on-line narration of events. *Cognitive Development, 7*, 133-170.

Trabasso, T. & van den Broek, P. W. (1985). Causal thinking and the representation of narrative events. *Journal of Memory and Language, 24,* 612-630.

Trabasso, T., van den Broek, P., & Suh, S.Y. (1989). Logical necessity and transivity of causal relations in stories. *Discourse Processes, 21,* 1-25.

van den Broek, P. (1989). Causal reasoning and inference-making in judging the importance of story statements. *Child Development, 60*, 286-297.

van den Broek, P. (1990). Causal inferences in the comprehension of narrative texts. In A.C. Graesser & G. H. Bowler (Eds.), *The psychology of learning and motivation: Inferences and text comprehension* (Vol. 25, pp. 175-194). San Diego, CA: Academic Press.

van den Broek, P. (1997). Discovering the cement of the universe: The development of event comprehension from childhood to adulthood. In P. W. van den Broek, P. J. Baur, & T. Bourg (Eds.), *Developmental spans in event comprehension and representation: Bridging fictional and actual events* (pp. 321-342). Mahway, NJ: Erlbaum.

van den Broek, P. W., Bauer, P. J., & Bourg, T. (Eds.). (1997). *Developmental spans in event comprehension and representation: Bridging fictional and actual events*. Mahwah, NJ: Erlbaum.

van den Broek, P., Lorch, E. P., & Thurlow, R. (1996). Children's and adults' memory for television stories: The role of causal factors, story-grammar categories and hierarchical level. *Child Development, 67,* 3010-3028.

Wagoner, G.A. (1983). Comprehension –monitoring: What it is and what we know about it. *Reading Research Quarterly, 43,* 328-346.

Whirley, K. S., Lorch, E. P., Lemberger, C. C., & Milich, R. (2003). Online cognitive engagement of boys with ADHD. *Journal of Attention Disorders 7*, 71-81.

Zentall, S.S. (1988). Production deficiencies in elicited language but not in the spontaneous verbalization of hyperactive children. *Journal of Abnormal Child Psychology, 16*, 657-673.

In: Attention Deficit Hyperactivity Disorder Research
Editor: Michelle P. Larimer, pp. 139-154
ISBN 1-59454-156-6

Chapter VI

Electrophysiologic Measures in Attention Deficit/Hyperactivity Disorder

Paulino Uclés[1].
Miguel Servet Hospital.
Zaragoza, Spain.

Abstract

Twenty seven children and adolescents, ages 4 to 18 years, fullfiling the DSM-IV diagnostic criteria for attention deficit hyperactivity disorder were included in this study. The diagnosis was determined by a paediatric neurologist, and a psychologist examined all 27 subjects with tests that included WISC-R, reading, writing, handedness, personality, and anxiety scores. Subjects with histories of epilepsy, head injury, drug abuse or psychotic disorders were excluded. Culturally based causes or emotional disorders were also excluded.

Transcranial magnetic stimulation was performed on all subjects, with recording of the motor evoked potential at the biceps brachii. Central motor conduction time was calculated by the method of cervical root stimulation. Due to the shape variability, the amplitude of the motor responses was not measured in the study. The mean value of central conduction time in the subjects group was very significantly increased ($p<0.001$) as compared to a group of normal controls, case-matched for IQ, age and sex. A central motor conduction time greater than 12 ms indicates abnormality. A second finding in the subjects was the significant difference of central conduction time on the side-to-side stimulation ($p=0.03$). These findings are correlated with delay in the maturation of the corticomotoneuronal system, and may provide neurophysiologic data for diagnosis.

[1] Correspomdence: Paulino Uclés M.D.Almagro, 11 7-B E-50004 Zaragoza. Spain Tel. +34 976 76 55 59. E-mail:doctorucles@inicia.es

Key words: Attention deficit hyperactivity disorder. Magnetic brain stimulation. Central motor conduction time.

A Search for Biological Markers

Attention deficit/hyperactivity disorder (ADHD) is the most common developmental disorder, affecting at least 5% of school-age children [1] and persisting into adulthood in 10% to 60% of the cases.[2, 3] The attention problems of ADHD children are described as distractibility and inability to sustain attention. An excessive level of activity is typically observed, taking place as restlessness, fidgeting and unnecesary body movements. A third group of symptoms, labeled as impulsiveness, such as precipitating answers and inability to await a turn, are increasingly seen as the greatest significance of the disorder. Individuals with ADHD present in childhood may continue to show symptoms as they enter adolescence and adult life.

Recorded prevalence rates for ADHD vary substantially, partly because of changing diagnostic criteria over time, and partly because of variations in ascertainment in different settings and the frequent use of referred samples to estimate rates. Practitioners of all types vary greatly in the degree to which they use Diagnostic and Statistical Manual of Mental Health Disorders, Fourth Edition (DSM-IV) criteria to diagnose ADHD.

Prevalence rates in school-aged community samples indicates rates vaying from 4% to 12%. In the general population, 9.2% (5.8%-13.6%) of males and 2.9 (1.9%-4.5%) of females are found to have behaviors consistent with ADHD.

The Causative Issue

ADHD is believed to be caused by genetic factors or environmentally acquired brain dysfunction contracted early in development [1], and a series of recent genetic studies have reported evidence of association of ADHD subjects with a dopamine transporter gene polymorphism.[6-9] Nevertheless, the acquired factors are frequently found in clinical practice, thereby opening a critical path for investigation. Public interest in ADHD has increased along with debate in the media concerning the diagnostic process and treatment strategies. Concern has been expresed about the over-diagnosis of ADHD by pointing to the several-fold increase in prescriptions for stimulant medication among children in the past decade. Practice surveys among primary care pediatricians and family physicians reveal wide variations in practice patterns about diagnostic criteria and methods.[5] But the most important thing is the different method used by pediatric neurologist, psichologist and other specialists in contrast to those used by primary care clinicians.

Nonetheless, whereas the possible root cause or causes of the disorder remain obscure, several imaging studies early this decade, using positron emission tomography (PET scan), reported focal cerebral dysfunction, mainly in the frontal lobes and the striatum;[8-10] and more recently, structural and functional magnetic resonance imaging (fMRI) investigations seem to confirm these focal dysfunctions.[11, 12] These approaches, viewed by many researchers as the neuroanatomical basis of the disorder, gave rise to severe criticism in recent months, arguing that the small differences in glucose metabolism or in frontal-striatal activation found between control groups and ADHD subjects are interpreted not as a mere correlation with hyperactivity and inattention, but rather as evidence that these symptoms may be caused by a brain abnormality, thereby confounding correlation and causation. A second important issue has been raised, as to whether these findings should or should not be proposed as biological markers for the clinical practice.[12, 13]

For some primary care pediatricians, brain imaging studies do not show raliable differences between children with ADHD and controls [5]. They argue that although some studies have demonstrated variation in brain morphology comparing children with and without ADHD, these findings do not discriminate reliable between children with and without this condition. In other words, although group means may differ significantly, the overlap in findings among children with and without ADHD creates high rates of false-positives and false-negatives. Similarly, the higher rates of certain electroencephalogram abnormalities among children with ADHD are not fully accepted for primary care clinicians because the overlap between children with and without ADHD and the lack of consistent findings among multiple reports.

Continuous performance tests have been designed to obtain samples of a child's behavior (generally measuring vigilance or or distractibility), which may correlate with behaviors associated with ADHD. Again, such tests are not accepted for diagnosis because all of these have a sensitivity and specificity <70%. Nevertheless, these criteria are based in a survey on articles published between 1980 and 1997. Later on, several papers have provided more evidence of electrophysiological finding in ADHD. This is specially true for quantitative EEG (qEEG), which has gained in recent years the strength of evidence as strong for developmental disorders. The same apply for event-related potentials, specially for cognitive P300, which is now a days reocognised as a precise biological measurement of the working memory, a keystone in the investigation of ADHD. The causative influence exerted now by cultural environmental factors upon a great deal of hyperactive/inattentive children is stressed by a number of psychologists, whereas the longstanding claim for the biological causes of the disorder still endures.

Cerebral Function

Abnormal cerebral function was a concept incorporated early in the 1960s into the cluster of symptoms of the then designed minimal brain dysfunction,[14] after the findings of abnormal electroencephalograms (EEG). Further correlational studies, with large cohorts of children, that utilized the Neurometric quantitative Electroencephalography (qEEG) technique, were performed.[15, 16] These findings have provided evidence that ADHD and specific learning disabilities show different subtypes of neurophysiological abnormality, that allow both groups to be distinguished from the normal population with a specificity of 88% and a sensitivity of 93.7% .[17] They studied behavioral and neurophyilogyc profiles of children with attention and learning disorders using qEEG developed by John and associates.[15] Medication-free, eyes-closed resting quantitative EEGs in large samples of normal children and children with attention deficit and specific learning disorders were examined. The majority of children with ADD showed evidence of neurophysiologic dysfunction, specially involving anterior cortical regions, with the patterns of qEEG abnormality suggesting a deviation from normal neurophysiologic development rather than a maturational lag. It is remarkable that the cortical and subcortical structures and pathways implicated by the quantitative EEG findings as showing neurophysiologic dysfunction are the same as those found to show structural abnormalities by positron emision tomography, magnetic resonance imaging, and regional cerebral blood flow studies.[8-12]

The types of quantitative EEG abnormality shown by children with ADD and by children with specific learning disorders also differed, with quantitative EEG showing a sensitivity of 97% and a specificity of 84.2% for distinguishing children with ADD from those with specific learning disorders.

Quantitative EEG also has been shown to be useful in the initial determination of whether or not pharmacologic intervention would be useful, and if so, in determining which medication is more appropriate. Quantitative EEG collected prior to treatment with methylphenidate showed a specificity of 81% and a sensitivity of 83% for distinguishing treatment responders from nonresponders. [16] It was found that 27.3% of the children in their sample previously had exhibited an adverse reaction to either dexanphetamine or metilphenidate, with 83.9% of these children correctly classified by a quantitative EEG discriminant function.

Given the serious implications of childhood disorders involving attention deficit, the endeavor for finding biological measures that externally validate the scores of current tests of hyperactivity and inattention [18-20] seems plausible, since it has been shown that these psychological measures alone are not fully reliable.[21, 22]

Another neurophysiological method proposed for testing the brain function of ADHD subjects is the transcranial magnetic stimulation (TMS). Magnetic stimulation is an ideal method for the maturational study of the motor pathways of man, since evidence indicates that it specifically excites the corticomotoneuronal system, which is presumably involved in the disorder. This technique has rarely been used for the investigation of developmental disorders.[23-25] We reported preliminary findings using TMS on ADHD children, and now a larger sample has been evaluated in order to confirm those findings.[26]

Neurophysiological Methods

Magnetic Stimulation and Quantitative EEG

Twenty seven children and adolescents, ages 4 to 18 years, seen between 3/97 and 5/99 were entered into this study. Twenty three were boys and four were girls, all having normal full scale IQ scores and being right handed, except for three boys. The diagnosis was determined by a pediatric neurologist. All 27 subjects fulfilled the DSM-IV diagnostic criteria for the inattention/hyperactive type of the disorder.[27] Information regarding perinatal illnesses or comorbid disorders was taken from the child´s medical records, and Fourier frequency analysis (qEEG) were compliant with the pattern reported for ADHD in all cases. Subjects with histories of epilepsy, head injury, drug abuse or psychotic disorders were excluded, as well as those with parental mood disorders which were responsible for the hyperactivity and inattention of the offsprings. None were receiving medication at the time of testing.

A psychologist examined all 27 subjects, with tests that included WISC-R,[28] reading-writing,[29] handedness,[30] personality,[31] and anxiety scores.[32] Table 1 summarizes the most relevant psychological tests.

Table 1. Relevant psychological scores and suspected causes of the disorder

n	Age (yrs)	WISC-R full-IQ	WISC-R digits subtet	Reading skill	Writing errors%	Familial integration	Anxiety level	Posible causes
1	4	106	-	-	-	good	middle	parental ADHD
2	5	86	low	low	45	good	low	tobacco/anoxia at birth
3	5	105	low	low	20	good	low	tobacco/anoxia at birth
4	6	98	low	low	30	good	low	adopted
5	6	100	low	middle	10	troubled	low	parental ADHD
6	6	105	low	good	5	good	low	tobacco/stress
7	6	100	middle	good	6	good	low	anoxia at birth
8	6	110	low	good	10	good	middle	parental ADHD/ß-adrenergics
9	6	127	middle	middle	20	good	low	parental ADHD
10	7	120	low	middle	30	good	low	parental ADHD
11	7	85	low	low	35	good	middle	parental ADHD
12	9	80	low	good	10	good	low	parental ADHD
13	9	100	low	low	50	good	low	parental ADHD
14	9	94	low	middle	8	good	low	adopted
15	10	10	low	middle	30	troubled	middle	parental ADHD/anoxia
16	10	90	low	low	20	good	low	anoxia at birth
17	10	110	low	good	10	good	low	bromocriptine
18	10	99	low	low	45	good	middle	adopted
19	10	95	low	low	40	good	middle	anoxia at birth
20	12	110	low	good	5	good	low	adopted
21	12	95	low	middle	6	good	low	hypermaturity
22	12	101	low	middle	30	good	low	tobacco
23	13	101	low	middle	12	good	low	anoxia at birth
24	13	121	middle	middle	20	good	high	parental ADHD
25	15	107	low	middle	20	troubled	low	parental ADHD
26	16	105	low	middle	10	troubled	low	adopted

The Weschler scale showed an overall IQ within the normal limits in all cases, though the digits subtest that measures attention and recent memory was remarkably abnormal in all subjects. Comorbidity is known to be frequent in ADHD, with special incidence in the reading and writting areas. Nine subjects had serious disabilities in reading and another nine had spelling mistakes that exceedes 20 % of the words; of these, six were coincident with dislexia. The heading Familial Integration in Table 1 is a condensation of a series of marital and societal circumstances, such as caregiving, emotional support and lifestyle, that may provide clues for causation. To this respect, traditional home characteristics were observed in all families, with the exception of difficulties derived from misconduct over several older children and adolescents. Similarly, the scores of the test on anxiety were not significant, except for one adolescent.

TMS was performed in morning sessions. The children were seated comfortably on a chair and disk surface electrodes were attached bilaterally to biceps brachii in a belly-to-tendon derivation. They were requested to tighten their fist in order to facilitate the response of the target muscle,[33] and one of us assured that facilitation reached a similar level for all the children. This activating manoeuvre has the effect of lowering the threshold of the anterior horn cells involved in the contraction of the target muscle and its agonists, so with just one single stimulus a muscle response can be elicited. Because of the nervousness of the children, the biceps brachii was found to be more convenient for the recording of the responses than hand muscles. Tightening the fist also exerted a slight contraction of the biceps muscle that avoided much background EMG, in addition to maintaining the child's concentration during a few seconds, which resulted in a maximal attainment of the responses.

A magnetoelectric stimulator delivered stimuli of a maximum magnetic field of 1.9 T, pulsed with a rise time of 100 μs and a total duration of 300 μs, with a monopolar pulse shape of the induced electrical field. The stimulator coil (diameter, 9.5 cm) was alternatively positioned 3 cm lateral to the vertex in the side-to-side stimulation.

Responses elicited at 80-90 % of the maximal intensity were usually weak, perhaps because cortical threshold remains high until well into the second decade,[33] so definite muscle responses were always attained at the full 1.9-T intensity, equivalent to 100% output. Stimuli were delivered every 5 to 10 seconds, and the MEPs were acquired and amplified by a Medelec MS-92 electromyograph with a band width of 20 Hz to 2 kHz (-3 dB) and an analysis time of 100 ms.

Twenty seven normal controls were recruited from local schools and these subjects had no known developmental, visual, hearing or neurologic disorder. The children were case-matched for IQ, sex, age, handedness, and socioeconomic status. They were tested with TMS, for comparison with the ADHD subjects. The latency of the evoked responses was measured in all subjects. The amplitude of the responses were not measured in this study because the MEP morphology usually changes with each stimulus, as a single spinal motoneuron is supplied by several corticomotoneurons that are spatially separated by several millimeters.[33]

Four MEPs on each muscle were recorded on photographic paper and stored for further analysis. The latency variability of the four consecutive MEPs of one muscle averaged less than 1 ms in both subjects and controls. The shortest of the four MEP latencies was measured at the onset.

Central motor conduction time (CMCT) was calculated by the method of magnetic stimulation of the spinal root. Three supramaximal stimuli were delivered on the Cv6 root site for eliciting well defined, replicable MEPs. The latency of these MEPs represent the peripheral segment of the total conduction time, and therefore was subtracted from the latency of the TMS potentials, in order to obtain the CMCT.

Statistics

For the study of the variables, an initial analysis of the normal distribution was performed using the Shapiro-Wilks and the Kolmogorov-Smirnov tests with an alpha=0.1; there was no normal distribution for the latency of the MEP to brachial biceps or the CMCT, either in the control or subject group. These tests were also used to relate CMCT values to height and then to age; there was no dependence of these variables on each other in any group. In this respect, a multiple linear regression test combining CMCT, height and age values resulted in a no linear relation (r=0).

Given these results, non-parametric tests were used for comparison of data between the two groups and between each brain hemisphere of a separate group. These included the U-test of Mann-Whitney for independent samples and the paired-data test of Wilcoxon for signs and for ranges, with an alpha=0.05.

Table 2. Central Conduction Time (ms)
ADHD Subjects

n°	AGE (yrs)	Left Stim.	Right Stim.
1	4	14.4	14.5
2	5	13	12.6
3	5	14.7	14.4
4	6	14.2	11.1
5	6	15	15
6	6	12.8	12.6
7	6	15.8	16.2
8	6	14.6	12.9
9	6	12.8	12.8
10	7	13.4	13.4
11	7	12.8	13.1
12	9	13.6	14.0
13	9	14.2	14.6
14	9	16.6	16.9
15	10	13.4	13.2
16	10	14.4	17.4
17	10	13.4	13.2
18	10	14	12.5
19	10	16.3	15.6
20	12	17.6	18.6
21	12	12.3	12.2
22	12	18.1	16.6
23	13	11.5	12.0
24	13	12.7	12.5
25	15	13.1	12.9
26	16	10.9	10.7
27	18	9.4	9.8
	9±3.2	13.6±1.8	13.7±2

Mean values and their standard deviations for the total latency to brachial biceps. the peripheral latency to root stimulation. and the CMCT of both sides were obtained.

Results

The ADHD subjects had. on left hemisphere stimulation. a mean total latency of 18.4±1.9 ms. and on right hemisphere stimulation of 18.2±1.9 ms. The peripheral latency had a mean value of 4.5 ±0.5 ms on both sides. The CMCT mean value was 13.6±1.8 ms on left stimulation (13 to 14.7 ms. 95 % confidence limits). and 13.7±2 ms on right stimulation (95 % confidence limits from 12.8 to 14.6 ms). See Table 2.

Table 3. Central Conduction Time (ms)
Controls

nº	Age yrs.	Left Stim.	Right Stim.
1	5	7.1	7.2
2	6	11.6	11.2
3	6	11.0	10.6
4	6	11.2	11.4
5	6	7.0	7.1
6	6	11.2	11.2
7	6	8.8	8.9
8	7	9.6	9.0
9	7	10.0	10.1
10	7	6.4	7.0
11	7	11.9	11.8
12	7	9.2	9.4
13	9	9.2	10.1
14	9	11.1	10.7
15	9	10.0	10.0
16	9	10.0	10.8
17	10	6.1	6.7
18	10	7.8	9.0
19	10	10.8	11.0
20	10	11.2	11.2
21	10	10.2	10.4
22	12	7.9	8.0
23	12	7.7	7.8
24	13	12.4	12.4
25	13	10.6	10.7
26	15	9.7	10
27	18	8.7	8.8
	9±3.1	9.5±1.7	9.7±1.5

The control group had a mean total latency on left stimulation of 13.8±1.7 ms, and on right stimulation had 13.9±1.7 ms. The peripheral latency averaged 4.2±0.5 ms on both sides. The CMCT mean value on left stimulation was 9.5±1.7 ms (8.8 to 10.3 ms, 95 % confidence limits), and on right stimulation was 9.7±1.5 ms (9 to 10.3 ms, 95% confidence limits). See Table 3.

The comparison of the CMCT values between groups, using the U-test of Mann Whitney and the Wilcoxon test resulted in a highly significant difference ($p<0.001$).

For the hemispheric symmetry analysis, the comparison of CMCT values on the side-to-side stimulation resulted in a significant difference for the ADHD group ($p=0.03$), while there was no significant difference for the controls ($p=0.68$). See Fig. 1.

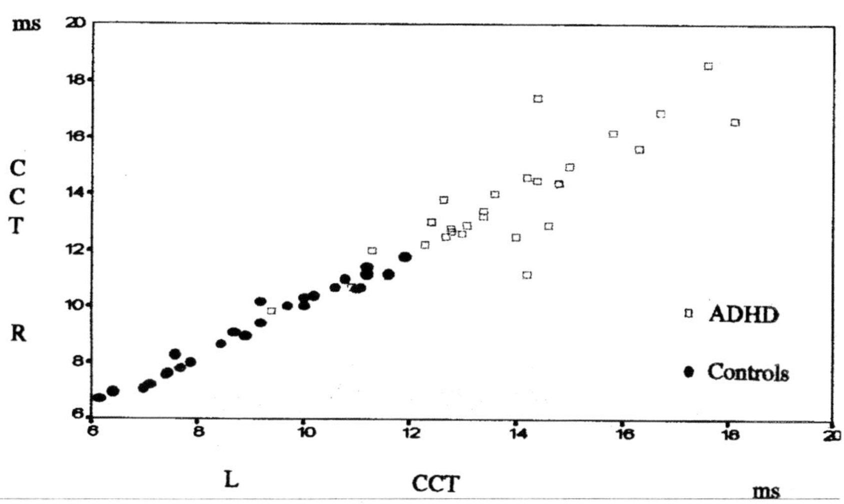

Fig. 1 Values of Central Conduction Time, corresponding to the side-to-side magnetic stimulation in each subject. Both groups are represented together. The controls show values under 12 ms, with a mean value statistically very significant from the mean for the ADHD subjects ($p<0.001$). Also, note the significant disper sion of the ADHD values ($p<0.05$), suggestive of hemispheric asimetry in the maturational process.

Evidence of a Biological Condition

In the early 1990s it was admitted that of the many techniques for measuring parameters of cerebral neurophysiology, no one had identified any neurological dysfunction specific to children diagnosed as hyperactive [34]. Subsequent developments in neuroimaging techniques, that have generated biological studies on the neural basis of the disorder, concluded that there was a dysfunction of the fronto-striatal structures. This statement is consistent with the theory proposed by Benson in 1991, that postulates a widespread delay in brain maturation, mostly in the frontal lobes, as the most likely source of the syndrome [35]. However, the results have lacked replication and reproduction in larger samples.

The increasing number of children diagnosed as ADHD over recent years has required that any study of this disorder today must address the underlaying major problem of causation. Early studies of children with hyperactivity often found an associated biological origin for hyperactivity, namely congenital defects of the brain, birth trauma, meningitis, postnatal head injury, epilepsy, or encephalopathy. Even findings of borderline abnormal or abnormal electroencephalograms (EEG) were incorporated into the syndrome.[14] The problem became more complicated when no minimal brain dysfunction could be localised, and then the causes were often believed to be environmental disturbances. Such disturbances have been more emphasized than the early biological ones, at least in North America, to the point that it has given rise to a grand theory that the disorder simply is a transformation of the human conciousness by the effects of a rapid-fire culture [13] . At the time when the controversy is at its peak, the idea that equates this disorder to the epileptic syndrome -with each form of seizure having its unique electrophysiologic, behavioral, neuroanatomic, and therapeutic implications- seems to reconcile both theories. However, as with epilepsy, the real cause is really unrevealed [36]. Culturally based causes are not so frequent in Europe; therefore, our study deals only with biologically suspected cases. The sample includes children whose parents relate that they themselves were hyperactive/inattentive children, with no other determining developmental events discovered in the offsprings. These data were derived from questions like marital status at the time of the child´s birth or the caregiving style; therefore we consider that the majority of questioned were genetically determined (Table 1).

However, those that postulate the rapid-fire culture theory admit the existence of a genetic background; the cultural influences would act only as contingent upon developmental changes.

There is a lack of information on the genetic background of the adopted children in this study, nevertheless they may be considered suspected of having genetically transmitted ADHD in the light of several studies [37, 38] For the rest of the cases, the attributed causes can be regarded as factors determining the disorder, either during pregnancy or at birth, as these act upon a genetic background. This genetic view is reinforced by the fact that most of the children were described by their parents as having been hyperactive since infants, though their temperament became clinically apparent about the age of 6 years.

ADHD is primarily a biological problem with an expresion amenable to neurophysiology, and therefore the application of a neurophysiological method like TMS seems a justified approach for identifying this type of behaviour in school-age children. According to Fuster, " we may rightfully consider the entire dorsolateral frontal cortex from the Rolandic fissure to the pole of the frontal lobe ' motor cortex '[39] These words are in agreement with his concept of ADHD as a type of frontal lobe-motor cortex disconnection. Related to it, repetitive TMS has been used to study the changes in cortical motor outputs associated with learning, and it is suggested that the dorsolateral prefrontal cortex plays a critical role in the induction of the appropriate plastic changes in motor cortical output [40] . The single stimulus TMS we have used for the measurement of CMCT shows very significant difference of the values obtained in ADHD subjects with respect to the controls ($p<0.001$), with CMCT above 12 ms indicating abnormality. This data reflect, in our view, a delay in the maturation of the corticomotoneuronal system. For a maturational problem like this, another approach would be the threshold studies but, since cortical threshold remains high until well into the second decade and adult values for central motor conduction are attained by about 8 years of age, the later parameter seems to be the method of choice. Also, the CMCT is the most reliable of the MEP characteristics that can be measured. The disparity between the attainment of adult values of central motor conducction velocity versus cortical threshold depends upon earlier central myelination versus later synaptogenesis. Hence, the delayed CMCT found in ADHD subjects might be regarded as a dysfunction of the cortical motor and premotor cells. Though evidence is not provided yet in humans, the age decline in cortical threshold correlates in non-human primates with increasing precision of hand and finger movements, i. e., the attainment of fractionated movement which requires completion of synaptogenesis [41].

Delay in laying down myelin is another posible explanation for the increased CMCT of the ADHD subjects, but this explanation is not likely to account for the steady increases found in older children and adolescents. Still, an approach to investigate the participation of the motor pathways in the delayed motor responses would be to use electric stimulation. This type of stimulus certainly acts upon the axon hillock downward; however this technique is undesirable in children because it is painful.

The side-to-side difference of CMCT in the ADHD group ($p=0.03$) is the second remarkable finding of the study (Fig. 1), which suggests hemispheric asymetry in the maturational process. Whether specific learning disabilities share the same TMS pattern with ADHD children or not is a matter that cannot now be stated, though further studies shall be done to disclose it.

Cognitive P300

In basic conditions, ADHD children have been shown to have both P300 amplitude and latency differences respect to controls, attributed to an impaired information processing in the subjects.[43] Yet, there are few studies upon the effect of methylphenidate on event-related potential P300.[44-45]

We conducted four years ago an investigation in our laboratory of clinical neurophysiology intended to corroborate the acute changes previously observed in P300 after methylphenidate intake.[45] A group of 22 children (males and females) with an age-range of 6-14 years, who fulfilled the DSM-IV critera for ADHD were included in the study. Both visual and auditory P300 were performed in all subjects before and 2 hours after a single dosis of 10 mg methylphenidate, together with a stroop test.

As we analysed the results of parameters that included amplitude, latency and scalp distribution of P300 it was shown, as principal finding, that 68% of the subjects had $\geq$ 30% enhancement of P300 amplitude respect to that obtained before methylphenidate administration ($p<0.05$),and that it was especially significant for auditory P300. (Fig. 2) It was also important that 100% of children performed fairly well the stroop test after methylphenidate. These findings suggest that cognitive P300 can be a good predictor for the clasification of methylphenidate responders and non-responders.

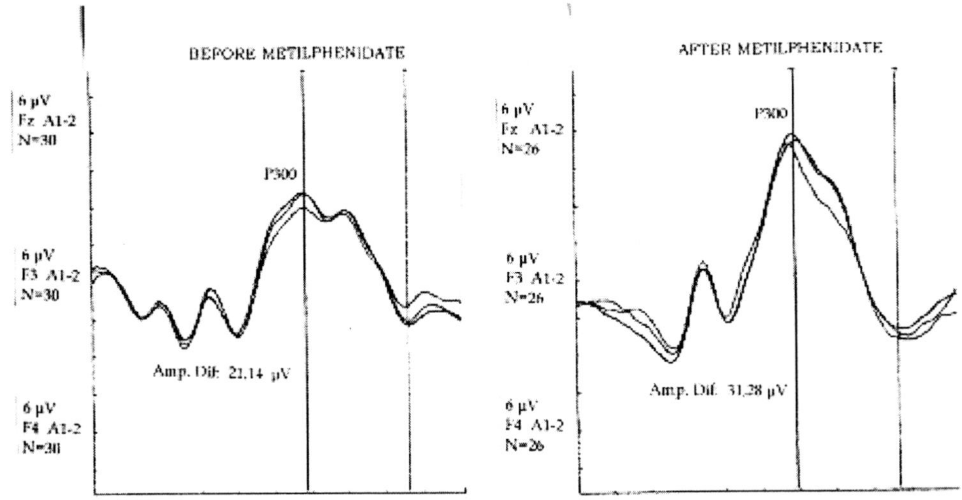

Fig. 2 This figure is an example of a case in our series. A 7 years old boy had an auditory P300 before and 2 hr after methylphenidate administration (MPH). Cursors highlight the increase in P300 amplitude.

Coexisting Conditions

The primary care clinician may not always be in a position to make a precise diagnosis of coexisting conditions. Nonetheless, extrinsic conditions such as problems with parent-child interaction or family violence should be detected. Oppositional defiant or conduct disorders coexist with ADHD in aproximatelly 35% of children. The diagnostic features of conduct disorder include "a repetitive and persistent pattern of behavior in which the basic rights of others or major age-appropiate social norms or rules are violated". Opositional defiant disorder, which is a less severe condition, includes persistent symptoms of negativistic, defiant, disobedient, and hostile behaviors toward authority figures". Frequently oppostional defiant disorder became a conduct disorder. Longitudinal follow-up for children with conduct disorders that coexist with ADHD indicates that these children fare more poorly in adulthood relative to their peers diagnosed with ADHD alone. One study has reported the highest rates of police contacts in children with ADHD and coexisting conduct disorder (30.8%) relative to their peers diagnosed with ADHD alone (3.4%) or conduct disorder alone (20.7 %). Preliminary studies suggest that this coexisting conditions are more frequent in children with the predominantly hyperactive-impulsive and combined subtypes.[42]

The coexistence of ADHD and mood disorders (major depressive disorders and dystimia) is aproximately 18%. Sometime, the family history of children with ADHD includes other family members with a history of major depresive disorder. In adolescence, they are at increased risk for suicide attempts. Several studies suggest that these coexisting conditions are more frequent in children with the predominantly innatentive and combined subtypes.

The coexisting association between ADHD and anxiety disorders has been estimated to be approximately 25%.[1] Here again, preliminary studies suggest that these coexisting conditions are more frequent in children with the predominantly inattentive and combined subtypes. Questionaries on anxiety performed by psychologists are in many cases mandatory.

The prevalence of learning disabilities as coexisting condition has been estimated in our series about 50%. [26] To date, no definitive data describe the differences among groups of children with different learning disabilities coexisting with ADHD in the areas of sociodemographyc characteristics, behavioral and emotional functioning, and response to various intervention. Nonetheless, for diagnostic purposes qEEG is very helpful to discriminate between ADHD alone and a coexixting learning disability.[15, 17]

The Need for an Interdisciplinary Team

The diagnostic process of ADHD requires collaborative task interventions of psychologists, pediatric neurologists, clinical neurophysiologists and teachers. Most times, parents firstly consult a psychologist; nevertheles, in light of the high prevalence of ADHD in pediatric practice, primary care clinicians frequently face diagnosis of this condition. DSM-IV has helped to define behavioral criteria for ADHD more specifically, but this questionary as a unique tool in the hands of the primary care clinicians is, in our view, clearly insufficient. Intelligence, personality, anxiety tests must be performed, as well as reading and writing measurements, and the cerebral function recordings. Follow up and treatment of an ADHD child also requires collaboration of educational psychologists, neurophysiologists and pediatric neurologists since specialiced cognitive-behavioral therapies have to be conducted, as well as modifications in the stimulant dosages according to changes in EEG patterns and P300 amplitude.

Conclusion

For clinical purposes, the increased CMCT together with side differences reproduce real, measured neurophysiologic data that provide a clue for the diagnosis. Magnetic stimulation is easier and even quicker to perform than other neurophysiological procedures, like qEEG or event related potentials (P300), an important factor to keep in mind for this type of restless subjects. Nonetheless, all these procedures are easily available complementary tests to the clinical history, DSM-IV, and the psychological testing.

References

[1] Barkley RA: Attention Deficit Hyperactivity Disorder: A Handbook for Diagnosis and Treatement. New York, *Guilford Press*, 1990.

[2] Weiss G, Hechtman L, Milroy T et al: Psychiatric status of hyperactives as adults: a controlled prospective 15-year follow-up of 63 hyperactive children. *J Am Acad Child Psychiatry* 1985;24:211-220.

[3] Manuzza S, Klein RG, Bessler A et al: Adult autcome of hyperactive boys:educational, achievement, occupational rank and psychiatric status. *Arch Gen Psychiatry* 1993;50:565-576.

[4] Diagnostic and Statistical Manual of Mental Disorders, 4th ed. Washington DC. *Am Psychiatr Assoc*, 1994.

[5] Clinical practice guideline: Diagnosis and evaluation of the child with attention deficit/hyperactivity disorder. *Pediatrics* 2000; 105 (5):1158-1170

[6] Cook EH, Stein MA, Krasowski MD et al: Association of attention deficit disorder and the dopamine transporter gene. *Am J Hum Genetics* 1995;56:993-998.

[7] La Hoste JL, Swanson JM, Wigal SB et al: Dopamine D4 receptor gene polymorphism is associated with attention deficit hyperactivity disorder. *Mol Psychiatry* 1996;1:121-124.

[8] Gill M, Daly G, Heron S et al: Confirmation of association between attention deficit hyperactivity disorder and dopamine transporter polymorphism. *Mol Psychiatry* 1997;2:311-313.

[9] Swanson JM, Sunohara GA, Kennedy JL et al: Association of the dopamine receptor D4 (DRD4) gene with a refined phenotype of attention deficit hyperactivity disorder (ADHD): a family-based approach. *Mol Psychiatry* 1998;3:38-41.

[10] Low HC, Henriksen L and Bruhn P: Focal cerebral dysfunction in developmental learning disabilities. *Lancet* 1990;335(8680):8-11.

[11] Zametkin AJ, Nordhal TE, Gross M et al: Cerebral glucose metabolism in adults with hyperactivity of childhood onset. *N Engl J Med* 1990;323 (20):1361-1366.

[12] Zametkin A, Liebenauer L, Fitzgerald G et al: Brain metabolism in teenagers with attention deficit hyperactivity disorder. *Arch Gen Psychiatry* 1993;50:333-340.

[13] Castellanos FX, Giedd JN, Marsh WL et al: Quantitative brain magnetic resonance imaging in attention deficit hyperactivity disorder. *Arch Gen Psychiatry* 1996; 53(7):509-601.

[14] Vaidya CJ, Austin G, Kirkorian G et al: Selective effects of methylphenidate in attention deficit hyperactivity disorder: A functional magnetic resonance study. *Proc Nat Acad Sci* USA 1998;95:14494-14499.

[15] DeGrandpre R and Hallowell E: Ritalin nation: rapid fire culture and the transformation of human consciousness. New York, *W.W. Norton*, 1999.

[16] Clements SD and Peters JE: Minimal brain dysfunction in the school-aged child. *Arch Gen Psychiatry* 1962;6:185-87.

[17] John ER, Karmel BZ, Corning WC et al: Neurometrics: numerical taxonomy identifies different profiles of brain functions within groups of behaviourally similar people. *Science* 1977;196:1383-1410.

[18] John ER, Prichep LS, Ahn H et al: Neurometric evaluation of cognitive dysfunctions and neurological disorders in children. *Progress Neurobiol* 1983;21:239-290

[19] Chabot RG, Merkin H, Wodd LM et al: Sensitivity and specificity of qEEG in children with attention deficit or specific developmental learning disorders. *Clin Electroenceph* 1996;27(1):26-34.

[20] Goyette CH, Conners CK, and Ulrich RF: Normative data on Revised Conners Parents and Teacher Rating Scales. *J Abn Child Psychology* 1978;6:221-236.

[21] Greenberg LM: T.O.V.A.(TM)Interpretation Manual.Minneapolis MN:*Author*, 1991.

[22] Dunn LM and Dunn LM: Peabody Picture Vocabulary Test-Revised. American Guidance Service. *Circle Pines* MN, 1981.

[23] Proceedings of the International ADHD Symposium on biological causes and trea tement. *Royal College Physicians*. London UK. Taylor E. (chairman). Nov. 1998.

[24] Gillberg C: Attention deficit hyperactivity disorder. *Editorial. Acta Paediatr* 1997;86:791-92.

[25] Koh THHG and Eire JA: Maturation of corticospinal tracts assessed by electromagnetic stimulation of the motor cortex. *Arch Dis Child* 1988;63:1347-1352.

[26] Müller K, Hömberg V and Lenard HG: Magnetic stimulation of motor cortex and nerve roots in children. Maturation of corticomotoneuronal projections. *Electro enceph Clin Neurophysiol* 1991;81:63-70.

[27] Nezu A, Kimura S, Uchara S et al: Magnetic stimulation of motor cortex in chil dren: maturity of corticospinal pathway and problem of clinical application. *Brain Dev* 1997;19:176-180.

[28] Uclés P and Lorente S: Electrophysiologic measures of delayed maturation in atten tion-deficit hyperactivity disorder. *J Child Neurol*, 1996;11(2):155-56.

[29] Escala de Inteligencia de Wechsler para Niños-Revisada. The psychological Corpo ration, New York. Spanish edition. *TEA Ediciones*. Madrid 1993.

[30] Prueba de lateralidad usual de M. Auzias. *TEA Ediciones*. Madrid, 1977.

[31] Coan RW and Castell RB: Cuestionario de personalidad para niños. Institute for Personality and Ability Testing (Illinois, U.S.A.). *TEA Ediciones*. Madrid, 1993.

[32] Gillis JS: Cuestionario de Ansiedad Infantil. Institute for Personality and Ability Testing (Illinois, U.S.A.). *TEA Ediciones*. Madrid, 1992.

[33] Castell MD: Cuestionario de personalidad para adolescentes.4ª ed. Institute for Personality and Ability Testing (Illinois,USA).*TEA Ediciones*.Madrid, 1988.

[34] Eisen A: Cortical and peripheral magnetic nerve stimulation, in Fuglsan-Frederik sen (ed): *Methods in Clinical Neurophysiology*. Copenhagen, 1992;3(4):70-71.

[35] Tyson K: Chilhood hyperactivity. *Smith College Studies in Social Work*,1991. Vol. 61:133-60.

[36] Benson DF: The role of frontal dysfunction in attention deficit hyperactivity disor der. *J Chil Neurol*, 1991;6(suppl):S9-S12.

[37] Weinberg WA and Brumback RA: The myth of attention deficit hyperactivity dis order: Symptoms resulting from multiple causes. *J Child Neurol*, 1992;7:43-45.

[38] Morrison JR and Stewart MA: The psychiatric status of the legal families of adopted hyperactive children. *Arch Gen Psychiatry*, 1973;28:888-891.

[39] Cantwell DP: Genetic of hyperactivity. *J Child Psychol Psychiatry*,1975;16:261-4.

[40] Fuster JM: Memory and planning: two temporal perspectives of frontal lobe function, in Jasper HH, Riggio S, Goldman-Rakic PS (eds): Epilepsy and Functional Anatomy of the Frontal Lobe. New York, *Raven Press*, 1995, pp 9-19.

[41] Pascual-Leone A, Grafman J, Cohen LG et al: Transcraneal magnetic stimulation. A new method for the study of higher cognitive functions in humans, in Grafman J and Boller F (eds): *Handbook of Neurophysiolog y* Vol. 10. Amsterdam, Elsevier Science Publishers, 1995.

[42] Flament DL, Hall EJ and Lemon RN: The development of corticomotoneuronal projections investigated using magnetic brain stimulation in the infant macaque. *J Physiol. London,* 1992;447:755-768.

[43] Wolraich ML, Hanna JN, Pinnock TY, Baumgaertel A, Brown J: Comparisosn of diagnostic criteria for attention deficit/hyperactivity disorder in a country-wide sample. *J Dev Behav Pediatr*. 1998; 19:162-168.

[44] Idiazábal M A, Palencia A B, Sangorrín J, Espadaler J M: Potenciales evocados cognitivos en el trastorno por déficit de atención/hiperactividad. *Rev Neurol*, 2002; 34:301-5.

[45] Winsberg BG, Javitt DC, Silipo GS: Electrophysiological indices of information proccesing in methylphenidate responders. *Biol Psychiatry*, 1997; 42:434-445.

[46] Young ES, Perros P, Prince GW, Sadler T : Acute challenge ERP as a prognostic of stimulant therapy outcome in attention deficit hyperactivity disorder. *Biol Psychiatry*, 1995; 37:25-33.

In: Attention Deficit Hyperactivity Disorder Research
Editor: Michelle P. Larimer, pp. 155-187
ISBN 1-59454-156-6

Chapter VII

Computational Strategies in the Evaluation of Attention Deficit/Hyperactivity Disorder (ADHD)

***Boris Kovatchev*[1]*, Jennifer Kim Penberthy*[1]*, Raina Robeva*[2]*, Marc Breton*[3] *and Daniel Cox*[1]**

[1]University of Virginia Health System, Charlottesville, Virginia
[2]Sweet Briar College, Sweet Briar, Virginia
[3]University of Virginia, Charlottesville, Virginia

Abstract

Attention Deficit/Hyperactivity Disorder (ADHD) is the most common developmental disorder of childhood, affecting 3 - 5% of children in the United States, and often continuing into adulthood. ADHD is associated with multiple serious complications, including poor school achievement, substance abuse, automobile accidents, etc. The symptoms of ADHD are manifestations of disruption of self-regulation, including dysregulation of inhibition and attention. These manifestations take the form of psychological symptoms, disturbances in cognitive performance, behavioral dysregulation, and electroencephalographic (EEG) deviations. Therefore, these manifestations are observed across various domains and time frames, and are proposed to be separate factors, or components, of an underlying disruption of self-regulation. These components are assessed by various tests, each with a different sensitivity and specificity. Currently there is no single objective procedure to diagnose and quantify ADHD, making it difficult to determine who does, and does not have, the disorder, what medication and what dose of medication is optimally effective, or whether the condition is changing with maturation.

This chapter presents several recently developed computational procedures that have been shown to improve the assessment of ADHD. The first set of procedures refers to

[1] Correspondence: Boris Kovatchev, Ph.D.University of Virginia Health System Box 800137 Charlottesville, VA 22908 E-mail: boris@virginia.edu

analysis of (EEG) data. Three distinct algorithms are discussed, each looking at the effect of ADHD on brain waves at a different time scale: the Engagement Index, originally developed by NASA and working on a time scale of seconds, the Alpha Blockade Index working on a scale of 2-3 minutes, and the Consistency Index working on a time scale of half hour. Further, we present a sequential probability model using Bayesian inference to combine disparate (biometric or psychometric) tests into a single assessment. This procedure allows for a stepwise increasingly precise evaluation and a concurrent decrease of the number of unclassified cases.

We illustrate the procedures using data from several studies conducted at the University of Virginia and Sweet Briar College. We conclude that advanced computational analysis of traditional data could result in an assessment of ADHD that is superior to the traditional assessment procedures.

Key Words: *Diagnostic Assessment, Attention deficit/Hyperactivity Disorder (ADHD), Bayesian Inference*

Introduction

The NIH Consensus Conferences [50] and Clinical Practice Guidelines [22] demonstrated that Attention Deficit/Hyperactivity Disorder (ADHD) is commonly diagnosed and associated with many negative consequences for the individual, family, and society. The DSM-IV [4] states: "The essential feature of ADHD is a persistent pattern of inattention and/or hyperactivity-impulsivity that is more frequent and severe than is typically observed in individuals in a comparable level of development." Evidence of six of nine inattentive behaviors and/or six of nine hyperactive-impulsive behaviors must have been present before age 7, and must clearly interfere with social, academic and/or occupational functioning. Consequently, the diagnosis of ADHD is highly dependent on a retrospective report of past behavior and subjective judgments on degree of relative impairment. Due to the subjective nature of assessment, precision in diagnosis has been elusive. Because ADHD cannot be strictly defined, and precisely and objectively measured, its true prevalence cannot be accurately determined [8]. While the DSM-IV [4] estimates the prevalence of ADHD in school-age children as between 3% and 5%, other community survey studies suggest it may be as high as 16% [74]. ADHD occurs more commonly in males than in females, with ratios ranging from 4:1 to 9:1 [47]. Of all child referrals for mental health services, one-third to one-half are thought to be attributable to ADHD [56].

The hallmarks of ADHD are hyperactivity, impulsivity, and an inability to sustain attention [8]. The DSM-IV distinguishes three types: predominantly inattentive type, predominantly hyperactive-impulsive type, and combined type. In addition to the core clinical symptoms of ADHD, high levels of co-morbidity have been found with learning, oppositional defiant, conduct, mood, and anxiety disorders [15]. Furthermore, it is estimated that the majority of children diagnosed with ADHD exhibit significant behavioral problems during adolescence [10], [32] [44] and manifest continuing functional deficits and psychopathology into adulthood [16], [39], [67], [71]. One real-life consequence of ADHD is a five-fold increase in automobile crashes [11]. In spite of these well-documented problems, the mechanisms and etiology of ADHD remain methodologically difficult to study, with different studies yielding inconsistent results. Most investigators accept that ADHD exists as a distinct clinical syndrome and suggest a multifactorial etiology that includes neurobiology as an important factor [3], [23]. For example, Zametkin and Rapoport [76] identified 11 separate neuroanatomical hypotheses that have been proposed for the etiology of ADHD.

In order to unite the multifactorial neuropsychological, behavioral, and physiological domains of ADHD, we conceptualize ADHD as a manifestation of irregularity in these domains, namely dysregulation of inhibition and self-regulation and a decrease in temporal stability of symptoms and performance. Existing theories of ADHD support this conceptualization, however, research to date has been conducted in separate field domains (e.g., biology, neuropsychology, cognitive sciences, behavioral sciences), and has yet to be tested within one comprehensive model. Below we review relevant literature within each domain of manifestation, briefly presenting how the theories and findings apply to the overall concept of disruption in self-regulation, inhibition, and attention.

Neuropsychological

An overview of neuropsychological literature reveals that research has focused on three theoretical mechanisms for the behavioral symptoms of poorly controlled attention in ADHD: response disinhibition, executive dyscontrol, and attentional disinhibition (failure of selective attention). Neurocognitive research on children with ADHD has reported deficits in executive functioning [7] and selective attention [18]. While these categories are not mutually exclusive, the tests used are typically characterized as belonging to one of these categories. Although, the neuropsychological patterns of ADHD are variable, in large part because of the variability among individuals with ADHD, most studies cite numerous cognitive impairments that cluster in the domains of attentional control, executive functioning, and both verbal and visual memory. Another subgroup of individuals with ADHD has definite neurocognitive deficits, which appear to be restricted to visuospatial attention and memory, and suggest a correlation with neuroimaging findings. A third group is characterized by impairment in continuous performance tests, suggesting that only such tests in a neuropsychological battery are sufficiently sensitive to the cognitive deficits of ADHD versus normal control samples, but may not discriminate individuals with ADHD from other disorders with related cognitive deficits [6]. Although the evidence is strong for deficits in some forms of executive response inhibition in ADHD, it remains unclear that this is the primary or mediating causal deficit. Some researchers [12] have argued that all of these deficits are secondary to a primary problem in "self-regulation." In a recent comprehensive review, Nigg [51] who concluded that ADHD children appear to have weak inhibition processes combined with low effort or alerting to stimuli, as assessed on measures of behavioral (the stop task), interference (Stroop task), cognitive (directed forgetting tasks), and oculomotor (anti-saccade task) inhibition, but that no single neuropsychological test was highly predictive of diagnosis of ADHD.

Behavioral

ADHD, presented in the DSM-IV [4], is typically characterized by inconsistency of behavior, cognitive functioning, and over-activity or impulsivity. Quay [57] proposes that ADHD stems from impairment in a neurologically based behavioral inhibition system. In an elaboration on this same theme, Barkley [9] proposes a compelling argument that problems with self-regulation underlie the majority of diagnostic symptoms in children with ADHD. He outlines a unifying model of ADHD that is founded on prior theories of the neuropsychological functions of the brains' prefrontal lobes. In this model, he specifies poor behavioral inhibition as the central deficiency in ADHD. He purports that most, if not all, of the cognitive deficits associated with ADHD seem to fall within the realm of self-regulation or executive functions. In addition, many others in the field share the view that behavioral inhibition deficits lie at the core of many ADHD symptoms [64],[66]. Barkley [9] summarizes that "the evidence that ADHD involves impaired behavioral inhibition seems compelling, arising as it does from multiple studies, methods, and sources." He further hypothesizes that self-regulation gives rise to the direction and persistence of behavior toward future goals and the ability to re-engage that behavior if disrupted. Overall, many researchers support the idea that a hallmark component of ADHD, in whichever form it is diagnosed, is the *inability to shift or transition* between tasks. Indeed, a study by McDonald, et al. [45] showed that ADHD subjects were able to "anchor" their attention in a task with muster, but that they were unable to easily shift their attention to an alternative location.

Biological

F.X. Castellanos [19], in his paper on the psychobiology of ADHD, defines ADHD as "a disorder of *deficient and delayed self-regulation*, due largely to genetic differences in the rate of development and functional integrity of brain systems. There is also evidence that the putative deviation in brain development interacts with genetic control of lateralization of brain function such that right sided circuits are those that are predominantly affected." Biederman [14], reviewing the literature on ADHD, moves the discussion from genetic and molecular paradigms into inconclusive results from imaging studies. He states, "Human studies of the catecholamine hypothesis of ADHD have produced conflicting results, perhaps due to the insensitivity of peripheral measures." Additionally, Sagvolden, et al. [60], note that ADHD boys displayed an inability to control their responses in a delayed reinforcement task. Grodzinsky & Barkley [33] suggest as Castellanos [20] and others do, that there is a problem with frontal cortex activation, which controls planning, anticipation of consequence, and sequencing. A theoretical paper presented by Pliszka, et al. [53] suggests that the cerebellum and the corpus callosum contribute to ADHD through the dysregulation of epinephrine. They postulate that epinephrine, which fuels the locus coeruleus, a portion of the brain that regulates visual attention and plays a part in emotional response, in addition to dopamine, is synthesized at an abnormally low level which may also contribute to ADHD patients' positive response to stimulant medications. Indeed, some studies have found that ADHD children have smaller corpus callosa, especially in the splenial area which is thought to be involved in the ability to sustain attention and smaller inferior posterior vermal cerebellum size [13], [36], [49], [65]. Abnormally low levels of the neurotransmitter dopamine were also implicated with ADHD [58]. Dopamine's role in the brain is to dampen electrical activity. In context, there are some neurotransmitters that cause the brain to be excited, for example, norepinephrine and glutamate. Dopamine helps balance out the excitation of the brain by helping an individual to focus on a task at hand. Among the areas of the brain where dopamine receptors are most prevalent are the pre-frontal cortex, the basal ganglia, and the portion of the limbic system that governs motivation, the nucleus accumbens [52]. Most physiological studies have concluded that either delayed maturation or defects in cortical activation play large roles in the pathophysiology of ADHD. For example, studies of cerebral blood flow determined by single-positron emission CT have demonstrated decreased metabolic activity in suspected attentional areas of the brain [27], [35], [75]. These, as well as additional neurophysiological findings, have been interpreted as evidence of delayed maturation and cortical hypoarousal in regions of the prefrontal and frontal cortex, two predominate etiological theories underlying ADHD

Electroencephalographic (EEG)

Unfortunately, while neuroanatomical findings lend support to the notion that ADHD is a distinct clinical syndrome and add to our understanding of the etiology of ADHD, neuroimaging techniques are too expensive, restricted to a few centers, and lack clear specificity and sensitivity in diagnosis of ADHD. For these reasons, EEG studies are of interest. There are a few basic methods of analyzing EEG data that have been employed in previous research – visual inspection of raw data and quantitative analyses of EEG data, including spectral and coherence methods of analysis. To date, none of these methods have revealed pervasive or consistent patterns of EEG abnormalities with sufficient specificity or sensitivity to separate children with ADHD from normal subjects. The first of these methods of analysis involves visual inspection of raw EEG data. As long ago as 1938, Jasper, Solomon, and Bradley [38], used this method and reported EEG abnormalities in children with minimal brain dysfunction (an outdated term used to describe children with hyperactivity and poor attentiveness as well as learning disabilities and conduct disorder). In parallel with the development of the computer, researchers have applied a second method of EEG analysis employing quantitative techniques. Quantitative EEG (Q-EEG) is a mathematical analysis of voltage-time series data with the intention of extracting useful information not readily apparent to visual inspection. Spectral analysis is a common technique of quantitative EEG. It mathematically transforms, via Fast Fourier Transform (FFT), raw amplitude-time data into its component frequencies. During the 1970s several laboratories utilized a combination of visual inspection and quantitative techniques, and reported differences between the EEGs of hyperactive and normal children [34], [62], [68], [72]. Among the differences discovered were: a higher percentage of abnormal EEG patterns (abnormal usually meaning excessive slow wave activity) in clinical subjects than in controls [62]; more power in the 0 to 8 Hz spectrum in hyperactive children compared to normal controls [61]; less power in the 10 Hz range for hyperactives than controls [48]; and less beta and weaker stimulus-locked alpha attenuation in hyperactive than in non-hyperactive children [34]. Many investigators have reported that only when subjects are engaged in behavioral paradigms (particularly those manipulating attention) do electrophysiological differences appear between normal and hyperactive or LD children. Dykman et al. [31] investigated the EEGs of four groups of boys (10 hyperactive, 10 learning-disabled, 10 with both hyperactivity and LD) engaged in a complex visual search task. Spectral analysis of EEG data indicated that LD boys, hyperactive boys, and boys with a mixed diagnosis displayed less beta and less stimulus-locked alpha attenuation than normal boys. Research in the 1980s-1990s began to address and correct issues of uniformity of diagnosis, methodology, and accuracy in EEG acquisition, both in terms of theoretical understanding and technical application. In an attempt to clarify some of the EEG differences between hyperactive and normal subjects, Satterfield et al [63] considered the impact of age upon EEG in two groups of normal (n = 60) and hyperactive, inattentive, and impulsive males (n = 138) ages 6-12, by examining follow-up EEGs on a subset of the hyperactive and normal subjects four years after the initial EEG. Their findings indicate "...electrophysiological differences between hyperactive and normal male children are complex and vary markedly with age." They further warn that "Computation of group averages which include data from children of a wide age range may obscure rather than clarify the electrophysiological correlates of this disorder."

More recent studies employing spectral analysis of EEG have also shown varying patterns of EEG activity in ADHD subjects. Janzen, et al. [37] compared EEG differences between eight ADD males and eight normal control males ages 9-12. Results demonstrated that the ADD males had higher theta amplitudes for all sites. Clarke, et al. [21] performed automated EEG on subjects (ages 8 -12) classified into groups of 20 ADHD-Combined Type, 20 ADHD-Predominantly Inattentive Type, and 20 controls. Overall, they found evidence of increased absolute and relative theta in all ADHD subjects, with the ADHD combined type showing a significantly greater amount of theta power than the predominantly inattentive-type. In addition, Clarke et al. found a decrease in alpha activity, but elevated theta present in all brain regions measured and not confined to frontal regions as previous studies had reported. In an interesting study by Ackerman, et al. [2] a group of 56 ADD/ADHD children who had normal reading skills were employed as a control group, and their EEGs compared to EEGs of 119 children with reading disorders (some of whom had a co-morbid diagnosis of ADD/ADHD). Subjects included 86 males and 33 females between the ages of 7.5 and 12 years. The major difference between groups was in the low beta band, where the ADD/ADHD group had greater power at the parietal and midline sites. The ADD/ADHD group also displayed marginally greater low beta at the right versus left temporal site. Conclusions drawn by Ackerman, et al. apply more to the impact of reading skill than to diagnosis of ADHD, and indicated that adequate readers (ADD/ADHD group) more actively processed the stimuli than did the poor readers, some of whom had co-morbid ADD/ADHD diagnoses. Crawford and Barabasz [28] found that 7 children with ADHD had more low alpha activity in their right than left hemispheres at frontal sites when listening to a story (with eyes closed) and at temporal and central sites while doing arithmetic, suggesting dysregulation in the right hemisphere because normally alpha activity is blocked during active processing. Mann, et al. [43] tested 25 nine to twelve year-old boys with predominantly inattentive-type ADHD, and found increased theta at both absolute and relative percent power calculations, and decreased beta in temporal and frontal sites. Monastra, et al [47] reported similar results from their large study on 482 subjects (ages 6-30). EEG data were used to test the hypothesis that prefrontal cortical slowing (excess theta) can differentiate ADHD subtypes from controls. Analysis of variance demonstrated cortical slowing that differentiated ADHD subjects, regardless of sex or age. Specifically, consistent with the presented hypothesis, statistical analysis revealed that the ADHD groups (inattentive and combined type) displayed significantly higher levels of slow-wave (theta) relative to fast-wave (beta) EEG activity. Consequently, Monastra, et al [47] derived an individual Attentional Index (AI) equal to the theta-beta power ratio of a subject. The AI was significantly higher in ADHD compared to control subjects. In terms of computing, the AI is the numerical inverse of a previously published beta/theta ratio, the Engagement Index used by NASA researchers to track attentional changes in pilots [54], [55].

Temporal Scales of EEG

The theory of dysregulation promotes the idea that EEG findings will generally reflect a difficulty in self-regulation, evident on various temporal scales, ranging from seconds (assessed by ratio of slow-to-fast wave activity), to minutes (e.g., degree of elevation of alpha activity during tasks on a temporal scale of 1-2 minutes), to half-hours (e.g., lack of coherent attentional transition between 10-15 minute tasks). The "fastest" measurement scale (seconds) is represented by NASA's Engagement Index, or its inverse, the Attentional Index [47]. In this chapter we present measures that cover the intermediate scale of 1-2 minutes (Alpha Blockade Index, ABI, [59] and the "slowest" measurement scale of half-hours (Consistency Index, CI, [25], [40], [46]. In our previous studies these measure proved to be sensitive to EEG impairments associated with ADHD.

Combined Psycho-Physiological Assessment of ADHD

It is now evident that manifestations of ADHD are observed at both psychological and physiological levels and assessed via various psychometric, EEG, and imaging tests. Consequently, diagnosing ADHD presents a challenge to traditional assessment paradigms because there is no single assessment tool or medical test that definitively establishes its presence. The recommended diagnostic procedure for ADHD relies on a multi-method assessment [22], [50]. Ideally, this assessment should consist of the following individual components: a) behavior rating scales, b) behavioral observations, c) parent and teacher interviews, d) neuropsychological assessment, e) academic screening, and f) EEG/brain imaging measures [8], [5]. However, the results from multiple measures and methods often do not clearly converge on a diagnosis, but rather provide contradictory information. Thus it is, most often, that the "best estimate" diagnosis is the subjective opinion of a clinician whose clinical judgment is influenced and limited by factors such as experience, resources, and prejudices. Thus a reliable and comprehensive assessment that is founded on and determined by objective and standardized methods would provide a welcome advantage to diagnosing

ADHD, as well as to evaluating the effectiveness of treatments for ADHD. In this chapter we discuss a stochastic assessment combining psychometric tests with EEG-based physiological markers of ADHD. The assessment utilizes classical Bayesian inference to refine after each step the probability of ADHD of each individual. In a pilot study involving 6 college females with ADHD and 6 matched controls, the assessment achieved correct classification for all ADHD and non-ADHD subjects. In comparison, the classification of ADHD vs. non-ADHD participants was <85% for any one of the tests separately [59]. Now, we present comprehensive data using a meta-analysis of several studies with 117 participants, which confirm the results of our pilot study. We conclude that this combined assessment procedure, designed to incorporate various tests and markers for ADHD none of which alone could claim perfect sensitivity and specificity, yields results superior to those of its components.

The Data

Subjects

During the past several years we have conducted a series of studies investigating EEG patterns associated with ADHD:

Study I: Four boys, ages 6-10, with ADHD (one primarily inattentive type, one primarily hyperactive/ impulsive type, and two combined type) and four age-matched control boys had their EEG data acquired during two 30-minute tasks (video and reading) separated by a 5-minute break. Parents completed the ADHD-SI [25]. ADHD subjects were regularly taking methylphenidate for their symptoms, but were off the medication during assessment. For the ADHD boys, this procedure was repeated three months later, to assess test-retest reliability. Two of the boys with ADHD were Caucasian, one was African-American, and one was Indian. All four of the control subjects were Caucasian. No subjects reported co-morbid diagnoses or learning disabilities. Results are reported by Cox, et al [25].

Study II: Seven ADHD males (four primarily inattentive type, and three combined type) and six non-ADHD males, ages 18-25, participated in a double-blind, placebo versus methylphenidate controlled crossover design study. ADHD subjects had to have previously taken methylphenidate but could not be taking any medication for their condition within the six months prior to the study. EEG data was acquired while the subjects were given four tasks of the Gordon Diagnostic System, two easy (auditory and visual) and two hard (auditory and visual). Subjects and their parents completed the ADHD-SI [25]. Two of the subjects were African- American, and one control subject was Asian, all others were Caucasian. No subjects had co-morbid diagnoses or learning disabilities. Results are reported by Merkel, et al [46] and Cox, et al [26].

Study III: Eighteen boys and 17 girls, ages 8-16, classified as either ADHD or non-ADHD (9 boys and 8 girls with ADHD-combined type and 9 boys and 9 girls without ADHD) had EEG data collected for 36 minutes while performing various tasks. Parents and teachers completed the Conners' Rating Scale [24], Achenbach Child Behavior Checklist [1], and the ADHD-SI [25]. All subjects were Caucasian with the exception of one child in the control group who was Hispanic. All ADHD subjects were taking a stimulant medication (with the exception of Cylert) to treat their symptoms, but were taken off their medication 24 hours prior to being tested. One ADHD subject reported having dyslexia, but no additional co-morbidities were reported or diagnosed. Results are reported by Kovatchev, et al [40].

Study IV was conducted at Sweet Briar College to study female college students with ADHD. The participants engage in a series of short concentration tasks (2-3 min.) with shorter resting intervals (1-2 min). Subjects are administered the ADHD-SI [25], and the Wender-Utah Rating Scale (WURS) [70], which is a 61-item retrospective self-report scale with adequate reliability and validity. We currently have collected data for 6 ADHD Caucasian females (all ADHD-combined type) and 6 non-ADHD Caucasian females. No subjects reported any co-morbid disorders or learning disabilities. Results are reported by Robeva, et al [59].

Study V: Seventy-seven children ages 8 - 12 (67 males and 10 females, 36 ADHD and 41 non-ADHD) were administered EEGs while watching a movie for 20 minutes, resting with eyes open for 5 minutes, reading silently for 10 minutes, resting with eyes open for 5 minutes, then performing creative drawing tasks for 10 minutes. This pattern was repeated once, for a total test time of 100 minutes. Parents and teachers were administered the DuPaul AD/HD Rating Scale-IV [30], and parents completed the ADHD-SI [25]. Subjects included two African-American males, one Indian male, and two subjects who did not specify their ethnicity. All other subjects were Caucasian. Twelve ADHD subjects were diagnosed as primarily inattentive type, one as primarily hyperactive/impulsive type, and the remainder (23) met criteria for ADHD-combined type. Co-morbid disorders in the ADHD groups included: specific phobia (7); oppositional defiant disorder (8); obsessive-compulsive disorder (1); enuresis (1): and 1 subject with separation anxiety disorder and ODD, and 1 subject with social phobia and GAD. Co-morbid disorders in the control group included: specific phobia (1) and enuresis (1). Results are first reported in this chapter.

Study VI: Six males diagnosed with ADHD (four primarily inattentive type and two combined type ADHD), were administered EEGs while on and off methylphenidate. The EEGs were acquired while the subjects viewed a movie for 20 minutes, rested with eyes open for 5 minutes, and read silently for 10 minutes. Parents and teachers were administered the DuPaul AD/HD Rating Scale-IV [30]. Subjects were between the ages of 16-21, and reported a previous positive response to methylphenidate. All subjects were Caucasian. One subject met diagnostic criteria for social phobia and one subject met criteria for oppositional defiant disorder. Three subjects reported that they had been diagnosed with learning disorders, such as dyslexia. Results are first reported in this chapter.

Procedure

Across all studies, subjects were placed in the *ADHD groups* if they: (a) met DSM-IV diagnostic criteria for ADHD (with or without hyperactivity) as assessed by an age-appropriate structured clinical interview such as the DICA, DISC-IV, or Structured Clinical Interview for DSM (SCID) administered by a clinical psychologist and/or psychiatrist who validated the diagnosis; (b) reported a history of a positive response to methylphenidate, whether they were currently on medication for ADHD or not, and no history of adverse reaction to methylphenidate, (c) did not meet diagnostic criteria for current co-morbid psychological disorders such as depression, psychosis, schizophrenia for which they were taking psychotropic medications; (d) did not meet criteria for current drug/alcohol abuse or addiction; and (e) did not have any significant health problems or disorders that might effect the brain or EEG recordings (e.g. Tourette's Syndrome, epilepsy). Participants in the *control groups* of the above studies were included if they (a) had no known history of ADHD or disruptive behavioral disorders; (b) did not currently meet criteria for any subtype of ADHD on the appropriate structured clinical interview administered to them by the clinical psychologist and psychiatrist; (c) had never been prescribed stimulant medication nor taken it for recreational purposes; (d) did not meet diagnostic criteria for current co-morbid psychological disorders, including depression, anxiety, psychosis, drug/alcohol abuse or addiction for which they were currently taking psychotropic medications; and (e) did not have any significant health problems or disorders that might effect the brain or EEG recordings (e.g. Tourette's Syndrome, epilepsy). All subjects were assessed by licensed clinical psychologists and psychiatrists, who had to both agree on the diagnosis, in order for a participant to be placed in an appropriate group.

EEG Data Acquisition

In all studies, individuals in the *ADHD groups were tested off of their ADHD medication* at least once. ADHD medications, if being taken, were discontinued under the supervision of a psychiatrist, at least 36 hours prior to the EEG testing. In Study I, II, and VI, subjects were also tested while on a therapeutic dose of methylphenidate. EEG acquisition was conducted for all individuals and involved the subjects being seated in front of the computer and an appropriately sized EEG cap placed over their heads. Electrode placement was in accordance with the international 10-20 system and the electrode sites were prepared with a ground in front of CZ, and a right earlobe reference electrode. EEG signals were amplified and processed by the Lexicor Neurosearch-24 system. The EEG data collection used standard settings of a clinical EEG acquisition with 5 KOhms impedance criterion measured by a Prep-Check electrode impedance meter. Specifics of the EEG acquisition procedure varied somewhat for each study, but always involved recording EEG across contiguous cognitive tasks at 4-8 electrode sites (either CZ, Pz, P3, P4 or CZ, Pz, P3, P4, F3, F4, T3, and T4).

Database

Although our studies were conducted sequentially over a period of years, each was conducted in the same laboratories and under the supervision of the same group of researchers. The data had similar structure and were organized in an interconnected database. In order to handle the large amount of the EEG data (thousands of records per EEG session per subject) and the structural complexity of the data coming from different studies, we have developed unified data structure that was applied to all available EEG data sets:

a) *EEG data pre-processing and normalization:* The raw EEG data (digitized amplitudes) are split into epochs with approximate duration of 2.5 seconds each. The data in each epoch are processed by Fast Fourier Transformation (FFT) software computing the power spectrum of brain waves for each epoch. The frequencies represented in this spectrum are, depending on the filter settings, between 0.5-2 and 80-100 Hz. This region includes four basic EEG frequency bands: Delta (0.5-4Hz), Theta (4-8 Hz), Alpha (8-13 Hz) and Beta (13-22 Hz). Separately recorded (and generally not included in further analysis) is High Beta + EMG (22-40 Hz) and the residual power, carried by frequencies above 40Hz.

b) *EEG data matrix record:* One record represents 2.5 seconds of EEG observation encoded as the relative power of theta, alpha, beta, and high beta computed separately for several EEG channels (electrodes). Depending on the study, we have used 4 or 8 EEG channels. Thus, a record contains 16 or 32 numbers. In addition, each epoch is stamped by a study index, time index, task index, and a subject key that contains ID number, diagnosis, and gender information. These records are structured in rectangular matrices, one matrix per subject per test, where each column is a time series tracking the power of a particular band at a particular channel during the study. We now have 162 such matrices for 117 subjects.

c) *Psychometric data pre-processing and normalization.* This procedure converts the scores of each psychometric test into a probability for ADHD. This is done in order to include the scores from disparate psychometric (and EEG) tests into a single assessment of ADHD. The procedure is described in detail in section 3.1.

d) *Finally*, the EEG data matrix is cross-referenced in the database with subjects' demographic and psychometric data.

Descriptive Characteristics of the Subjects

The rate of co-morbid psychiatric disorders or learning disorders was approximately 21% in our ADHD group, and 2% in the control group. We excluded subjects with co-morbid depression, psychosis, schizophrenia, or mental retardation. Therefore, the majority of co-morbid disorders in the ADHD group were Opposition Defiant Disorder (10 of 24 subjects with co-morbid disorders) and anxiety disorders (10 of 24 subjects with co-morbid disorders). Overall, female subjects made up approximately 25% of the sample, due in large part to preferential recruiting of males in many of the studies. This ratio approximately matches the overall prevalence of ADHD, with boys outnumbering girls by approximately 4:1 to 9:1 [4]. The race/ethnic composition of the database is presented in Table 1:

Table 1: Race/Ethnic Composition of the Database

	Asian or Pacific Islander	Black, not of Hispanic Origin	Hispanic	White, not of Hispanic Origin	Other, or Unknown
Subjects	1	5	1	106	4
% of total	0.9%	4.3%	0.9%	90.5%	3.4%

The majority of ADHD subjects met criteria for ADHD-Combined Type (61%), with approximately 36% diagnosed as Primarily Inattentive Type, and only 3% meeting diagnosis for Primarily Hyperactive/Impulsive Type. This appears to be reflective of the distribution in the DSM-IV clinical field trials [41].

Electroencephalographic (EEG) Measures of ADHD

Our studies have concentrated on the physiological manifestations of dysregulation in the form of EEG irregularities observed at different temporal scales. In particular, our six consecutive studies investigated NASA's Engagement Index relative to ADHD, and introduced and investigated the EEG Consistency Index [25], [40], [46] and the Alpha Blockade Index [59] quantifying EEG dsyregulation when transitioning from one cognitive task to another at different time scales. The results from these studies are described below and in separate published articles listed under each study.

Power of Theta & Theta/Beta Ratio (Temporal Scale of Seconds)

As presented in the Introduction, one important consistency is the finding of patterns of higher levels of theta relative to beta in children with ADHD, or higher average power of theta [17], [42], [43], [47]. Therefore, we utilized our database to replicate these findings. Since the published research in the area involved male subjects only, we conducted separate analyses for males and females. In addition, we investigated all available EEG channels (CZ, Pz, F3, F4, P3, P4, T3, T4) separately and found that the best separation between ADHD and non-ADHD subjects is achieved from data acquired by CZ only. The results for this particular channel were as follows: We found a mildly elevated power of theta in ADHD boys compared to matched controls ($p=0.05$). Although this difference was statistically significant, it did not have diagnostic utility (i.e. it was not useful for ADHD – non-ADHD classification). There was no statistical difference in power of theta between ADHD girls and controls, or for EEG channels other than CZ. The ratio of theta/beta was significantly elevated in ADHD boys and girls, compared to controls ($p<0.001$). This difference was preserved over the course of the entire EEG data acquisition. *Figure 1* presents the dynamics (averaged across all subjects) of the theta/beta ratio as acquired by CZ over 1000 epochs (approximately 40 minutes of EEG). Since the unit of resolution of the theta/beta ratio is approximately 2.5 seconds (one EEG epoch), we can conclude that any ADHD-induced irregularities in this ratio represent events taking place at a temporal scale of seconds. This result confirms the utility of the Attentional Index introduced by Monastra, et al [47]. However, despite its overall good statistical significance, the AI was insufficient to clearly classify ADHD subjects vs. controls in any of the six studies that we have conducted.

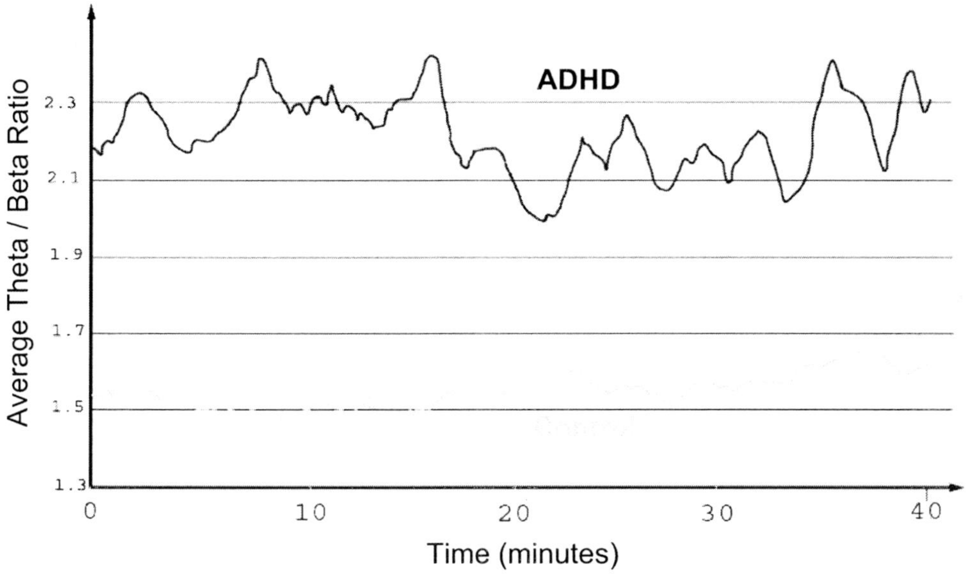

Figure 1: Dynamics of the Ratio of Theta/Beta in ADHD Subjects and Controls

Alpha Blockade Index (Temporal Scale of 1-2 Minutes)

Activities of the waking EEG in alpha frequencies have special significance in that they form the "alpha rhythm," a posteriorly-dominant activity that attenuates (or "blocks") with eye opening. This rhythm first emerges at age 3-4 month and gradually increases in frequency until adult levels are attained in late childhood. Since the alpha rhythm is slowed or absent during heightened anxiety or extremely low arousal such as drowsiness, attaining alpha enhancement (increasing power of alpha) is more difficult for both over-aroused subjects (such as ADHD subjects) and for under-aroused subjects (again, such as ADHD subjects or other persons suffering from inattention). This theory supports the results of our clinical studies, in which ADHD subjects demonstrated similar alpha powers when shifting from a short cognitive task to rest, while control subjects demonstrated a significant difference in the power of alpha, with a higher power during rest and a lower power of alpha during cognitive tasks (*Figures 2A, 2B*).

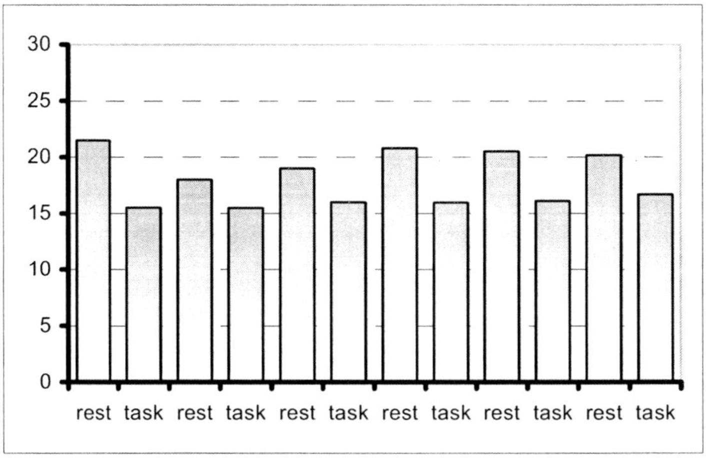

A: Power of Alpha – ADHD Subjects

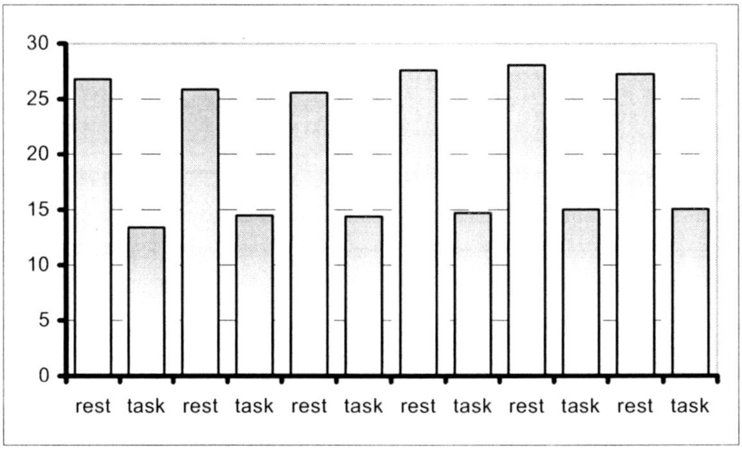

B: Power of Alpha – Control Subjects

Figure 2: Changes in alpha during a rapid sequence of task and rest periods

We used EEG data from the six tasks and the five separating rest periods to quantify the suggested weaker attenuation of alpha in ADHD. Each task in *Figures 2A and 2B* has a duration of 1-2 minutes, and each rest period is approximately 1 minute. Thus, the observed phenomenon takes place in a temporal scale of minutes. Specifically, our initial analysis indicates that a rapid succession of 1-minute cognitive tasks differentiates adults with attentional deficits from adults without attention deficits. The analysis of the series of short tasks separated by short rest periods performed in the second half of the data collection during Study IV revealed previously unknown, but very significant inconsistencies in the EEGs of female college students with ADHD relative to non-ADHD controls. ADHD subjects had (i) Less elevated alpha activity (vigilance) during rest periods, and (ii) Less suppressed alpha activity during tasks. These differences classified correctly 5 out of 6 ADHD subjects and 5 out of 6 non-ADHD control subjects [59]. This finding was also observed in some of our original data, involving young male children with and without the diagnosis of ADHD, but with less strength of the effect. This result served as a base for the development and investigation of the Alpha Blockade Index. The ABI was designed as a measure that quantifies the attenuation of alpha waves of a person going through a rapid sequence of task and rest periods. It was expected that a person with ADHD would display less alpha attenuation, compared to a control.

In numerical terms this translates into a lower average absolute difference between the alpha powers in sequential task and rest periods. In particular, during the EEG session a sequence of high-alpha powers $\alpha_1, \alpha_2, \ldots \alpha_k$ is obtained for each person, corresponding to the sequence of rapidly changing tasks and rest periods. Then the ABI for a person is computed using the formula: $ABI = \frac{10}{k-1} \cdot \sum_{2}^{k} \left| \alpha_k - \alpha_{k-1} \right|$, where k is the total number of task and rest periods. ABI values which are greater than 100 are reset to 100, which results in an index expressed in percentage points between 0 and 100%. A lower ABI is associated with weaker attenuation of alpha during active periods, as compared to rest periods and could therefore be indicative of ADHD. Based on the results in this study, we suggest a cutoff of 20%, i.e. ABI<20% would indicate ADHD.

A brief justification of this formula follows: The ABI is essentially equal to the average of the absolute values of the differences in alpha power between two consecutive tasks/rest periods, i.e. the ABI is essentially equal to $\frac{1}{k-1} \sum_{2}^{k} \left| \alpha_k - \alpha_{k-1} \right|$, where k is the total number of tasks and rests. The coefficient 10 and the reset of values above 100 to 100 are only used to calibrate the ABI to the range 0-100, similarly to the calibration of the Consistency Index [40]. This calibration does not alter the classification of ADHD/non-ADHD based on the ABI (with a suggested cut-off of 20), or any statistical tests reflecting the power of that classification. Note also, that the formula could be applied to any sequence of short tasks separated by short breaks with suggested length 3 and 2 minutes, respectively.

In Study IV k = 6(tasks) + 5(rest periods) = 11. The average ABI for ADHD subjects was 23% vs. 33% for controls. With a cutoff of 20%, the ABI misclassifies one ADHD subject and one control subject. The Fisher's exact test showed a significant classification ability, p=0.04 [59]. Based on physiology and these pilot data, we conclude that the ABI maybe a valid EEG marker of ADHD.

Consistency Index (Temporal Scale of ½ Hour)

This section presents our most detailed results to date, confirmed in all of our previous studies. We found that the EEG power patterns of boys with and without ADHD differed substantially when the boys transitioned between two contiguous cognitive tasks. It became apparent that the EEG power shift from one task to another by non-ADHD boys was more "consistent" as compared to the ADHD boys. The problem then was to create a measure that would quantify the EEG power consistency during subjects' transition from one cognitive task to another. During our pilot studies, we created such a measure through the development of a mathematical model of EEG transition consistency and called it the Consistency Index

(CI). This was based upon quantitative representation of the idea that ADHD is reflected by chaotic changes in the EEG power spectrum when subjects shift from one cognitive task to another. The CI uses a rigid mathematical frame that incorporates this idea [40]. This frame is based on our notion that the EEG data stream can be represented by a three-dimensional numeric array - at any given moment one dimension is frequency of brain waves, another is spatial - the location of the electrode on a subject's head, and the third is time. ADHD can cause inconsistency in the frequency or spatial dimension, or in both, when shifting across cognitive tasks.

Mathematical Modeling Of EEG Consistency

As described in Section 2.3, the EEG assessment procedure begins with a standard EEG data acquisition, followed by pre-processing of the EEG data (Section 2.4). The basic CI uses 8 electrodes, F3, F4, CZ, PZ, C3, C4, P3, P4, however this model is flexible enough to accommodate experiments with other locations, such as FZ, F7, F8, P7, P8, T7, T8, and any number of electrodes. FFT and artifact rejection procedures are commercially available. We will now explain the computing of EEG consistency in detail, relying on our past experience that the best way to present this mathematical paradigm is to use a series of figures depicting the sequential steps leading to the computation of the CI.

EEG Frequency Dimension: Figure 3 presents the basis of our idea of consistent EEG in the frequency dimension. The black line is the power spectrum of a subject performing a task; the gray line is the power spectrum of the same subject while performing an adjacent task. In Figure 3-A the black line is above the gray line at lower frequencies and mostly below the gray line at higher frequencies (above 16 Hz). This shows that a shift from one task to another (from black to gray) results in an increase of higher frequencies and a decrease of lower frequencies. In contrast, in Figure 3-B no specific change in the frequency distribution over is observed.

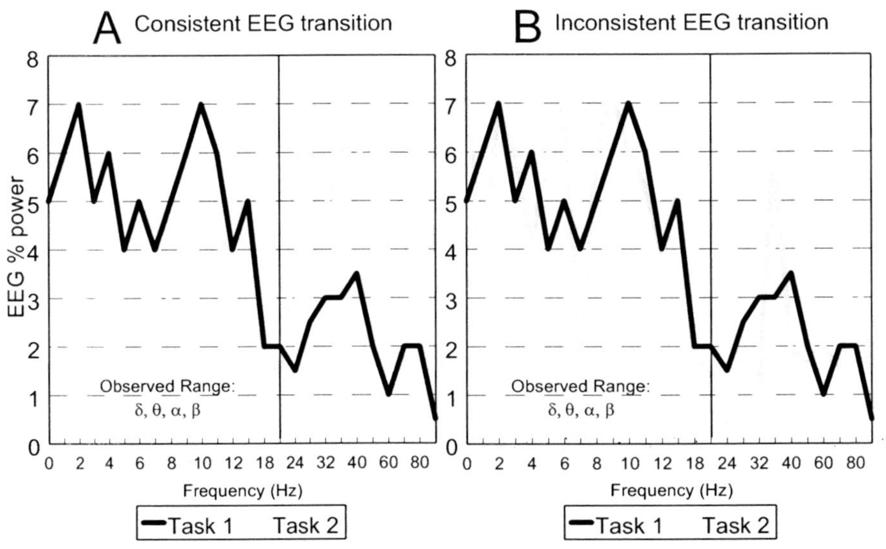

Figure 3: EEG Power Spectrum at Two Cognitive Tasks

The term "consistent" is best defined by looking at mean differences of power spectra from task-to-task (Figure 4). In Figure 4-A this difference is mostly positive at lower frequencies and mostly negative at higher frequencies. In Figure 4-B the power differences are scattered below and above the frequency axis. Visually, a consistent shift between two tasks will be presented by an uninterrupted domain (Figure 4-A) while an inconsistent shift would result in sporadic power changes along the EEG spectrum as in Figure 4-B.

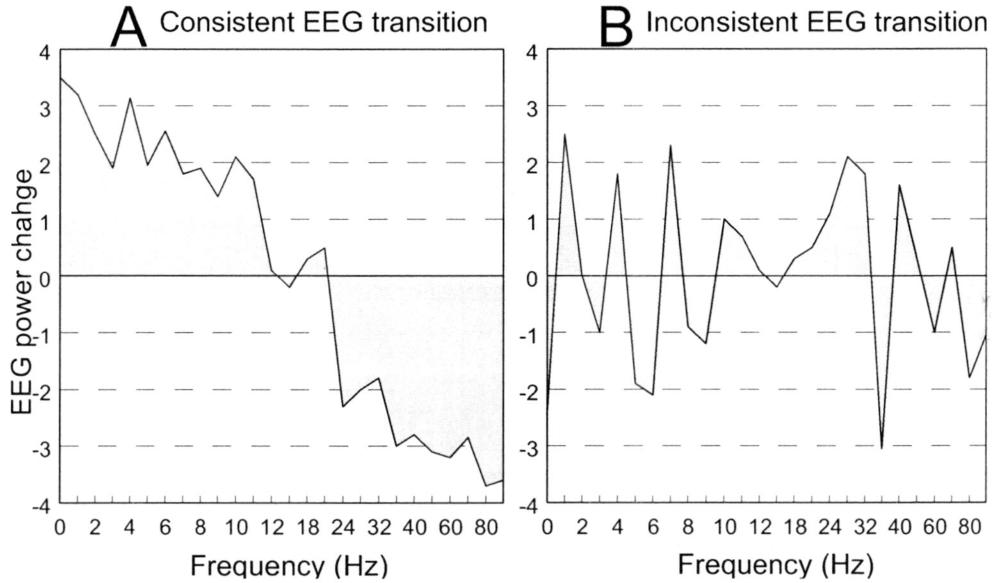

Figure 4: EEG Transition Consistency-Frequency Dimension

EEG spatial dimension - the location of electrodes: As opposed to the frequency dimension, the presentation of spatial EEG consistency is based on a discrete presentation of the power spectrum at several EEG channels. Figure 5 presents an 8-channel (electrode) setting and spatially consistent / inconsistent shifts between two tasks. The continuous spectrum at each electrode is integrated into [four in this example] frequency bands. A consistent shift would mean that at a particular frequency band most channels would display similar, unidirectional readings (Figure 5-A), while an inconsistent shift would result in scattered power changes across the electrode sites (Figure 5-B).

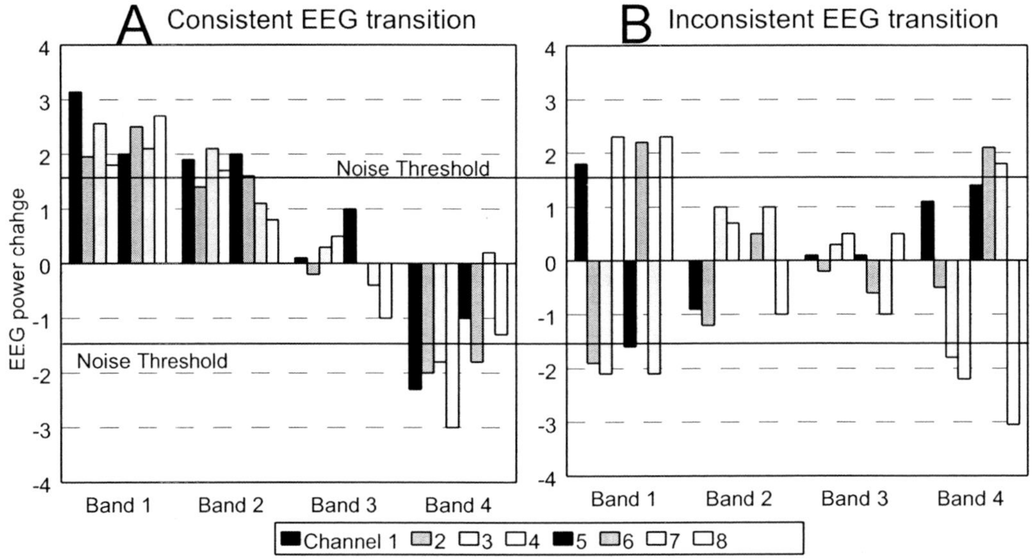

Figure 5: EEG Transition Consistency-Spatial Dimension

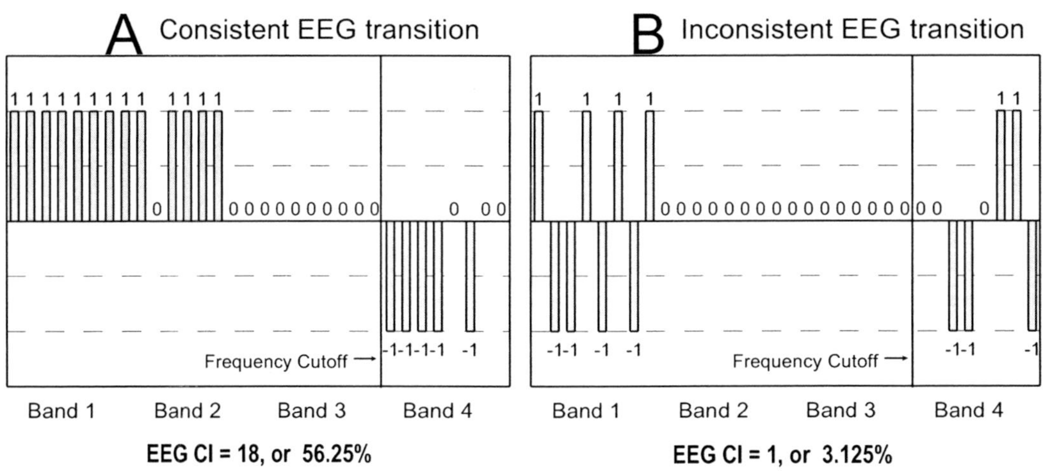

Figure 6: Computation of the EEG Consistency Index

Algorithmic Definition of the EEG Consistency Index: The concept of EEG consistency (Figures 3-5) was used to develop an algorithm that computes the CI, which works as follows:

1) Discrete spectra, including residual power, are calculated for all EEG channels.

2) *Power change distances* (PCD) between two contiguous tasks are computed for each EEG band and channel. Each PCD is normalized using the formula $PCD = \dfrac{M1 - M2}{\sqrt{\dfrac{SD\,1^2}{N1} + \dfrac{SD\,2^2}{N2}}}$, where *M1* and *M2* are the mean powers at two contiguous tasks,

SD1 and *SD2* are their standard deviation, and *N1* and *N2* are the epoch counts at these tasks. Normalization allows changes in one channel/frequency band to be directly comparable to another.

3) PCD are filtered to eliminate changes below a "noise threshold". The *noise threshold*, presented by horizontal lines in Figure 5, works as follows: The PCD that are larger by an absolute value than the threshold are marked with 1 or –1 depending on their direction, while all PCD below threshold are marked by zero. In Figure 5 noise thresholds of $\pm$ 1.65 are presented by black lines. These thresholds transform the PCD of Figure 5 into a sequence of 1, 0, -1 that indicates, for each EEG band and channel, whether a significant power change was observed while the person shifted from one task to another. The filtered set of PCD is presented in Figure 6. Since the PCD have a distribution close to Student t-distribution, a threshold of 1.65 is equivalent to making an one-tailed t-test comparing the average EEG power at Task 1 and 2 at p=0.05. Once again, this is just an association provided to clarify our methods. No conclusions based on t-test or any other parametric technique are involved in the computation of the CI. The threshold value, although based on the normal distribution of EEG spectra, is adjustable and can be empirically derived from population data. Thus, further studies of normal and ADHD children may provide gains in specificity and sensitivity of the CI.

4) Intuitively, the shift from Task 1 to Task 2 would be consistent if most of the filtered PCD below some *cutoff frequency* are positive, while most of the indicators above this cutoff frequency are negative, or vice versa. In contrast, the shift would be inconsistent if the PCD vary greatly by magnitude and/or sign. Thus, Figure 6-A and 6-B present a consistent and an inconsistent EEG at a cutoff frequency between beta and high beta.

5) The final pass of the computation is a simple addition of the filtered PCD below and above the cutoff value: $CI = 100.\left|\frac{1}{N}\sum_{i,j}\delta_{ij}\right|\%, where\delta_{ij} = -1,0,1; N = i.j$

For example, in Figure 6-A, we have a sum of 13 below the cutoff and a sum of –5 above the cutoff. Reversing the sign of PCD above the cutoff, the CI of the consistent shift presented in Figure6-A will be 18. In contrast the CI of the inconsistent shift in Figure 6-B will be 1 (0 below the cutoff and –1 above the cutoff). The maximum CI equals the number of EEG channels multiplied by the number of EEG bands used during spectrum discretization. For example, with 8-channel EEG equipment and 4 bands the CI ranges from 0 to 32. In order to make the results comparable across different experiments, the CI is expressed in terms of percentage from its maximum value. For example, the CI in Figure 6-A is 56.25%, while in Figure 6-B it is 3.125%.

Results

The CI clearly separated ADHD from control subjects, demonstrating consistent findings from all studies involving different subjects, different age groups, different sexes, and data collected by different research assistants. Specifically, meta-analysis of variance with independent factors ADHD vs. Control, Gender and Age group revealed that: a) The average CI of ADHD subjects was 29% vs. 50% for controls, $F = 43.7$, $p < .0001$; b) There was a significant Gender effect with males having a higher CI, $F = 4.1$, $p < .05$; c) There was an age trend with younger subjects having higher CI, $F = 3.7$, $p = .06$, and d) There was a significant interaction between ADHD-control and gender effects with males displaying stronger CI differences between ADHD and controls, $F = 5.6$, $p < .05$. On the basis of the CI, a logistic regression model classified correctly 82% of all ADHD subjects and 77% of all control subjects with an overall classification accuracy of 80%. This model was statistically significant, $p< .0001$. The classification power of the logistic model increased to 90% if only younger male subjects were included in the analysis. In addition, a Boolean decision-making rule based on the CI classified all but one of younger ADHD boys vs. their age-gender-matched controls, a 96% correct classification.

The results of these studies are reported in several publications [25], [40], [46], which have repeatedly demonstrated that a CI<40% is a sign of ADHD, and can be summarized as follows: a) The CI clearly differentiates ADHD from control subjects and correctly classifies over 80% of all subjects; b) discriminates, with almost no overlap, ADHD male subjects (age<16 years) from controls; c) correlates significantly with psychometric measures of ADHD; and d) is reliable over time and is positively influenced by methylphenidate. Thus, the CI is a highly significant discriminant of ADHD versus control subjects. In addition, with the specific subgroup of younger males it works extremely well on case-by-case basis classifying accurately almost all of these subjects in our pilot studies.

Summary Of Biological Manifestations Of ADHD-Related Dysregulation

After analyzing more than 160 EEG data matrices accumulated in 6 consecutive studies, we arrive at the following conclusions:

A: Attentional deficits influence EEG records in a different way at different levels of resolution in terms of time. More precisely: power of Theta and Theta/Beta ratio are measured on a temporal scale of the order of seconds; the Alpha Blockade Index is measured on time scale of one to two minutes; and the Consistency Index is measured on a time scale of the order of ½ hour.

B: Any one of the existing EEG measures is not powerful enough to make a clear distinction between individuals with and without ADHD.

The latter conclusion leads us to the idea that a carefully weighted combination of several measures would work best for assessment of ADHD. Thus, in the next section we discuss a sequential stochastic model using Bayesian inference to combine psychometric and EEG measures in a single assessment of ADHD. In general, this procedure is especially useful in situations where there is no single conclusive assessment, but a number of imperfect tests that marginally address the outcome of interest are available. In addition, this procedure is capable of superior handling of missing data, a very important feature in any practical situation.

Sequential Psycho-Physiological Assessment of ADHD

The diagnosis of many mental health disorders can be difficult and controversial to make, primarily because the majority of diagnostic approaches to mental disorders are based upon subjective reports of symptoms. Although almost all mental disorders are considered to be manifestations of biological, psychological, and environmental components within one individual, all of these domains are rarely thoroughly assessed and simultaneously incorporated into the diagnostic process. Even if all domains are assessed, the evaluations often lead to incomplete or conflicting data or "gray zones," where the diagnosis is not clear, and where clinicians are forced to make a dichotomous diagnosis, based primarily upon their own subjective clinical judgment. This is a particular problem when diagnosing ADHD, since no laboratory or psychological test or battery is available that provides sufficient sensitivity and specificity of diagnosis. This problem is made more urgent by the fact that early recognition, assessment, and management of this condition can redirect the educational and psychosocial development of most children with ADHD, thereby having a significant impact upon the well-being of a child accurately diagnosed with ADHD. In this section we present a probabilistic method using a sequential Bayesian decision-making procedure, which allows the results of multiple tests to be combined in a single assessment that is more precise and with a smaller gray zone of unclassified cases than its individual components. The procedure is designed in a way that keeps the probability for a misclassification below certain pre-fixed level.

Gray Zone and Misclassification Rate of a Test

Let's assume that a test of a condition produces a certain score for each tested individual, and a higher score implies a greater likelihood of that condition, a lower score indicates that the condition is unlikely, and a score between certain numbers x, y indicates that the diagnosis is inconclusive. In this setting, the interval $[x, y]$ is the "gray zone" of the test. β is the relative size of the gray zone of our test, e.g. β is the probability that a person may remain unclassified after administering the test because his/her score is between x and y. Another important characteristic of the test is its probability for a misclassification α; in our setting α is the probability that a person with a high score would be classified as not having the condition, or a person with low score would be classified as having the condition. It is intuitively clear that α and β are inversely related – if we want to hold the misclassification rate α below a certain number, the likelihood that a person cannot be classified β increases. In other words, if we insist on certainty of the classification $(1- \alpha)$, the percentage of cases β that cannot be classified with that certainty will increase. Thus at a fixed error rate α, a test with a larger gray zone probability β would be less comprehensive than a test with a smaller β. Consequently, if a combination of tests results in an assessment with a smaller than each individual test gray zone, while keeping the error rate below a fixed α, such a combination would be more comprehensive than each of its individual components.

Standardizing the Scores of Different Tests

In order to integrate the various study data from the psychometric tests and the CI results into a single assessment of ADHD, we first need to standardize the output of these tests using a previously reported methodology [59]. In order to do so, we translate the output of each test into a *probability for ADHD*. The idea is that at each step of the overall assessment, each subject receives a certain test score and the magnitude of this score depends on whether the subject has ADHD, as well as on the severity of the disorder. In other words, the probability of earning a certain score depends on the subjects' condition, ADHD or non-ADHD. In addition, each test has a suggested cutoff value, and scores greater (or lower) than this cutoff value are accepted as indicators of ADHD. Thus, for each test we can define a function that represents the conditional probability of earning the specified score given ADHD. In this chapter we use linear mappings of a test score into a [conditional] probability ranging from 0 to 1 with the test cutoff value mapped to 0.5, and the test maximal (or minimal) value indicating ADHD mapped to 1. If the test has a gray zone, then the entire gray zone is mapped to a probability of 0.5. Several examples will clarify the test score standardization:

1. ADHD-Symptom Inventory [25]: The score on the ADHD-SI ranges from 0 to 36 with scores >12 indicating ADHD. The mapping formula is then: $$\begin{cases} x \le 12 & P(ADHD \mid x) = \dfrac{x}{24} \\ x > 12 & P(ADHD \mid x) = \dfrac{x}{48} + \dfrac{1}{4} \end{cases}$$
2. DuPaul AD/HD Rating Scale-IV Inattentive Type [30]: The score ranges from 0 to 100 with scores >93 indicating ADHD. The mapping formula is then: $$\begin{cases} x \le 93 & P(ADHD \mid x) = \dfrac{x}{186} \\ x > 93 & P(ADHD \mid x) = \dfrac{x}{14} - \dfrac{43}{7} \end{cases}$$
3. DuPaul AD/HD Rating Scale-IV Hyperactive/ Impulsive Type [30] ranges from 0 to 100 with scores >98 indicating ADHD. Thus: $$\begin{cases} x \le 98 & P(ADHD \mid x) = \dfrac{x}{196} \\ x > 98 & P(ADHD \mid x) = \dfrac{x}{4} - 24 \end{cases}$$
4. WURS scale [70]: The score ranges from 0 to 100 with scores >30 indicating ADHD. The mapping formula is then: $$\begin{cases} x \le 30 & P(ADHD \mid x) = \dfrac{x}{60} \\ x > 30 & P(ADHD \mid x) = \dfrac{x}{140} + \dfrac{2}{7} \end{cases}$$

5. The Alpha Blockade Index [59] ranges from 0 to 100% with a ABI<20% indicating ADHD. The mapping formula is then: $\begin{cases} x \le 20 & P(ADHD \mid x) = 1 - \dfrac{x}{40} \\ x > 20 & P(ADHD \mid x) = \dfrac{5}{8} - \dfrac{x}{160} \end{cases}$
6. The Consisteny Index [40] ranges from 0 to 100% with a CI<40% indicating ADHD. The mapping formula is then: $\begin{cases} x \le 40 & P(ADHD \mid x) = 1 - \dfrac{x}{80} \\ x > 40 & P(ADHD \mid x) = \dfrac{5}{6} - \dfrac{x}{120} \end{cases}$

In order to visualize these procedures, Figure 7 illustrated the standardization of the WURS and the CI.

Combining the Scores of Different Tests

Once the standardization of measures is completed, the results from the individual assessments in each study are linked following the Bayesian algorithm described by Robeva, et al [59] to calculate the combined probability for ADHD for each individual. The algorithm works as follows: At step 0, a prior probability for ADHD $P^0_{ADHD} = 0.5$ is assigned to each subject regardless of whether she is ADHD or control. Then, after the first test P_1^{test} = *P(ADHD / test score)* and $P_2^{test} = 1 - P_1$ are used to calculate a posterior probability P^1_{ADHD} for ADHD, using the formula:

$$P^1_{ADHD} = \frac{P_1^{test} \cdot P^0_{ADHD}}{P_1^{test} \cdot P^0_{ADHD} + P_2^{test} \cdot (1 - P^0_{ADHD})}$$

From here on the procedure is recursive - after each step the posterior probability becomes a prior probability for the next step; e.g. in the formula above P^0_{ADHD} is replaced by P^1_{ADHD}, P_1^{test} and P_2^{test} derived from the second test, etc [59]. In general, the posterior probability from step (n-1) is becomes a prior probability in step (n) and then posterior probability is computed for step (n) using the results from the assessment at step (n-1). At each step we may have a "gray zone" of a non-definitive assessment, however, at each sequential step the gray zone will become smaller and the final result is an assessment that is substantially more precise than any of its individual steps. The final outcome is a probability for ADHD assigned to each subject (0 to 100%), e.g. a placement of each subject on a continuum of disruption, with greater number and severity of disruptions resulting in placement on the high extreme end of the continuum. Since the final outcome is based upon the combination of all of the above psycho-physiological data, it has increased specificity/sensitivity beyond any single measure.

A: Calibration of the WURS Scale

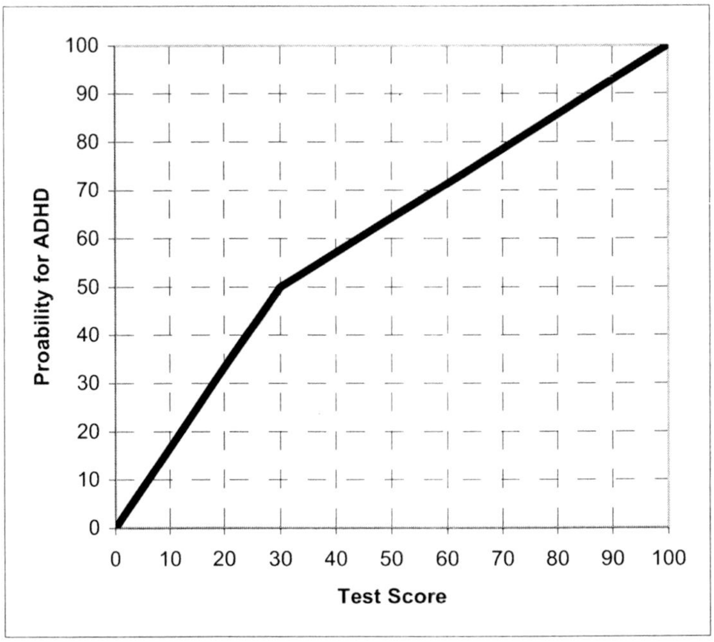

B: Calibration of the CI

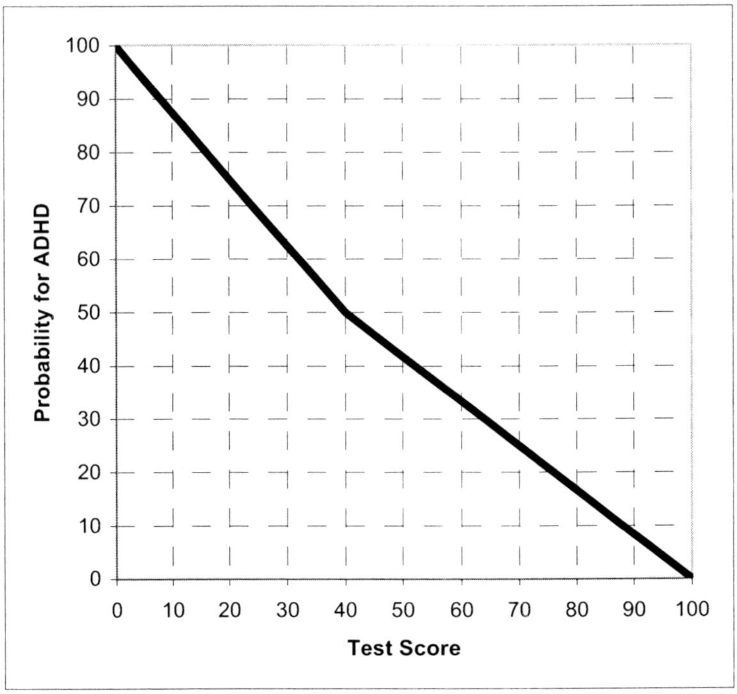

Figure 7: Examples of Test Score Standardization

Figure 8 presents the general structure of the sequential assessment of ADHD. Each module of the assessment has the unified internal structure presented in Figure 8A. The screening module would typically include input from demographic characteristics (e.g. age, gender) and several questionnaires screening for ADHD, such as ADHD SI, parent survey, teacher report, etc. The screening module produces an initial estimate of the probability for ADHD of the screened person even if only one of the questionnaires is completed. Each additional questionnaire will update and refine this estimate using our Bayesian model. The short-term behavioral assessment would typically include questionnaires and neuropsychological tests, which would allow for testing of the effectiveness of a medication, dose adjustment, etc. The EEG assessment would include several potential markers of ADHD, in particular our Consistency Index [40], the Alpha Blockade Index [59] and the Attentional Index (ratio of theta/beta, which is reported in the literature as a marker of ADHD [47]. The combination of the results from different tests within each module follows the Bayesian algorithm described above.

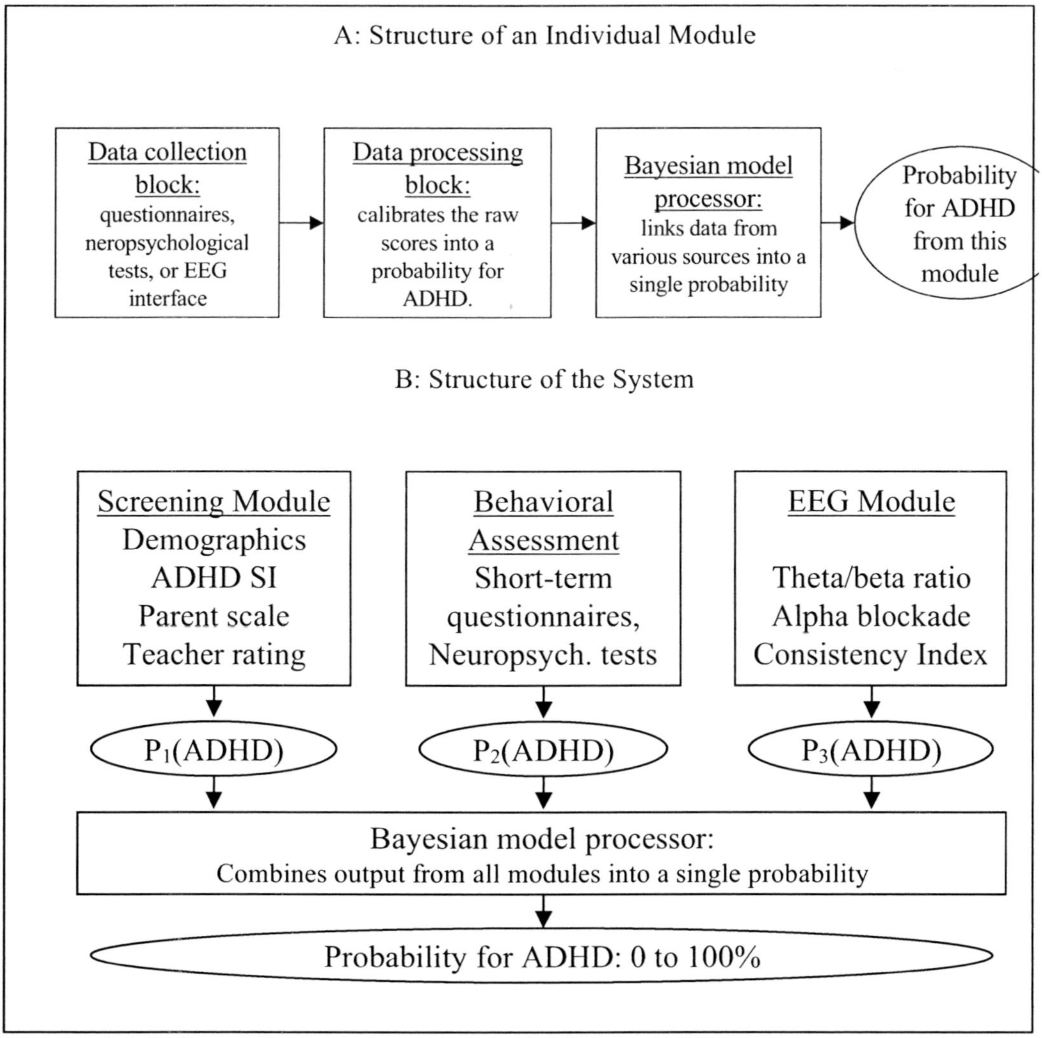

Figure 8: Modular System Evaluating a Person's Probability for ADHD

The result of each module is a probability for ADHD. Then, as presented in Figure 8B, the combination of results across all modules into a single assessment of ADHD.

The modular design of this system allows for a separate utilization of a screening, or screening + behavioral assessment modules, if EEG system is unavailable in some settings. This design also allows for inclusion of future ADHD screening technologies. For example, data from a motion detector recording the movement of a subject's head during a task could be included if proven valuable in the assessment of ADHD.

Results of Combining the Scores of Different Tests

We applied this method to the data from studies I-V described in Section 2, including behavioral rating scales and EEG assessments. Table 2 presents the probabilities for ADHD estimated by each test for ADHD vs. Control subjects. T-tests compare these probabilities within each study. As evident from Table 2, although a number of tests reach significance in most studies, a correction for the significance level accounting for multiple parallel tests would eliminate many significant results. The last column of Table 2 (Combined probability) presents the joint results from ADHD questionnaire plus EEG assessment within each study, computed using our Bayesian algorithm. It is evident that a combination of tests within a study generally provides a better ADHD-control separation than each individual test (in terms of a smaller p-value).

Table 2. Probabilities for ADHD within each study for each test

Study		ADHD-SI	WURS	DuPaul (I)	CI	Combined probability
I	ADHD	0.63	-	-	0.79	0.78
	Control	0.04			0.24	0.014
	p-level	0.0146			0.01	0.0009
II	ADHD	0.7	-	-	0.88	0.93
	Control	0.16			0.57	0.21
	p-level	0.0008			0.095	0.0024
III	ADHD	0.86	-	-	0.81	0.94
	Control	0.19			0.51	0.24
	p-level	0			0.0019	<0.0005
IV	ADHD	-	0.56	-	0.83	0.84
	Control		0.18		0.18	0.033
	p-level		0.0029		0.0019	<0.0005
V	ADHD	-	-	0.68	0.65	0.74
	Control			0.19	0.54	0.29
	p-level			<0.0005	0.19	<0.0005

Combining the Results from Different Studies

As described in Section 2, most studies alone had a small sample focused on a specific age/gender group, e.g. 8 boys ages 6-10. Thus, some analyses, such as gender or age comparisons, were not possible within any particular study. However, the standardization of each study results into the same scale, probability for ADHD, allows for combination of the data across studies. When standardized and combined, the data resulted in a clear separation between ADHD vs. non-ADHD groups in males below the age of 16 ($p<0.001$), males above the age of 16, ($p=0.015$), females below the age of 16, ($p=0.0014$), and females above the age of 16, ($p=0.0022$). Specifically, Table 3 presents the means and the standard deviations for each cross-section of the combined across studies population. The black bars in the second row of Table 3 indicate subject groups that cannot be differentiated at $P=0.05$ It is evident that the control population were quite homogeneous – there are no groups different in terms of their probabilities for ADHD. The ADHD population, however was not internally homogeneous: while boys and girls under the age of 16 were similar, and girls under 16 were similar to boys above 16, girls above 16 stand alone as a separate subgroup, which is somewhat closer to controls in terms of its probability for ADHD. Such previously unrecognized results were made possible by the use of cross-study standardization of the data.

Table 3: Cross-Sectional Probabilities for ADHD and Cross-Sectional Similarities

	ADHD				Control			
	Age < 16 years		Age > 16 years		Age < 16 years		Age > 16 years	
	Boy	Girl	Boy	Girl	Boy	Girl	Boy	Girl
Probability for ADHD (%)	80%	87%	93%	67%	23%	32%	21%	30%
Cross-Sectional Similarities	■	■						
		■	■					
					■	■	■	■

Finally, Figure 9 presents the process of increasing of the precision of assessment along the steps of the Bayesian model across all studies. This standard Box plot presents the median, 50% of the distribution, and outliers. It is evident that with the application of consecutive test the differentiation between ADHD and No-ADHD groups increases, achieving a best separation at the end of the procedure.

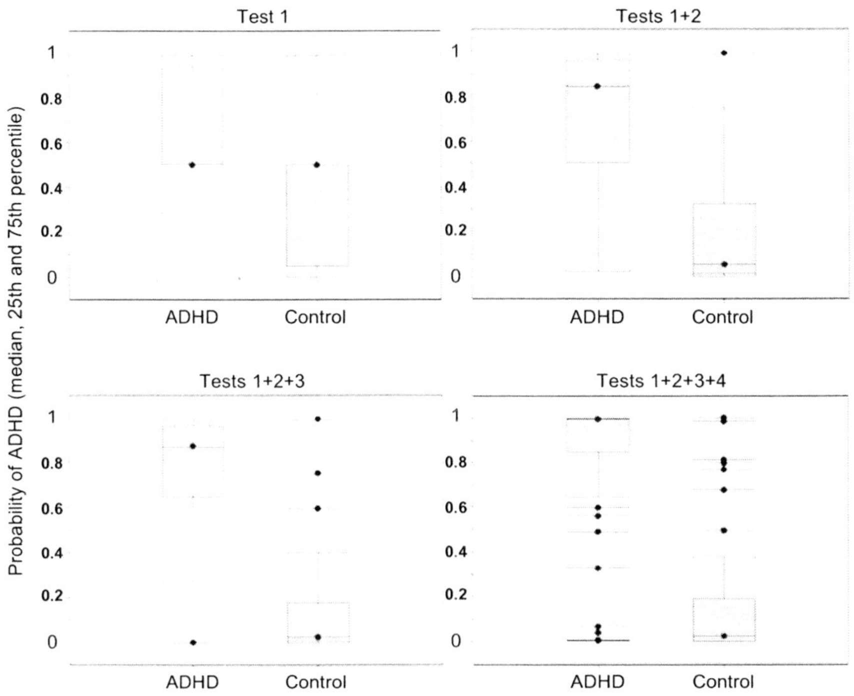

Figure 9: Sequential Improvement in the Assessment of ADHD with the Application of Consecutive Tests

Conclusion

This chapter presents several mathematical models and the results from six consecutive studies revealing various parameters of ADHD-related disruption at psychological, behavioral, and physiological levels. Overall, we feel that we have optimized both our data acquisition procedures with respect to EEG, our theoretical development of mathematical models of EEG consistency, and our choice and method of psychological and behavioral assessments. The first set of models discussed here refers to procedures maximizing the assessment of inconsistency in EEG waves on a temporal level of half-hour, minutes, and seconds. Various data sets (ours and by others) support the utility of each of these scales in various subpopulations. For example, the Consistency Index works best in boys below the age of 16, while the Alpha Blockade Index is a good marker of ADHD in college-age females. However, none of these individual measures, and none of the widely used psychometric measures, achieve a perfect assessment of ADHD when used in isolation, nor do they adequately evaluate the impact of a medication. For this reason we have developed and successfully pilot tested a sequential stochastic model combining behavioral and biologic data for classification of participants with and without ADHD, and demonstrated that several imperfect tests can successfully be combined into a comprehensive assessment that is more powerful than its individual components. Thus, we now have an integrated multi-method psycho-physiological ADHD assessment procedure, based upon a theoretical model of disruption of self-regulation and empirically supported by research experience and findings.

References

[1] Achenbauch, T.M., & Edelbrock, C. *Manual for the child behavior checklist*. Burlington, VT: University of Vermont Department of Psychiatry, 1983.

[2] Ackerman, P.T., Dykman, R.A., Oglesvy, D.M., & Newton, J.E.O. EEG Power Spectra of Children with Dyslexia, Slow Learners, and Normally Reading Children with ADD During Verbal Processing. *Journal of Learning Disabilities*, 27 (10), 619-630, 1994.

[3] Ahn, H., Prichep, L., John, E. R., Baird, H., Treptin, M. & Kaye, H. Developmental equations reflect brain dysfunctions. *Science,* 210, 1259-1262, 1980

[4] American Psychiatric Association. *Diagnostic and statistical manual of mental disorders* (4th ed.). Washington, DC: American Psychiatric Association, 1994.

[5] Anastopoulous, A.D., & Shelton, T.L. *Assessing Attention deficit/Hyperactivity Disorder.* New York, Kluwer Academic/Plenum Publishers, 2001.

[6] Armstrong, C.L., Hayes, K.M., Martin, R. Neurocognitive problems in attention deficit disorder. Alternative concepts and evidence for impairment in inhibition of selective attention. *Ann.N.Y Acad.Sci.* 931:196-215, 2001.

[7] Barkley, R.A. Grodzinsky G, DuPaul GJ: Frontal lobe functions in attention deficit disorder with and without hyperactivity: a review and research report. *J.Abnorm.Child Psychol*. 20:163-188, 1992.

[8] Barkley, R.A. *Attention deficit hyperactivity disorder: A handbook for diagnosis and treatment.* New York, Guilford press, 2002.

[9] Barkley, R.A. Attention deficit/hyperactivity disorder, self-regulation, and time: toward a more comprehensive theory. *J.Dev.Behav.Pediatr.* 18:271-279, 1997,

[10] Barkley, R.A., Fischer, M., Edelbrock, C.S., & Smallish, L. The adolescent outcome of hyperactive children diagnosed by research criteria: I. An 8-year prospective follow-up study. *Journal of the American Academy of Child and Adolescent Psychiatry, 29,* 546-57, 1990..

[11] Barkley, R.A., Guevremont, D.C., Anastopoulos, A.D., DuPaul, G.J., & Shelton, T.L. Driving-related risks and outcomes of attention deficit hyperactivity disorder in adolescents and young adults: a 3- to 5-year follow-up survey. *Pediatrics*, 92, 212-218, 1993.

[12] Berman T, Douglas VI, Barr RG: Effects of methylphenidate on complex cognitive processing in attention- deficit hyperactivity disorder. *J.Abnorm.Psychol.* 108:90-105, 1999.

[13] Berquin PC, Giedd JN, Jacobsen LK, Hamburger SD, Krain AL, Rapoport JL , Castellanos FX: Cerebellum in attention deficit hyperactivity disorder: a morphometric MRI study. *Neurology* 50:1087-1093, 1998.

[14] Biederman J: Attention deficit/hyperactivity disorder: a life-span perspective. *J.Clin.Psychiatry* 59 Suppl 7:4-16, 1998.

[15] Biederman, J., Newcorn, J., & Sprich, S. Comorbidity of attention deficit hyperactivity disorder with conduct, depressive, anxiety, and other disorders. *American Journal of Psychiatry*, 148, 564-77, 1991.

[16] Biederman, J., Wilen, T.E., Spence, T.J. & Faraone, S. Diagnosis and treatment of adult attention- deficit/hyperactivity disorder. In M.H. Pollack, M.W. Otto, J.F. Rosenbaum (Eds.) *Challenges in clinical practice: Pharmacologic and psychosocial strategies*, 380-407. New York: Guilford Press, 1996.

[17] Bresnahan, S.M., Anderson, J.W., Barry, R.J. Age-related changes in quantitative EEG in attention- deficit/hyperactivity disorder. *Biol.Psychiatry* 46:1690-1697, 1999

[18] Carter CS, Krener P, Chaderjian M, Northcutt C, Wolfe V: Abnormal processing of irrelevant information in attention deficit hyperactivity disorder. *Psychiatry Res.* 56:59-70, 1995.

[19] Castellanos FX, Lau E, Tayebi N, Lee P, Long RE, Giedd JN, Sharp W, Marsh WL, Walter JM, Hamburger SD, Ginns EI, Rapoport JL, Sidransky E. Lack of an association between a dopamine-4 receptor polymorphism and attention deficit/hyperactivity disorder: genetic and brain morphometric analyses. *Mol.Psychiatry* 3:431-434, 1998.

[20] Castellanos FX: Toward a pathophysiology of attention deficit/hyperactivity disorder. *Clin.Pediatr.(Phila)* 36:381-393, 1997.

[21] Clarke, A.R., Barry, R.J., McCarthy, R., Selikowitz, M. EEG analysis in Attention deficit/Hyperactivity Disorder: a comparative study of two subtypes. *Psychiatry Research, 81,* 19-29, 1998.

[22] Clinical practice guideline: diagnosis and evaluation of the child with attention deficit/hyperactivity disorder. American Academy of Pediatrics. *Pediatrics* 105:1158-1170, 2000.

[23] Comings, D.E. Genetic aspects of childhood behavioral disorders. *Child Psychiatry and Human Development*, 27, 139-150, 1997.

[24] Conners CK. *Conners' Rating Scales – Revised; technical manual.* North Tonawanda, NY: Multi-Health Systems, 1997.

[25] Cox DJ, Kovatchev BP, Morris JB, Jr., Phillips C, Hill RJ, Merkel L: Electroencephalographic and psychometric differences between boys with and without attention deficit/Hyperactivity disorder (ADHD): a pilot study. *Appl. Psychophysiol .Biofeedback* 23:179-188, 1998.

[26] Cox DJ, Merkel R L, Kovatchev B, Seward R. Effect of stimulant medication on driving performance of young adults with attention deficit hyperactivity disorder: A preliminary double-blind placebo controlled trial. *Journal of Nervous and Mental Disorders*, 188, 230-234, 2000.

[27] Crawford HJ, Corby JC, Kopell BS: Auditory event-related potentials while ignoring tone stimuli: attentional differences reflected in stimulus intensity and latency responses in low and highly hypnotizable persons. *Int.J.Neurosci.* 85:57-69, 1996.

[28] Crawford, H. & Barabasz, M. Automated EEG magnitudes in children with and without attention deficit disorder during neurological screening and cognitive tasks. *Child Study Journal*, 26, 71-86, 1996.

[29] DeGrandpre, R. *Ritalin nation: Rapid-fire culture and its transformation of human consciousness.* New York: Norton, 1998.

[30] DuPaul GJ, Power TJ, Anastopoulos AD, Reid R. *Manual for the AD/HD Rating Scale-IV.* New York: Guildford Press, 1998.

[31] Dykman, R.A., Holcomb, P.J., Oglesby, D.M., & Ackerman, P.T. Electrocortical Frequencies in Hyperactive, Learning-Disabled, Mixed, and Normal Children. *Biological Psychiatry,* 17(6), 675-685, 1982.

[32] Gittleman, R. Mannuzza, S., Shenker, R., & Bonagura, N. Hyperactive boys almost grown up: I Psychiatric status. *Archives of General Psychiatry, 42*, 937-947, 1985.

[33] Grodzinsky GM, Barkley RA: Predictive power of frontal lobe tests in the diagnosis of attention deficit hyperactivity disorder. *Clin.Neuropsychol.* 13:12-21, 1999.

[34] Grunewald-Zuerbier, E., Grunewald, G., & Rask, A. Hyperactive behavior and EEG arousal reactions in children. *Electroencephalographic Clinical Neurophysiology*, 38, 149-159, 1975.

[35] Heilman KM, Voeller KK, Nadeau SE: A possible pathophysiologic substrate of attention deficit hyperactivity disorder. *J.Child Neurol.* 6 Suppl:S76-S81, 1991.

[36] Hynd GW, Semrud-Clikeman M, Lorys AR, Novey ES, Eliopulos D, Lyytinen H: Corpus callosum morphology in attention deficit-hyperactivity disorder: morphometric analysis of MRI. *J.Learn.Disabil.* 24:141-146, 1991.

[37] Janzen, T., Graap, K., Stephanson, S., Marshall, W., Fitzsimmons, G. Differences in Baseline EEG Measures for ADD and Normally Achieving Preadolescent Males. *Biofeedback and Self-Regulation,* 20(1), 65-82, 1995.

[38] Jasper, H.H., Solomon, P., & Bradley, C. Electroencephalographic analysis of behavior problems in children. *American Journal of Psychiatry,* 95, 641-658, 1938.

[39] Klein, R.G. & Mannuzza, S. Long-term outcome of hyperactive children: a review. *Journal of the American Academy of Child and Adolescent Psychiatry,*_30, 383-387, 1991.

[40] Kovatchev B, Cox D, Hill R, Reeve R, Robeva R, Loboschefski T: A psychophysiological marker of attention deficit/hyperactivity disorder (ADHD)--defining the EEG consistency index. *Appl.Psychophysiol.Biofeedback* 26:127-140, 2001.

[41] Lahey BB, Applegate B, McBurnett K, Biederman J, Greenhill L, Hynd GW, Barkely RA, Newcorn J, Jensen P, Richter J, Garfinkel B, Kerdyk L, Frick PJ, Ollendick T, Perez D, Hart E, Waldman I, Shaffer D. *DSM-IV* field trials for attention deficit/hyperactivity disorder in children and adolescents. *American Journal of Psychiatry*, 151, 1673-1685, 1994.

[42] Lazzaro I, Gordon E, Whitmont S, Plahn M , Li W, Clarke S, Dosen A, Meares R: Quantified EEG activity in adolescent attention deficit hyperactivity disorder. *Clin.Electroencephalogr.* 29:37-42, 1998.

[43] Mann CA, Lubar JF, Zimmerman AW, Miller CA, Muenchen RA: Quantitative analysis of EEG in boys with attention deficit- hyperactivity disorder: controlled study with clinical implications. *Pediatr.Neurol.* 8:30-36, 1992.

[44] Mannuzza, S., Klein, R.G., Bonagura, N., Malloy, P., Giampino, T.L., & Addalli, K.A. Hyperactive boys almost grown up. V. Replication of psychiatric status. *Archives of General Psychiatry,* 48, 77-83, 1991.

[45] McDonald S, Bennett KM, Chambers H, Castiello U: Covert orienting and focusing of attention in children with attention deficit hyperactivity disorder. *Neuropsychologia* 37:345-356, 1999.

[46] Merkel RL, Cox DJ, Kovatchev B, Morris J, Jr., Seward R, Hill R, Reeve R: The EEG consistency index as a measure of ADHD and responsiveness to medication. *Appl.Psychophysiol.Biofeedback* 25:133-142, 2000.

[47] Monastra VJ, Lubar JF, Linden M, VanDeusen P, Green G, Wing W, Phillips A, Fenger TN: Assessing attention deficit hyperactivity disorder via quantitative electroencephalography: an initial validation study. *Neuropsychology* 13:424-433, 1999.

[48] Montagu, J.D. The hyperactive child: A behavioral, electrodermal and EEG investigation. *Developmental Medicine and Child Neurology,* 17, 299-305, 1975.

[49] Mostofsky SH, Reiss AL, Lockhart P, Denckla MB: Evaluation of cerebellar size in attention deficit hyperactivity disorder. *J.Child Neurol.* 13:434-439, 1998.

[50] National Institutes of Health Consensus Development Conference Statement: diagnosis and treatment of attention deficit/hyperactivity disorder (ADHD). *J.Am.Acad.Child Adolesc.Psychiatry* 39:182-193, 2000.

[51] Nigg JT: Is ADHD a disinhibitory disorder? *Psychol.Bull.* 127:571-598, 2001.

[52] Pennartz CM, Groenewegen HJ, Lopes da Silva FH: The nucleus accumbens as a complex of functionally distinct neuronal ensembles: an integration of behavioural, electrophysiological and anatomical data. *Prog.Neurobiol.* 42:719-761, 1994.

[53] Pliszka SR, McCracken JT, Maas JW: Catecholamines in attention deficit hyperactivity disorder: current perspectives. *J.Am.Acad.Child Adolesc.Psychiatry* 35:264-272, 1996.

[54] Pope AT, Bogart EH: Extended attention span training. *Proceedings of Technology 2001 Conference* 1:368-304, 1991.

[55] Pope AT, Comstock JR, Bartolome DS, Bogart EH, Burdette DW: Biocybernetic system validates index of operator engagement in automated tasks. In *Human Performance in Automated Systems: Current Research and Trends.* Mouloua M, Parasuraman R, Eds. Hillsdale, NJ, Lawrence Erlbaum Associates, 1994, p. 300-306.

[56] Popper CW: Disorders usually first evident in infancy, childhood, or adolescence. In *Textbook of Psychiatry.* Talbot JA, Hales RE, Yudofsky SC, Eds. Washington, DC, American Psychiatric Press, 1988, p. 649-735.

[57] Quay HC. Inhibition and attention deficit hyperactivity disorder. *Journal of Abnormal Child Psychology, 25,* 7-13, 1997.

[58] Raskin LA, Shaywitz SE, Shaywitz BA, Anderson GM, Cohen DJ: Neurochemical correlates of attention deficit disorder. *Pediatr.Clin.North Am.* 31:387-396, 1984.

[59] Robeva R, Penberthy JK, Loboschefski T, Cox D, Kovatchev B. Sequential Psycho-Physiological Assessment of ADHD: A Pilot Study of Bayesian Probability Approach Illustrated by Appraisal of ADHD in Female College Students, *Applied Psychophysiology and Biofeedback,* 28, 2003.

[60] Sagvolden T, Aase H, Zeiner P, Berger D: Altered reinforcement mechanisms in attention deficit/hyperactivity disorder. *Behav.Brain Res.* 94:61-71, 1998.

[61] Satterfield, J., Cantwell, D., Lesser, L., & Podosin, R. Psychophysiological studies of the hyperkinetic child. *American Journal of Psychiatry,* 128, 102-108, 1972.

[62] Satterfield, J., Lesser, L.I., Saul, R., & Cantwell, D. EEG aspects in the diagnosis and treatmetn of minimal brain dysfunction. *Annals of the N.Y. Academy of Science,* 205, 274-282, 1973.

[63] Satterfield, J., Schell, A., Backs, R., & Hidaka, K. A Cross-sectional and longitudinal study of age effects of electrophysiological measures in hyperactive and normal children. *Biological Psychiatry*, 19(7), 973-990, 1984.

[64] Schachar RJ, Tannock R, Logan G. Deficient inhibitory control in attention deficit hyperactivity disorder. *Journal of Abnormal Child Psychology*, 23, 411-438, 1993.

[65] Semrud-Clikeman M, Filipek PA, Biederman J, Steingard R, Kennedy D, Renshaw P, Bekken K: Attention deficit hyperactivity disorder: magnetic resonance imaging morphometric analysis of the corpus callosum. *J.Am.Acad.Child Adolesc.Psychiatry* 33:875-881, 1994.

[66] Sergeant JA. Hyperkinetic disorder revisited. In JA Sergeant (Ed.) *Eunnethydis: European approaches to hyperkinetic disorder* (pp 7-17). Amsterdam: JA Sergeant, 1995.

[67] Shaffer, D. Attention deficit disorder in adults. *American Journal of Psychiatry,* 151, 633-638, 1994.

[68] Sheer, D.E. Focused arousal and the 40 Hz EEG. In *The Neurophysiology of Learning Disabilities,* R. Knights & D. Baker (Eds.). University Park Press: Baltimore, MD.

[69] Stein, M.A. Sandoval, R., Szumowski, E., Roizen, N., Reinecke, M.A., Blondis, T.A., & Klein, Z. Psychometric characteristics of the Wender Utah Rating Scale (WURS): Reliability and factor structure for men and women. *Psychopharmacology Bulletin,* 31, 425-433, 1976.

[70] Ward MF, Wender PH, Reimherr FW: The Wender Utah Rating Scale: an aid in the retrospective diagnosis of childhood attention deficit hyperactivity disorder. *Am.J.Psychiatry* 150:885-890, 1993.

[71] Weiss, G. & Hechtman, L. *Hyperactive children grown up (2nd ed.).* New York: Guilford Press, 1993.

[72] Wikler, A., Dizon, J., & Parkes, J. Brain function in problem children and controls: Psychometric, neurological, and electroencephalograph comparisons. *American Journal of Psychiatry,* 127, 634-645, 1970.

[73] Wolraich ML, Baumgaertel A: The practical aspects of diagnosing and managing children with attention deficit hyperactivity disorder. *Clin.Pediatr.(Phila)* 36:497-504, 1997.

[74] Wolraich, M.L. & Baumgaertel, A. The prevalence of Attention Deficit Hyperactivity Disorder based on the new DSM-IV criteria. *Peabody Journal of Education,* 71, 168-186, 1996.

[75] Zametkin AJ, Nordahl TE, Gross M, King AC, Semple WE, Rumsey J, Hamburger S, Cohen RM: Cerebral glucose metabolism in adults with hyperactivity of childhood onset. *N.Engl.J.Med.* 323:1361-1366, 1990.

[76] Zametkin, A.J. & Rapoport, J.L. Neurobiology of attention deficit disorder with hyperactivity: where have we come in 50 years? *Journal of the American Academy of Child and Adolescent Psychiatry,* 26, 676-686, 1987.

In: Attention Deficit Hyperactivity Disorder Research
Editor: Michelle P. Larimer, pp. 189-205
ISBN 1-59454-156-6

Chapter VIII

Treatment of Attention Deficit/ Hyperactivity Disorder with Monoamine Oxidase Inhibitors from Childhood to Adulthood

Daniel Bailly[1] and Guillaume Vaiva[2]
[1]Institut des Neurosciences Cognitives de la Méditerranée UMR 6193 CNRS & Fédération de psychiatrie de l'enfant et de l'adolescent, Centre hospitalier universitaire Sainte-Marguerite, 270 boulevard Sainte-Marguerite, 13009 Marseille, France
[2]INSERM U513 & Centre d'Accueil et de Crise Pierre Janet, Centre hospitalier régional universitaire de Lille, Clinique Fontan, 6 rue du Professeur Laguesse, 59037 Lille cedex, France

Abstract

Several findings support the model of a multisystem dysfunction underlying ADHD pathophysiology: low dopaminergic tone could mediate overall symptom severity, abnormal noradrenergic tone impairment in attention, and serotoninergic activity impulsivity. In addition, studies have reported abnormal MAO activity in children with ADHD and in individuals with high impulsivity, ADHD with conduct disorder, and thrill-seeking personality characteristics. Although the stimulants are the most established treatment for ADHD, as many as 30 % of affected individuals do not respond or may not tolerate such treatments. In the same way, ADHD is a heterogeneous disorder with a considerable incidence of comorbid psychiatric disorders including conduct, substance use, affective, and tic disorders, and the question remains whether these complex conditions respond preferentially or not to different psychotropic agents. According to the data above mentioned, the MAOI antidepressants may be an alternative to psychostimulants in such patients. From this point of view, several studies have shown that the MAOIs may be effective in the treatment of children with ADHD, ADHD with tic disorders, and in the treatment of adults with residual ADHD symptoms. However, because of potentially severe reactions in most MAOIs due to dietetic restrictions and potential drug-drug interactions, their use as a mainline treatment of ADHD has been discouraged. The availability of new MAOIs (reversible MAO-A inhibitors) that do not require dietary restriction has recently given rise to new clinical trials. Several studies show that MAO-A inhibitors improve the condition of children and adults with ADHD. Clinical reports also confirm the effectiveness of MAO-A inhibitors in adolescents with ADHD and aggressive behaviors, and in adults with comorbid ADHD and addictive disorders. Although most reports are uncontrolled and nonblind studies, these findings show that MAO-A inhibitors may be important to consider in treatment ADHD individuals and suggest that they may become a viable alternative to psychostimulants. They also should prompt further research of reversible MAOIs in ADHD.

Introduction

Although the stimulants are the most established treatment for attention deficit / hyperactivity disorder (ADHD), as many as 30 % of affected individuals do not respond or may not tolerate such treatments (Spencer et al., 1996). Several possible reasons exist for lack of response.

ADHD is defined by a large variety of symptoms which can be divided into several major categories (inattention, hyperactivity, impulsivity). Different neurotransmitters may underlie these subtypes of ADHD, and some individuals may have no response or only a partial response to stimulants according to the symptom spectrum observed (Hunt, 1997; Pliszka et al., 1996). In addition, ADHD is a heterogeneous disorder with a considerable incidence of comorbid psychiatric disorders (Hornig, 1998; Pliszka, 1998). These include oppositional defiant / conduct and antisocial personality disorders, substance use disorders, mood and anxiety disorders, tic and learning disorders. These ADHD subgroups may also be underlain by differing risk factors and neurobiological dysfunctions, and, furthermore, may have differing pharmacological responses (Hornig, 1998; Hunt, 1997). Lastly, because of these comorbid psychiatric disorders, some individuals may have difficulty tolerating the side effects of stimulants (for example, ADHD individuals with anxiety or tic disorder may have a less satisfactory response to stimulants, which can increase anxiety or tics).

For these reasons there is a need for viable alternatives to stimulants. In the last two decades, a considerable research literature has emerged addressing the effectiveness, tolerability, and safety of other medications. Among these, medications traditionally considered antidepressants, including monoamine oxidase inhibitors (MAOIs), were the most studied.

It should be noted that MAOIs are not licensed for the treatment of ADHD, and their administration remains the personal responsibility of the prescribing physician. However, the lack of license does not limit physician prescribing of a drug for an off-label indication if rational scientific theory, expert medical opinion, or evidence from controlled clinical trials exist that the drug may be effective and safe for the unapproved condition.

Rationale for the Use of MAOIs in the Treatment of ADHD

Pharmacological Effects of MAOIs

MAOIs are a class of antidepressant defined by function rather than structure. All drugs in this class either reversibly or irreversibly inhibit the ubiquitous mitochondrial enzyme monoamine oxidase (MAO). This enzyme deaminates a variety of substrates, including serotonin, epinephrine, norepinephrine, tyramine, and dopamine. MAO exists in at least two forms (A and B), which differ in substrate preference, systemic distribution, and sensitivity to specific MAOIs. Both forms metabolize tyramine and dopamine. However, MAO-B predominates in the central nervous system and accounts for most of the dopamine metabolism in the striatum, while cortical dopamine is primarily metabolized by MAO-A (Glover and Sandler, 1986; Kalaria et al., 1988). MAO-A also metabolizes epinephrine, norepinephrine and serotonin. However that may be, MAO-B predominates in the serotonergic neurons, while MAO-A predominates in the catecholaminergic neurons (Levitt et al., 1982; Westlund et al., 1988).

The MAOIs differ regarding their selectivity. Some are nonselective, inhibiting both forms of the enzyme, others are selective, inhibiting MAO-A or MAO-B (Table 1). Experimental use of selective MAOIs has revealed functional differences between MAO subtypes. Selective MAO-B inhibitors have a greater effect on dopamine levels. They are less effective in depression, probably because they do not change the norepinephrine and serotonin concentrations, and are not sensitive to dietary tyramine. This suggest that the antidepressant and pressor effects of MAOIs are mediated by MAO-A inhibition (Pickar et al., 1981). Furthermore, MAO-A inhibitors increase the intra- and extra-neuronal concentrations of norepinephrine and serotonin preferentially, and have an antidepressant effect (Larsen, 1988). These functional differences between MAO subtypes were demonstrated in several trials using L-deprenyl (selegiline). At low doses (10-15 mg/day), selegiline is a selective MAO-B inhibitor, and shows no antidepressant effect and no tyramine pressor effect. At higher doses (30-60 mg daily), the drug is less selective, inhibiting both MAO-A and MAO-B, and does show significant antidepressant properties and may induce hypertensive crises by reacting with dietary tyramine (Mann et al., 1989; Schulz et al., 1989; Sunderland et al., 1985).

The MAOIs also differ regarding their reversibility (Table 1). The classic MAOIs are irreversible. Once the drug binds to MAO, the enzyme is effectively removed from the system. The resulting reduction in MAO activity persists for as long as two weeks after the drug has been metabolized, while new enzyme is synthesized. The long duration of irreversible MAOIs action is associated with a waste of selectivity and raises the potential for a number of dietary and drug interactions (Larsen, 1988; McDaniel, 1986). On the contrary, reversible MAOIs have a shorter duration of action, even if their elimination half-lives vary to a greater degree than do the classic agents and may be as long as 12-15 hours. They are also more selective and less sensitive to dietary interactions. The pharmacodynamic distinction between reversible and irreversible MAOIs was demonstrated in studies comparing the activities of tranylcypromine (irreversible, nonspecific) and moclobemide (reversible MAOI-A). Both are eliminated quickly, with half-lives of approximately 2 hours, but MAO activity returns to normal 24 hours after the discontinuation of moclobemide (Amrein et al., 1989).

Table 1. Pharmacodynamics and pharmacokinetics of monoamine oxidase inhibitors (from Bourin, 1993 and 1995)

MAOIs / selectivity	Reversibility	Tmax (hours)	t ½ (hours)	Vd (l/kg)
Nonselective				
Iproniazid	No			
Isocarboxazid	No			
Nialamide	No	0.5	1.5	
Phenelzine	No	2-4	1.2	
Tranylcypromine	No (2)	0.7-3.5	1.5-3.1	1.1-5.7
Selective MAO-A				
Clorgyline (1)	No			
Moclobemide	Yes	0.3-1	1.3-2.2	0.9-1.3
Toloxatone	Yes	0.3-1	1.2	1.2
Selective MAO-B				
L-Deprenyl (1)	No			
Pargyline (1)	No			

(1) Nonselective at higher doses
(2) Partially reversible in vitro
Abbreviations:Tmax – time of maximum plasma level;
t1/2 – elimination half-life;
Vd – volume of distribution

Administration of an MAOI initially increases the intracellular concentrations of both central nervous system and peripheral substrates. Chronic administration is associated with the return of these neurotransmitters levels to baseline, but with long-term changes in receptor populations (down-regulation) (McDaniel, 1986). This change in receptor density, similar to the one observed with the tricyclic antidepressants, is thought to mediate the clinical effects of MAOIs. Therefore, like the tricyclic agents, the MAOIs require 2 to 4 weeks of administration before producing clinical benefit.

Some data suggest that a threshold level of MAO inhibition is required for these drugs to be effective for depression. Correlations with symptom response to treatment with phenelzine suggest a clinical threshold at 60 % (Davidson et al., 1978) to 80-90 % platelet MAO inhibition (Ravaris et al., 1976; Robinson et al., 1973). In addition, biochemical studies with iproniazid detect significant changes in neurotransmitters and metabolites with greater than 80 % inhibition of platelet MAO (Ganrot et al., 1962). However, it is difficult to know whether platelet MAO inhibition reflects central enzyme inhibition, and the use of platelet MAO activity to assess adequate MAO inhibition is not applicable to newer selective MAO-

A inhibitors since platelet MAO is type B. Plasma level of 3,4-dihydroxyphenylglycol (DHPG) may be a better index of MAO inhibition (MAO-A) since DHPG principally reflects the norepinephrine intraneuronal disposition. In a clinical trial of phenelzine in depressed subjects, a good correlation was found between decrease in plasma DHPG level and symptom response (Robinson et al., 1983). More recent studies show that the MAOI-A, moclobemide, at a mean dose of 450 mg/day has an antidepressant effect similar to the one observed with the tricyclic agents, and that this daily dose results in a 50-60 % MAO inhibition (Berlin et al., 1990; Wiesel et al., 1985).

Neurobiology of ADHD

ADHD is most often thought of as a disorder of catecholamine underactivity. The catecholamine neurotransmitters norepinephrine and dopamine play crucial roles in attentional and intentional behaviors. Both neurotransmitters play a role in working memory, and both are involved in developmental neuronal plasticity (Voeller, 1998). In a synthesis of thinking on the neurobiology of ADHD, McCracken (1991) notes that all medications shown to be efficacious in ADHD share the properties of increased dopamine release and increased inhibition of the noradrenergic locus coeruleus. If studies using blood and urinary metabolites of brain neurotransmitters have been in general interpreted as inconclusive (Shaywitz et al., 1983; Zametkin and Rapoport, 1987a), some direct evidence from studies of cerebral spinal fluid in ADHD and normal children indicates decreased brain dopamine in ADHD children (Raskin et al., 1984). On the other hand, some correlations have been noted between monoamines and relevant behavioral dimensions (Castellanos et al., 1994), and the pathophysiology of ADHD appears more complex and varying according to the symptom spectrum observed.

From neurobiological, neurochemical, and neurobehavioral findings, Hunt (1997) has evolved a heuristic schema in wich the wide variety of ADHD symptoms is divided into four major categories, each of these categories being associated with a specific neurotransmitter dysfunction (table 2). In the same way, some other authors (McCracken, 1991; Mefford and Potter, 1989; Pliszka et al., 1996) have propounded a model of a multisystem dysfunction underlying the ADHD pathophysiology, including some degree of specialization in the role of the various neurotransmitter systems in behavior (Ernst et al., 1997): low dopaminergic tone could mediate overall symptom severity, abnormal noradrenergic tone impairment in attention, and serotoninergic activity impulsivity.These models also include many of the conditions frequently comorbid with ADHD (Table 2).

Since the MAOIs take effect on a large variety of substrates, they may be potentially useful in the treatment of ADHD. More particularly, as mounting evidence suggests both that impulse control disorders may be improved by agents with serotonin effects and that the putative dopamine component of the impaired behavioral inhibition symptom cluster (i.e., response selection abnormalities) might be addressed through the use of a psychostimulant in addition, Hunt (1997) suggests that agents with serotonin and dopamine-enhancing effects, such as the MAOIs, may be indicated in the treatment of this specific ADHD subtype.

Table 2. A categorical schema for ADHD symptoms (from Hunt, 1997)

ADHD subtype	Major symptoms	Comorbid conditions	Neurotransmitter dysfunction
Cognitive-processing deficit system	Deficit in selective attention and information processing	Learning disabilities, mental retardation	Hypoactivity of the dopamine system
Excessive arousal system	Increased motor activity, difficulties with sustained attention, impulsivity, aggression	Conduct disorder, mania	Hyperactivity of the noradrenergic system
Impaired behavioral inhibition system	Impulsivity, difficulties with response selection		Dysfunction of the serotonergic and dopaminergic systems
Deficient reward system	Difficulties in affect regulation leading to emotional remoteness and indifference to reward or punishment, faulty cognitive analysis and integration of information		Dopamine, endorphins and other neuropeptides

In addition, even if a direct relationship between platelet MAO activity and central nervous system MAO has not been established, several studies have reported abnormal platelet MAO activity in ADHD and related disorders. Therefore, studies have reported both high and low platelet MAO activity in children and adolescents with ADHD (Shekim et al., 1982, 1986; Young et al., 1980), and ADHD with conduct disorder (Bowden et al., 1988), and in individuals with high impulsivity (Shekim et al., 1984; Stoff et al., 1989), and thrill-seeking personality characteristics (Af Klinteberg et al., 1987ab; Perris et al., 1980). In a small study, Shekim et al. (1982) showed that treatment with d-amphetamine returned MAO activity to normal in children with ADHD. Whatever the significance of these findings (abnormal platelet MAO activity may be a manifestation rather than a biological marker of hyperactivity and impulsivity), they also suggest that the MAOIs may be helpful in the treatment of ADHD.

Evidence of the MAOIs Efficacy in the Treatment of ADHD

Studies in Children and Adolescents

To explore the basis for stimulant drug efficacy in ADHD, Zametkin et al. (1985ab) at the National Institute of Mental Health (NIMH) have compared psychostimulants with several medications that alter catecholamine metabolism. After inconclusive trials with pharmacological agents considered relatively selective in their immediate action and prompted by the hypothesis that MAOIs should have an effect on catecholamine systems comparable to that of psychostimulants, this group conducted a 12-week double-blind cross-over study, including a 2-week placebo washout between active drug periods, comparing the efficacy of MAOIs and dextroamphetamine in 14 boys, aged 8 to 12 years, with ADHD. Four of the children also met diagnostic criteria for conduct disorder, and four others had a specific developmental disability in reading or language. All 14 children received dextroamphetamine (mean daily maintenance dose: 13.2 +/- 2.5 mg), 6 received clorgyline, a selective MAO-A inhibitor (12.1 +/- 4.5 mg), and 8 received tranylcypromine, a nonselective MAO-A and MAO-B inhibitor (10.4 +/- 1.1 mg). The Conners Abbreviated Teacher Rating Scale and a 48-item Parent Questionnaire were completed weekly. A modification of the Continuous Performance Test (CPT) was given during placebo week 2 and treatment week 4. All patients were on a low-monoamine diet. Most children responded to both stimulant and MAOIs. The MAOIs had immediate, clinically significant benefit (indicating a different mechanism from that mediating antidepressant effect), and were clinically indistinguishable from dextroamphetamine. Sustained attention (measured by the CPT) was also significantly improved. Both dextroamphetamine and MAOIs produced persistent changes in monoamines and metabolites, which were most marked and consistent for norepinephrine and its metabolite 3-methoxy-4-hydroxyphenylglycol. However, these changes did not correlate in a consistent fashion with clinical response during drug treatment. Moreover, there was rapid clinical relapse following cessation of either treatment while the alterations in norepinephrine metabolism remained during the 2 weeks following drug, suggesting the independence of these changes from clinical state. Side effects, monitored with the Treatment Emergent Symptom Scale, were minimal with MAOIs. Drowsiness was the only striking side effect. Interestingly, in contrast with these findings, a study conducted by Donnelly (cited by Zametkin and Rapoport, 1987b) showed that L-deprenyl at doses of 15 mg/day (a dose thought to inhibit selectively MAO-B) had relatively little therapeutic effect in 14 hyperactive children. Other data also suggest that L-deprenyl is inferior to clorgyline and tranylcypromine in the treatment of ADHD (Rapoport et al., 1985).

If the NIMH group has discouraged the use of MAOIs as a mainline treatment of ADHD, this hesitancy was based on the strict dietary restrictions and potentially serious side effects of irreversible MAOIs. However, the data above-mentioned suggest that the therapeutic effects of MAOIs on ADHD are mediated by MAO-A. If reversible MAO-A inhibitors (which do not require dietary restriction) prove efficacious, they may become a viable alternative to psychostimulants.

Two open trials were conducted with the reversible MAO-A inhibitor, moclobemide. Trott et al. (1992) administered moclobemide at doses of 100 to 200 mg/day to 12 ADHD children (11 boys and 1 girl), aged 6 to 13 years, in a 4-week study. All children had previously discontinued treatment with methylphenidate due to side effects. A 40 % improvement in parental assessment of children's behavior as measured on the Abbreviated Conners Rating Scale occurred among those who received moclobemide as outpatients (N = 7), and a 31 % improvement among the inpatients (N = 5). There was also a general increase in concentration and attention span at the end of the trial (with a 117 % improvement in the concentration check test scores). Even if mood changes and explosive behavior continued to be present at a low level, the children's psychological status, as determined by the Clinical

Global Impression, improved from "seriously ill" to "moderately ill". Moclobemide was well tolerated by the patients, although 2 complained of mild gastrointestinal disturbances during the first week of treatment. In the second study, Antkowiak and Rajewski (1998) administered moclobemide at doses of 75 to 225 mg/day to 15 ADHD children (13 boys and 2 girls), aged 6 to 13 years, during a period of 8 weeks. Efficacy was being estimated with psychometric, questionnaire, and experimental methods.After 4 weeks, the drug was discontinued in 2 patients because of a complete lack of improvement or a deterioration in functioning. In the other 13 patients, a significant improvement in attention and hyperactivity functioning was observed at the end of the trial. Moclobemide was well tolerated, with rare and mild undesirable effects. In addition to these findings, one of us reported the use of toloxatone, an other reversible MAO-A inhibitor, in a 16-year-old female adolescent with ADHD and conduct disorder (Parquet et al., 1988). All previous treatments proved ineffective and she was out of school because of her behavioral disorders. Toloxatone was administered at a dose of 600 mg/day. Severity of symptoms was assessed by means of an observational scale, derived from the Conners Rating Scale (CRS) and adapted for adolescents and young adults. After 40 days of treatment, a significant improvement was observed in the quantification of all the dimensional problems inherent in ADHD as measured on the CRS. No aggressive behavior was observed. This improvement allowed her to return to school. Toloxatone was well tolerated, with no clinically significant undesirable effect.

One side effect of stimulant medications that receive serious attention from clinicians is the possible increase in motor or vocal tics. It is known that stimulant medication can exacerbate preexisting motor tics or result in the de novo onset of tics, including those observed in Tourette's syndrome, even if these findings are somewhat controversial (Barkley, 1988; Erenberg et al., 1984; Golden, 1974; Weiner et al., 1978). It has been estimated that about 1 % of children with ADHD who are treated with stimulants will develop a tic disorder and that in 13 % of the cases, the medication may exacerbate preexisting tics (Caine et al., 1984). Even if there is reassuring evidence that such exacerbations may have little long-term consequence (Castellanos et al., 1997), until more is known, most authorities advise against using stimulants in children and adolescents with tic disorders.

According to this, Jankovic (1993) reported the use of L-deprenyl in 29 children and adolescents (25 boys and 4 girls), aged 6 to 18 years, with comorbid ADHD and Tourette's syndrome. All patients were enrolled in this open trial after they became refractory to conventional treatments for ADHD. Deprenyl was administered at a mean daily dose of 8 mg during 3 to 15 months. Twenty-six patients (89.6 %) reported clinically meaningful improvement in their ADHD. There were no serious adverse side effects and only 2 patients (6.9 %) noted exacerbation of their tics. In a double-blind, placebo-controlled, cross-over study of L-deprenyl in 24 children with Tourette's syndrome and ADHD, Feigin et al. (1996) reported more moderate results: on the one hand, the improvement observed in ADHD as measured by means of the ADHD Rating Scale-IV appeared not statistically significant, while on the other hand, the improvement in Yale Global Tic Severity Scale scores was substantial. According to the fact that L-deprenyl does not seem to be the most effective MAOI in ADHD, these findings suggest that the MAO-A inhibitors, such as moclobemide, may be a safe and effective treatment in patients with comorbid ADHD and Tourette's syndrome.

Studies in Adults

The rate of persistence of ADHD into adulthood varies as a function of the study and the methods used to determine presence of the diagnosis. However, despite a decrease in ADHD symptom intensity, especially hyperactivity, over time, follow-up studies show that hyperactivity and attention deficit, as well as the full ADHD syndrome, persist into early adulthood in about 30-65 % of children with ADHD (Lie, 1992; Weiss and Hechtman, 1993). There may be even cases of unrecognized ADHD until adulthood. In adults, the symptoms of ADHD are seen in the workplace, and also have to be present in one other setting, such as at home, according to the DSM-IV critetria. Studies in adults with ADHD show that they have comparable educational and social histories, comorbid psychiatric diagnoses, and adaptive functioning impairments as do children with ADHD followed into adulthood (Murphy and Barkley, 1996a; Wender, 1995).

Just like in children, the management of ADHD in adults should combine pharmacotherapy with psychotherapeutic approaches. However, trials of pharmacologic treatments in adults with ADHD have produced mixed results due to considerable variability in diagnostic criteria, dosing, and response. If most studies were conducted with stimulants, there are also some trials with other medications, including MAOIs (Adler and Chua, 2002; Wender, 1998).

Two open trials in adults with residual ADHD symptoms were conducted with the MAO-B inhibitors, pargyline (N = 22) (Wender et al., 1983) and selegiline (N = 11) (Wood et al., 1983), administered in low doses. Both drugs produced moderate-to-marked improvement in about 60 % of the patients. More recently, Ernst et al. (1996) examined the clinical effects of low-dose (selective MAO-B inhibition) and high-dose (mixed MAO-A and MAO-B inhibition) selegiline treatment in 36 carefully screened ADHD adults, 24 men and 12 women (mean age: 37.6 +/- 7.1 years), without any other psychiatric diagnoses. The study used a double-blind randomized three-arm parallel-groups design with a 2-week placebo baseline followed by 6 weeks of treatment (placebo, 20 mg/day, or 60 mg/day selegiline) and then by 2 weeks of placebo post-treatment. Behavioral variables included self-rated scores on the Conners Abbreviated Teacher Rating Scale (Conners-ATRS) and performance on a Continuous Performance Task (CPT). Significant reductions in severity of symptoms from baseline to end of treatment were shown in the low-dose and high-dose selegiline groups. However, these changes were not significantly different from the decreases observed in the placebo group. Side effects were more severe in the high-dose selegiline group than in either of the two other groups. Twenty-seven subjects continued into an additional 6-week 20 mg/day or 60 mg/day selegiline period. The subjects who had been initially randomized to placebo were subsequently randomized to either low-dose or high-dose treatment. In addition to the behavioral variables, plasma monoamines and monoamine metabolites were assessed (blood samples were obtained at the end of the initial 2-week placebo baseline, first 6-week treatment, and second 6-week treatment periods) (Ernst et al., 1997). The results showed that selegiline treatment produced dose-dependent changes in monoaminergic plasma levels, and correlations were found between biochemical and behavioral measures: dopaminergic indices were associated with ADHD symptom severity (Conners-ATRS), noradrenergic indices with CPT performance, and serotonergic metabolism correlated with clinical changes.

These findings must be interpretated with caution because of methodological limitations and because studies in children showed that the MAO-B inhibitors had little therapeutic effect in ADHD. However, they support the model of a multisystem dysfunction underlying ADHD pathophysiology, and suggest that the response to MAOIs may differ according to the subtypes of ADHD.

Estimates of the comorbidity of mood disorders with ADHD in adults run from 16 % to 31 % (Barkley et al., 1996; Biederman et al., 1993; Murphy and Barkley, 1996b; Roy-Byrne et al., 1997; Tzelepis et al., 1995). In an early report, Wender et al. (1981) noted that the mood disorders accompanying ADHD in adults often appeared consistent with so-called "atypical depression". As such atypical depressions may respond exceptionally well to agents with potent dopaminergic activity, Wender et al. (1981) suggest that patients with comorbid ADHD and atypical depression may be selective responders to MAOIs, with benefit for symptoms of both disorders. However, pharmacologic treatment of adults with comorbid ADHD and mood disorders has not been systematically evaluated.

Even if there are conflictual approaches attempting to specify the nature of the relationship between ADHD and substance abuse, a number of studies report that ADHD is a frequent antecedent of or a risk factor for substance abuse in either adolescence or adulthood (Bukstein et al., 1989; Kaminer, 1992). More recent longitudinal prospective studies show that ADHD does not increase the exposure to drugs of abuse, but facilitates and accelerates the transition from drug use to drug abuse (Klein and Mannuzza, 1999), and that childhood ADHD predicts substance abuse if only at least one of the primary symptoms of ADHD (inattention, impulsivity or hyperactivity) is retained into adolescence or early adulthood (Kaminer, 1992). Therefore, studies find lifetime rates of alcohol use disorders ranging between 32 % and 53 % of adults with ADHD, whereas 8 % to 32 % may manifest some other form of substance use disorders (Barkley et al., 1996; Biederman et al., 1993; Murphy and Barkley, 1996b; Roy-Byrne et al., 1997; Shekim et al., 1990; Tzelepis et al., 1995).

Although there are no data to support the view that stimulants lead to an increased drug abuse, there is general agreement that the use of stimulants is somewhat dangerous in patients at particularly high risk for substance abuse (Gadow, 1981). According to this, open trials with the reversible MAO-A inhibitor, moclobemide, were conducted in adult patients with comorbid addictive disorder and ADHD.

Chamorro and Lopez (1995) reported the use of moclobemide in a 25-year-old male patient with comorbid alcohol dependence, pathological gambling and ADHD, and without any affective disorder. Treatment with moclobemide was initiated at a dose of 450 mg/day. During the 3 months of the follow-up, a remarkable change in the patient's behavior was observed: hyperactivity, impulsiveness, alcohol intake and pathological gambling disappeared, an adequate stress tolerance was achieved, and his concentration on tasks was improved. More recently, we described the use of moclobemide in a 27-year-old male patient with comorbid opiate addiction and ADHD, and without any associated mood or anxiety disorder (Vaiva et al., 2002). The patient was first successfully withdrawn using clonidine.

After 3 weeks of abstinence, he reported difficulties in his work. He could not tolerate the frustrations and daily stress caused by his work, which led to impulsive behaviors and frequent confrontations with his superiors and colleagues. He started use cannabis and sometimes heroin again during the weekends. Treatment with moclobemide was then initiated at a dose of 450 mg/day. After 1 week of treatment, the patient felt well, but he had headaches and was nervous. The dose of moclobemide was reduced to 300 mg/day. After 2 weeks, he reported that his work was now well executed. He did not relapse, but he was still nervous. Treatment with moclobemide was continued at a dose of 150 mg/day. An observational scale, derived from the Conners Rating Scale (CRS) and adapted for adolescents and young adults, was used to assess the responsivity of ADHD to medication. From day 0 to day 42 of treatment, the CRS scores showed a significant decrease in the quantification of all the dimensional problems inherent in ADHD. After this period, the patient was examined again every month during 2 years. Treatment with moclobemide was well tolerated. The patient reported significant improvements on his social, familial, and professional activities. No relapse in drug use was observed.

As suggested by Cocores et al. (1987), it is possible that drug use improves the condition of individuals with ADHD by correcting the neurobiological dysfunctions underlying ADHD. This hypothesis is consistent with the conceptual model of the self-medication theory of addictive disorders evolved by Khantzian (1985). In such a case, effective treatment of ADHD should cure these individuals of substance abuse. Another hypothesis is that ADHD (McCracken, 1991) and drug dependence (Koob and Bloom, 1988) may share a common neurobiological pattern, including more particularly a mesolimbic / mesocortical dopaminergic dysregulation. In ADHD (Bowden et al., 1988; Shekim et al., 1982, 1986; Young et al., 1980) as well as in drug dependence (Ades, 1994), data suggest that this deficit may be related to an abnormal MAO activity. If this is the case, MAOIs may be a treatment particularly well adapted to patients with comorbid substance dependence and ADHD. By enhancing the dopaminergic function, they should improve both disorders.

Conclusions

A total of 180 ADHD patients, 109 children or adolescents and 71 adults, have been included in MAOI treatment studies, including 3 controlled studies, 6 open trials, and 3 case reports. Although the results of these studies are inconsistent, they bring some interesting data.

The comparison between studies with selective MAO-B inhibitors and studies with selective MAO-A or mixed MAO-A / MAO-B inhibitors suggests that the therapeutic effects of MAOIs on ADHD are mediated by MAO-A. This is all the more interesting because the new reversible selective MAO-A inhibitors, such as moclobemide and toloxatone, are more safe and do not require dietary restriction. In addition, the MAO-A inhibitors seem to have clinically significant benefit at relatively low doses (moclobemide appears to be most effective when used at a dose of 150 mg daily).

If the mechanism of action of MAOIs on ADHD is still unknown, the short delay and low doses required to obtain a therapeutic effect suggest a different mechanism from that mediating antidepressant effect. The results of the studies including measurement of plasma and urinary monoamines and metabolites also indicate that the functional alterations of the activity of dopamine, serotonin and norepinephrine systems are, together, crucial mediators of the therapeutic effect. By this way, future researches should include specific assessment of all the dimensional problems inherent in ADHD in order to determine selective responders to MAOIs and to help to get rational pharmacologic approaches to the complex symptom spectrum observed in ADHD.

In the same way, future researches should take comorbid psychiatric disorders into account. The available data suggest that the MAOIs may be particularly helpful in patients with comorbid ADHD and tic disorders or substance use disorders, that are conditions in which the use of stimulants may be somewhat dangerous. From a theoretical point of view, patients with comorbid ADHD and atypical depression may also be selective responders to MAOIs. Since ADHD patients with comorbid anxiety disorders, such as generalized anxiety disorder, may not respond satisfactorily to stimulants and the MAOIs have proved their effectiveness in anxiety states, it will be also interesting to examine their usefulness in such a condition.

In summary, this critical review shows that the MAOIs, and more particularly the new reversible selective MAO-A inhibitors, are important to consider in the treatment of ADHD patients and suggests that they may become a viable alternative to psychostimulants. These findings also should prompt further research, including controlled studies, in order to specify more closely their indications.

References

Ades J. Conduites de dépendance et recherche de sensations. In: Bailly D, Venisse JL eds. Dépendance et conduites de dépendance. Paris: *Masson* 1994; p. 147-166.

Adler LA, Chua HC. Management of ADHD in adults. *J Clin Psychiatry* 2002; 63 (suppl 12): 29-35.

Af Klinteberg B, Levander SE, Oreland L, et al. Neuropsycholocical correlates of platelet monoamine oxidase (MAO) activity in female and male subjects. *Biol Psychol* 1987a; 24: 237-252.

Af Klinteberg B, Schlling D, Edman G, et al. Personality correlates of platelet monoamine oxidase (MAO) activity in female and male subjects. *Neuropsychobiology* 1987b; 18: 89-96.

Amrein R, Allen SR, Guentert TW, et al. The pharmacology of reversible monoamine oxidase inhibitors. *Br J Psychiatry* 1989; 6 (suppl): 66-71.

Antkowiak R, Rajewski A. Administration of moclobemide in children with attention deficit hyperactivity disorder. *Psychiatr P*ol 1998; 32: 751-757.

Barkley RA. Tic disorders and Gilles de la Tourette syndrome. In: Mash EJ, Terdal LA eds. Behavioral assessment of childhood disorders (2nd edn). New York: *Guilford Press* 1988; p. 69-104.

Barkley RA, Murphy KR, Kwasnik D. Motor vehicle driving competencies and risks in teens and young adults with ADHD. *Pediatrics* 1996; 98: 1089-1095.

Berlin I, Zimmer R, Thiede HM, et al. Comparison of the monoamine oxidase inhibiting properties of two reversible and selective monoamine oxidase-A inhibitors moclobemide and toloxatone, and assessment of their effect on psychometric performance in healthy subjects. *Br J Clin Pharmacol* 1990; 30: 805-816.

Biederman J, Faraone S, Spencer T, et al. Patterns of psychiatric comorbidity, cognition, and psychosocial functioning in adults with attention deficit hyperactivity disorder. *Am J Psychiatry* 1993; 150: 1792-1798.

Bourin M. Les I.M.A.O. Paris: *Ellipses* 1993.

Bourin M. Antidépresseurs. In: Senon JL, Sechter D, Richard D eds. Thérapeutique psychiatrique. Paris: *Hermann* 1995; p. 299-325.

Bowden CL, Deutsch CK, Swanson JM. Plasma dopamine-beta-hydroxylase and platelet monoamine oxidase in attention deficit disorder and conduct disorder. *J Am Acad Child Adolesc Psychiatry* 1988; 27: 171-174.

Bukstein OG, Brent DA, Kaminer Y. Comorbidity of substance abuse and other psychiatric disorders in adolescents. *Am J Psychiatry* 1989; 146: 1131-1141.

Caine ED, Ludlow CL, Polinsky RJ, et al. Provocative drug testing in Tourette's syndrome: D- and L-amphetamine and haloperidol. *J Am Acad Child Psychiatry* 1984; 23: 147-152.

Castellanos FX, Elia J, Kruesi M, et al. Cerebrospinal fluid monoamine metabolites in boys with attention deficit hyperactivity disorder. *Psychiatry Res* 1994; 52: 305-316.

Castellanos F, Giedd J, Elia J, et al. Controlled stimulant treatment of ADHD and comorbid Tourette's syndrome: effects of stimulant and dose. *J Am Acad Child Adolesc Psychiatry* 1997; 36: 589-596.

Chamorro L, Lopez I. Treatment of the attention deficit disorder (residual type) with moclobemide. *Eur Psychiatry* 1995; 10: 112.

Cocores JA, Davies RK, Mueller PS. Cocaine abuse and adult attention deficit disorder. *J Clin Psychiatry* 1987; 48: 376-377.

Davidson J, McLeod MN, White HL. Inhibition of platelet monoamine oxidase in depressed subjects treated with phenelzine. *Am J Psychiatry* 1978; 135: 470-472.

Erenberg G, Cruse RP, Rothner AD. The effect of stimulant drugs on Tourette syndrome. *Neurology* 1984; 34: 84.

Ernst M, Liebenauer LL, Jons PH, et al. Selegiline in adults with attention deficit hyperactivity disorder: clinical efficacy and safety. *Psychopharmacol Bull* 1996; 32: 327-334.

Ernst M, Liebenauer LL, Tebeka D, et al. Selegiline in ADHD adults: plasma monoamines and monoamine metabolites. *Neuropsychopharmacology* 1997; 16: 276-284.

Feigin A, Kurlan R, McDermott MP, et al. A controlled trial of deprenyl in children with Tourette's syndrome and attention deficit hyperactivity disorder. *Neurology* 1996; 46: 965-968.

Gadow KD. Prevalence of drug treatment for hyperactivity and other childhood behavior disorders. In: Gadow KD, Loney J eds. Psychosocial aspects of drug treatment for hyperactivity. Boulder CO: *Westview Press* 1981; p. 13-70.

Ganrot PO, Rossengren E, Gottfries CG. Effect of iproniazid on monoamines and monoamine oxidase in human brain. *Experientia* 1962; 18: 260-261.

Glover V, Sandler M. Clinical chemistry of monoamine oxidase. *Cell Biochem Func* 1986; 4: 89-97.

Golden GS. Gilles de la Tourette's syndrome following methylphenidate administration. *Develop Med Child Neurol* 1974; 16: 76-78.

Hornig M. Addressing comorbidity in adults with attention deficit / hyperactivity disorder. *J Clin Psychiatry* 1998; 59 (suppl 7): 69-75.

Hunt RD. Nosology, neurobiology, and clinical patterns of ADHD in adults. *Psychiatric Annals* 1997; 27: 572-581.

Jankovic J. Deprenyl in attention deficit associated with Tourette's syndrome. *Arch Neurol* 1993; 50: 286-288.

Kalaria RN, Mitchell MJ, Harik SI. Monoamine oxidases of the human brain and liver. *Brain* 1988; 111: 1441-1451.

Kaminer Y. Clinical implications of the relationship between attention deficit hyperactivity disorder and psychoactive substance use disorders. *Am J Addict* 1992; 1: 257-264.

Khantzian EJ. The self-medication hypothesis of addictive disorders: focus on heroin and cocaine dependence. *Am J Psychiatry* 1985; 142: 1259-1264.

Klein RG, Mannuzza S. Importance de l'hyperactivité de l'enfance dans le développement des troubles liés à l'utilisation de substances. In: Bailly D, Venisse JL eds. Addictions et psychiatrie. Paris: *Masson* 1999; p. 107-122.

Koob GF, Bloom FE. Cellular and molecular mechanisms of drug dependence. *Science* 1988; 242: 715-723.

Larsen JK. MAO inhibitors: pharmacodynamic aspects and clinical implications. *Acta Psychiatr Scand* 1988; 345 (suppl): 74-80.

Levitt P, Pintar JE, Breakefield XO. Immunocytochemical demonstration of monoamine oxidase B in brain astrocytes and serotonergic neurons. *Proc Nat Acad Sci* USA 1982; 79: 6385-6389.

Lie N. Follow-ups of children with attention deficit hyperactivity disorder (ADHD). Review of literature. *Acta Psychiatr Scand* 1992; 368 (suppl 1): 1-40.

Mann JJ, Aarons SF, Wilner PJ, et al. A controlled study of the antidepressant efficacy and side effects of (-)-deprenyl. *Arch Gen Psychiatry* 1989; 46: 45-50.

McCracken JT. A two-part model of stimulant action on attention deficit hyperactivity disorder in children. *J Neuropsychiatry Clin Neurosci* 1991; 3: 201-209.

McDaniel KD. Clinical pharmacology of monoamine oxidase inhibitors. *Clin Neuropharmacol* 1986; 9: 207-234.

Mefford IN, Potter WZ. A neuroanatomical and biochemical basis for attention deficit disorder with hyperactivity in children: a defect in tonic adrenaline mediated inhibition of locus coeruleus stimulation. *Med Hypotheses* 1989; 29: 33-42.

Murphy K, Barkley RA. Attention deficit hyperactivity disorder adults: comorbidities and adaptive impairments. *Compr Psychiatry* 1996a; 37: 393-401.

Murphy K, Barkley RA. Prevalence of DSM-IV symptoms of ADHD in adult licensed drivers: implications for clinical diagnosis. *J Attention Disord* 1996b; 1: 147-161.

Parquet PJ, Servant D, Bailly D, et al. Inhibiteur de la monoamine oxydase dans le traitement du trouble déficitaire de l'attention – type résiduel. A propos d'une observation. *L'Encéphale* 1988; XIV: 4439-441.

Perris C, Jacobsson L, von Knorring L, et al. Enzymes related to biogenic amine metabolism and personality characteristics in depressed patients. *Acta Psychiatr Scand* 1980; 61: 477-484.

Pickar D, Cohen RM, Jimerson DC, et al. Tyramine infusions and selective monoamine oxidase inhibitor treatment II. Interrelationships among pressor sensitivity changes, platelet MAO inhibition, and plasma MHPG reduction. *Psychopharmacology* 1981; 74: 8-12.

Pliszka SR. Comorbidity of attention deficit / hyperactivity disorder with psychiatric disorder: an overview. *J Clin Psychiatry* 1998; 59 (suppl 7): 50-58.

Pliszka SR, McCracken JT, Maas JW. Catecholamines in attention deficit hyperactivity disorder: current perspectives. *J Am Acad Child Adolesc Psychiatry* 1996; 35: 264-272.

Rapoport JL, Zametkin A, Donnelly M, et al. New drug trials in attention deficit disorder. *Psychopharmacol Bull* 1985; 21: 232-236.

Raskin LA, Shaywitz SE, Shaywitz BA, et al. Neurochemical correlates of attention deficit disorder. *Pediatr Clin North Am* 1984; 31: 387-396.

Ravaris CL, Nies A, Robinson DS, et al. A multiple dose controlled study of phenelzine in depression-anxiety states. *Arch Gen Psychiatry* 1976; 33: 347-352.

Robinson DS, Nies A, Ravaris CL, et al. The monoamine oxidase inhibitor, phenelzine, in the treatment of depressive-anxiety states. *Arch Gen Psychiatry* 1973; 29: 407-413.

Robinson DS, Johnson GA, Nies A, et al. Plasma levels of catecholamines and dihydroxyphenylglycol during antidepressant drug treatment. *J Clin Psychopharmacol* 1983; 3: 282-287.

Roy-Byrne P, Scheele L, Brinkley J, et al. Adult attention deficit hyperactivity disorder: assessment guidelines based on clinical presentation to a specialty clinic. *Compr Psychiatry* 1997; 38: 133-140.

Schulz R, Antonin KH, Hoffman E, et al. Tyramine kinetics and pressor sensitivity during monoamine oxidase inhibition by selegiline. *Clin Pharmacol Ther* 1989; 46: 528-536.

Shaywitz SE, Shaywitz BA, Cohen DJ, et al. Monoaminergic mechanisms in hyperactivity. In: Rutter M ed. Developmental neuropsychiatry. New York: *Guilford Press* 1983; p. 330-347.

Shekim W, Asarnow RF, Hess E, et al. An evaluation of attention deficit disorder – residual type. *Compr Psychiatry* 1990; 31: 416-425.

Shekim WO, Bylund DB, Alexson J, et al. Platelet MAO and measures of attention and impulsivity in boys with attention deficit disorder and hyperactivity. *Psychiatry Res* 1986; 18: 179-188.

Shekim WO, Davis LG, Bylund DB, et al. Platelet MAO in children with attention deficit disorder and hyperactivity: a pilot study. *Am J Psychiatry* 1982; 139: 936-938.

Shekim WO, Hodges K, Horwitz E, et al. Psychoeducational and impulsivity correlates of platelet MAO in normal children. *Psychiatry Res* 1984; 11: 99-106.

Spencer TJ, Biederman J, Wilens T, et al. Pharmacotherapy of ADHD across the lifecycle: a literature review. J Am Acad Child Adolesc *Psychiatry* 1996; 35: 409-432.

Stoff DM, Friedman E, Pollock L, et al. Elevated platelet MAO is related to impulsivity in disruptive behavior disorders. *J Am Acad Child Adolesc Psychiatry* 1989; 28: 754-760.

Sunderland T, Mueller EA, Cohen RM, et al. Tyramine pressor sensitivity changes during deprenyl treatment. *Psychopharmacology* 1985; 86: 432-437.

Trott GE, Friese HJ, Menzel M, et al. Use of moclobemide in children with attention deficit hyperactivity disorder. *Psychopharmacology* 1992; 106 (suppl): 134-136.

Tzelepis A, Schubiner H, Warbasse LH. Differential diagnosis and psychiatric comorbidity patterns in adult attention deficit disorder. In: Nadeau K ed. A comprehensive guide to attention deficit disorder in adults: research, diagnosis, treatment. New York: *Bruner / Mazel* 1995; p. 35-57.

Vaiva G, de Chouly de Lenclave MB, Bailly D. Treatment of comorbid opiate addiction and attention deficit hyperactivity disorder (residual type) with moclobemide. A case report. *Progress Neuro-Psychopharmacol Biol Psychiatry* 2002; 26: 609-611.

Voeller KKS. Attention deficit / hyperactivity disorder I: neurobiological and clinical aspects of attention and disorders of attention. In: Coffey CE, Brumback RA eds. Textbook of pediatric neuropsychiatry. Washington DC: *American Psychiatric Press* 1998; p. 449-482.

Weiner WJ, Nauseida PJ, Klawans HL. Methylphenidate-induced chorea: case report and pharmacologic implications. *Neurology* 1978; 28: 1041-1044.

Weiss G, Hechtman L. Hyperactive children grown up (2nd ed). New York: *Guilford Press* 1993.

Wender P. Attention deficit hyperactivity disorder in adults. New York: *Oxford University Press* 1995.

Wender PH. Pharmacotherapy of attention deficit / hyperactivity disorder in adults. *J Clin Psychiatry* 1998; 59 (suppl 7): 76-79.

Wender PH, Reimherr FW, Wood DR. Attention deficit disorder ("minimal brain dysfunction") in adults: a replication study of diagnosis and drug treatment. *Arch Gen Psychiatry* 1981; 38: 449-456.

Wender PH, Wood DR, Reimherr FW, et al. An open trial of pargyline in the treatment of attention deficit disorder, residual type. *Psychiatry Res* 1983; 9: 329-336.

Westlund KN, Denney RM, Rose RM, et al. Localization of distinct monoamine oxidase A and monoamine oxidase B cell populations in human brainstem. *Neurosci* 1988; 25: 439-456.

Wiesel FA, Raaflaub J, Kettler R. Pharmacokinetics of oral moclobemide in healthy human subjects and effects on MAO-activity in platelets and excretion of urine monoamine metabolites.*Eur J Clin Pharmacol* 1985; 28: 89-95.

Wood DR, Reimherr FW, Wender PH. The use of L-deprenyl in the treatment of attention deficit disorder, residual type. *Psychopharmacol Bull* 1983; 19: 627-629.

Young JG, Cohen DJ, Waldo MD. Platelet monoamine oxidase activity in children and adolescents with psychiatric disorders. *Schizophr Bull* 1980; 6: 324-333.

Zametkin AJ, Rapoport JL. Neurobiology of attention deficit disorder with hyperactivity: where have we come in 50 years ? *J Am Acad Child Adolesc Psychiatry* 1987a; 26: 676-686.

Zametkin AJ, Rapoport JL. Noradrenergic hypothesis of attention deficit disorder with hyperactivity: a critical review. In: Meltzer HY ed. Psychopharmacology. The third generation of progress. New York: *Raven Press* 1987b; p. 837-842.

Zametkin A, Rapoport JL, Murphy DL, et al. Treatment of hyperactive children with monoamine oxidase inhibitors. I. Clinical efficacy. *Arch Gen Psychiatry* 1985a; 42: 962-966.

Zametkin A, Rapoport JL, Murphy DL, et al. Treatment of hyperactive children with monoamine oxidase inhibitors. II. Plasma and urinary monoamine findings after treatment. *Arch Gen Psychiatry* 1985b; 42: 969-973.

In: Attention Deficit Hyperactivity Disorder Research
Editor: Michelle P. Larimer, pp. 207-226

ISBN 1-59454-156-6

Chapter IX

Stimulant Dosing in Adults with Attention Deficit Hyperactivity Disorder

Julian N. Trollor[1] and Perminder S. Sachdev

[1] School of Psychiatry, University of New South Wales and Neuropsychiatric Institute, Prince of Wales Hospital, Sydney.

Abstract

The authors review the literature on the efficacy of stimulants in adults, particularly in relation to dose. The pharmacokinetics and behavioural pharmacology of stimulants are examined in order to better identify factors that may assist in determine an appropriate stimulant dose for adults. The potential risks of using high doses of stimulant are explored.

Introduction

Even though it is often considered to be disorder of childhood, attention deficit hyperactivity disorder (ADHD) is recognized to persist well into adulthood. An age-dependent decline in retention of diagnosis [1, 2] has been noted, with approximately one-third of ADHD children experiencing ADHD symptoms persistent into adulthood. As the current cohort of children and teenagers treated with psychostimulants is maturing, increasing numbers are seeking continuation of treatment in adulthood. Popularization of ADHD has also resulted in a large number of individuals coming forward for assessment for the first time in adulthood. However, despite its increasing recognition, concerns remain regarding the validity of the adult diagnosis and the appropriateness of long-term management with psychostimulants.

[1] Correspondence: Dr J. Trollor, Neuropsychiatric Institute, Euroa Centre, Prince of Wales Hospital, Randwick, NSW 2031.Tel 61-2-93823763; Fax: 61-2-93823774; Email: Trollor@unsw.edu.au

Treatment with stimulants in adulthood raises a number of issues peculiar to this age group. In patients who are continuing treatment from childhood and in those commencing treatment for the first time as adults, an endpoint for stimulant treatment can be difficult to identify. The potentially open-ended nature of the treatment therefore provokes concerns about long-term exposure to stimulant medication, in terms of its efficacy, toxicity and the potential for psychological 'dependence' on the drug. Whether age renders individuals more susceptible to adverse effects is an unanswered question. As with the use of stimulants in adolescence, there is concern about the potential for abuse in adults. As society demands a 'quick fix' to most problems, there is pressure on both clinicians and patients to use the most rapidly effective treatment, often at the expense of development of non-pharmacological methods of symptom control (for example skills training or cognitive behavioural strategies). Despite these obvious issues, there are as yet no widely adopted guidelines for stimulant prescription and dosing in adults with ADHD.

In this chapter, we review the literature on the efficacy of stimulants in adults, particularly in relation to dose. The pharmacokinetics and behavioural pharmacology of stimulants are examined in order to better identify factors that may assist in determine an appropriate stimulant dose for adults. The potential risks of using high doses of stimulant are explored. We present some clinical guidelines for the use of stimulants in adults, focusing on dosing strategies. We define stimulant dose in units of milligram per kilogram per day (mg/kg/day), with low dose stimulant treatment as equal to or less than 0.5mg/kg/day of dexamphetamine or 1.0mg/kg/day of methylphenidate; high dose as between 0.5.0 mg/kg/day of dexamphetamine or 1.0-2.0 mg/kg/day of methylphenidate; and very high as equal to or greater than 1.0 mg/kg/day of dexamphetamine or 2.0mg/kg/day of methylphenidate. This arbitrary definition is derived from what are generally considered low, high and very high dose in the human and animal literature.

Context of Stimulant Use in Adults

The treatment of adult ADHD with psychostimulants is a growing phenomenon in clinical practice [3]. Most psychiatrists approach the prescription of stimulants with some trepidation. Stimulants are more commonly thought of as drugs of abuse rather than therapy, their long-term effects are not known and beneficial effects are hard to quantify objectively. When a patient makes a request for an increasing dose of the drug for the treatment of ADHD, it immediately arouses the suspicion of abuse or fear of adverse consequences. The problem is particularly acute in adults because the validity of the diagnosis of ADHD in adults is often questioned [4], the empirical basis for treatment is less well-established than for children [3, 4], the co-occurrence of drug abuse is common [5] and many patients have the additional diagnosis of personality disorder [5]. If one does accept the legitimacy of stimulant drug treatment in adult ADHD, is there a maximum daily dosage that should not be exceeded? The answer to this question needs to be sought from the efficacy data available, the neuroscientific information that underpins the treatment, the pharmacokinetics and bioavailability data on stimulants in adults in comparison with children and the differential likelihood of long-term side effects with higher doses.

In contradistinction to this clinical imperative is the limited data on the long-term use of psychostimulants in ADHD adults. The majority of studies are short or medium term and the issue of long-term tolerability and safety in adults has not been systematically addressed. As yet, there are no well-defined clinical guidelines regarding the doses of stimulants appropriate to the adult population. In Australia as in other parts of the world, the degree of regulation of stimulant prescription varies. In a phenomenon mirrored in other parts of the world, some Australian regulatory authorities notionally specify maximum permissible dose for use in adults but the regulations concerning stimulant prescription vary markedly from State to State. In the absence of clear guidelines, the titration and dosing process with stimulants is likely to vary considerably from clinician to clinician. This chapter aims to puts forward some of the theoretical and practical issues pertaining to stimulant dosing in adults with ADHD.

Studies of Efficacy

The treatment of ADHD with stimulants has been extensively investigated in children. A recent meta-analysis of the effect of methylphenidate in children included 62 randomised trials with a total of 2897 participants [6]. This review highlighted the short duration of most studies, which had an average duration of just over three weeks. Less than 15% of studies lasted longer than four weeks. Overall, the quality of these trials was assessed as low. Significant effects of methylphenidate were demonstrated as rated by teachers and parents of affected children. Positive effect sizes were seen for core features of ADHD, and were highest for hyperactivity and a combined inattention and overactivity rating. Other features such as aggression and conduct problems also showed a favorable response. For both teacher and parent estimates, there was no significant effect of methylphenidate demonstrable on separate attention ratings. The most prominent adverse effects were decreased appetite, insomnia and stomach ache. Across these trials, various dosing schedules were used and no conclusions could be drawn regarding relationship between dose and efficacy or side effects.

The effectiveness of stimulant treatment in adults with ADHD has been studied in a very limited manner. The efficacy of stimulants, in particular methylphenidate, in adult ADHD has been examined in at least seven studies (N=193 subjects), five of which were controlled, with an overall report of significant reduction of symptoms of ADHD [7]. Within these studies, there was considerable variability in response rates ranging from 25% to 73%. Some of this variability could be explained by differences in methodology between studies, such as poorly standardized diagnostic procedures, variability in stimulant dose, variable rates of comorbidity and differing methods in determining efficacy of medication. Convincing evidence for dose effect is not apparent in these initial studies. For example, the highest response rate in the fixed dose studies was seen in the study in which the lowest milligram per kilogram dose of methylphenidate was used [8]. The majority of these studies used a relatively low dose of methylphenidate. In four of the five controlled studies [8, 9, 10, 11], the average daily dose of methylphenidate used was 0.6 mg/kg and the average response rate was about 50%. A double-blind placebo-controlled randomized crossover trial by Spencer et al [12] utilized a variety of doses of methylphenidate in the same patient in a crossover design. An average daily dose of methylphenidate in the initial week of 0.51 mg/kg was used, followed by a second week dose of 0.75 mg/kg and a final week dose of 0.92 mg/kg. A significant effect of methylphenidate on ADHD symptoms was apparent as well as a significant interaction between time and drug response. An overall response rate of 78% (versus 4% for placebo) was observed as determined by a reduction of at least 30% in individual rating scale scores. Average one hour serum methylphenidate levels were 4.6 +/- 0.8 ng/mL, a level approximately half that of levels reported in pediatric samples. No clear association between serum level and clinical response was observed, although the authors argue for the prescription of higher doses on the basis of their overall high response rates. However, there is an obvious limitation of such data i.e. differential improvement rates in studies utilizing different doses in the same patients cannot be accepted as evidence that higher doses are more efficacious. For this to be shown, a direct head-to head comparison of different doses is required. Furthermore, the maximum dose examined in the Spencer et al study [12] was 1 mg/kg, thereby providing no information on even higher doses, the question that is raised by many clinicians and patients.

Higher doses were used in one open study treating predominantly children [13], with the daily dosage range for dexamphetamine being 1.6 to 3.6 mg/kg and for methylphenidate 1.4 to 7.7 mg/kg. The highest dose of dexamphetamine used in this report was 230 mg/day. The open nature of this report is a serious limitation and makes it an unlikely basis to guide therapy [14]. More recently, Bouffard et al [15] undertook a direct comparison of the efficacy of two different doses of methylphenidate in 30 adult ADHD subjects. This study was a double blind placebo crossover trial administered 10 mg of methylphenidate t.i.d. for two weeks, followed by 15 mg t.i.d. for two weeks. Following a one week washout, the process was repeated with either placebo or methylphenidate. Although significant improvements in ADHD symptoms were noted and there were significant improvements on computerised tests, there was no difference between the two doses.

There has been only one controlled trial of dexamphetamine in adult ADHD [16]. This randomized double-blind placebo-controlled trial (N=45; mean age 35.5 years, range 19-57 years) used a number of efficacy measures including self and relative's reports, clinician ratings and a general measure of psychological well-being. Compliance was monitored by urinalysis. Dexamphetamine was gradually increased over a three week period to 15 mg/day and then titrated by the patient up to a maximum of 30 mg/day in weeks four to six. Patients were reviewed at the end of week six. The mean titrated daily dose of the dexamphetamine was 23.85 mg (0.34 mg/kg). Although both groups improved significantly, the dexamphetamine group had lower self ratings of symptoms, and performed better on the Global Improvement Scale and measures of patient satisfaction. No patients ceased dexamphetamine as a result of side effects. This study and some anecdotal reports [17] support the proposition that dexamphetamine shares similar efficacy to methylphenidate in ADHD adults. Furthermore, the effective dose of dexamphetamine, if usage in children is a guide, is about one-half the methylphenidate dose [18, 19].

Horrigan et al [20] examined the effectiveness of mixed amphetamine salt (i.e. a mix of *d*-amphetamine and *l*-amphetamine) in an open label study of 24 ADHD adults. Treatment was commenced at 5 mg twice daily and titrated according to clinical response over a 16 week period. Fifty four percent of patients were classified as responders based on the clinical global impression improvement scale. Mean dose for responders was very small at 10.77 mg/day (0.14 mg/kg/day). Significant reductions in other measures of ADHD symptoms including the Copeland symptom checklist and Brown Attention Deficit Disorder scales were noted. This study provides preliminary evidence of the effectiveness of mixed amphetamine salt in adult ADHD.

The above studies suggest that chronic low-dose stimulant treatment is as effective in adult ADHD as in the childhood disorder, and that methyphenidate and dexamphetamine have similar efficacy. There is no empirical evidence to suggest that the use of high dose stimulant treatment in adults is superior to the average dose. There are however deficiencies in the literature including no head-to-head comparison of different stimulant doses, a lack of correlation of efficacy with serum stimulant levels, and in many studies a lack of comprehensive assessment of stimulant response on neuropsychological measures.

Behavioural Pharmacology

An examination of the behavioural pharmacology of dopaminomimetic drugs is instructive in determining the theoretical rationale for stimulant dosing. It has been hypothesised that stimulants such as methylphenidate and dexamphetamine have a biphasic response in animals. At lower doses these drugs are thought to reduce locomomotor activity, whereas at high doses they stimulate locomotor activity [21, 22, 23]. The dose of amphetamine that reduces activity in mice is in the range of 0.5 to 1.0 mg/kg, with activity levels increasing progressively with doses from 1.0 to 5.0 mg/kg [23]. The same biphasic response is seen in humans. However, the precise doses required to produce an increase in locomotor activity is uncertain and is subject to individual variation. The commonly used clinical dose of dexamphetamine (0.2 to 0.6 mg/kg) is in the same range as that of the hypo-locomotor animal model, and in the vast majority of patients does not produce significant increase in motor activity or agitation. Furthermore, as it is common practice to titrate the dose of stimulant medication at the time of initiation, (e.g. by introducing a dose of approximately 0.15 mg/kg/day of dexamphetamine or 0.30 mg/kg/day of methylphenidate), an increase in locomotor activity is unlikely to be seen.

The activation of postsynaptic dopamine receptors is thought to mediate most of the locomotor activating effects of stimulant medications. However, there is some debate regarding how the reduction in locomotor activity in hyperactive animal models and ADHD humans may be mediated. Both methylphenidate and dexamphetamine are indirectly acting stimulants. They augment catecholaminergic transmission through the blockade of catecholamine uptake at high affinity uptake sites. Dexamphetamine also promotes the release of newly synthesized dopamine from catecholaminergic terminals, the resulting dopamine being free to act on both presynaptic and postsynaptic receptors. Low-dose directly acting dopamine agonists such as apomorphine preferentially activate autoreceptors leading to a reduction in dopamine release. At high doses, this is overridden by stimulation of postsynaptic receptors [24, 25]. This differential responsiveness for directly acting dopamine agonists may explain why a biphasic behavioral response is seen with these agents. While the above observation has been used to argue for the biphasic response to stimulant medication

[26], there are several problems in applying this theory to indirectly acting stimulants such as methylphenidate and dexamphetamine.

The first difficulty with this theory is that not all investigators have demonstrated a reduction in locomotor activity in response to stimulant medication in animal models. Although supported by some studies of spontaneously active rodents [27], other investigators have demonstrated a failure of low doses of dexamphetamine to reduce locomotion scores in normal animals [28, 29]. However, in studies of rats made hyperactive with a neonatal dopaminergic lesion [30], support for a biphasic response is evident. An additional problem is that some electrophysiological studies of the effect of dexamphetamine suggest that there is no differential between its presynaptic and postsynaptic effects [25, 31] in the healthy state.

Another theory, put forward by Seeman and Madras [32], suggests that the differential effects of dexamphetamine are due to relative rather than absolute increases in synaptic dopamine levels. There is a differential effect of the drug on the resting level of extracellular dopamine compared to the increase it produces in pulsatile dopamine release associated with the nerve impulse [32]. In a drug-free condition, a nerve impulse produces a transient 60-fold rise in synaptic dopamine level above the baseline level of about 4 nM [33]. Methylphenidate and dexamphetamine, like cocaine, block the dopamine transporter, and dexamphetamine additionally has a direct dopamine releasing action [34]. These drugs therefore raise the baseline level of extracellular dopamine as well as the nerve impulse-associated rise. At low doses of stimulants in the rat, the rise in baseline values is about six-fold and that in the impulse-related values two-fold [35, 36]. The relative rise of dopamine, when expressed as a percentage of the baseline value, is therefore lowered by stimulants at low doses. At higher doses of dexamphetamine (> 1 mg/kg), the rise in baseline is 7 to 35-fold and that in the pulsatile output about 7-fold [37]. This differential effect of low and high doses may account for the biphasic response of stimulants. However, this explanation has been criticized by Ruskin et al [31] on the basis that the effect would require a differential sensitivity of presynaptic and postsynaptic dopamine receptors, which in their opinion does not exist.

It is possible that there is a differential effect of stimulants on dopamine neurotransmission in the healthy versus diseased states. Abnormalities of the structure and function of the basal ganglia in ADHD subjects [38] raises the possibility that in humans, as in hyperactive animal models, there may be alterations in pre or postsynaptic dopamine receptor sensitivity. Direct measurement of dopaminergic function in humans with and without ADHD would be required to consolidate this theory. However, the biphasic response model in ADHD continues to be a useful one. It could be argued that higher dexamphetamine doses (for example greater than 1 mg/kg) will have a stimulating effect and could possibly worsen the features of ADHD.

Functional Imaging Studies

The above argument can be further informed by recent work using positron emission tomography (PET) and single photon emission computerised tomography (SPECT). The effects of methylphenidate have been extensively studied in the brains of healthy adults. At oral doses of approximately 0.8 mg/kg, methylphenidate significantly increases the extracellular dopamine concentrations in the striatum [39]. Commonly used doses of methylphenidate result in blockade of at least 50% of dopamine transporters and the peak concentration of methylphenidate in the brain is reached after 60 min [40]. Plasma levels of methylphenidate correspond to the dopamine transporter occupancy [40]. Methylphenidate produces a 50% blockade at an oral dose of 0.25 mg/kg. Clinical doses of methylphenidate, therefore, can be expected to produce a greater than 50% occupancy which should be pharmacologically meaningful. At a dose of 1 mg/kg, 80% or greater occupancy should be expected [40], arguing against the value of further increases in clinical doses. In fact, adverse effects are likely to outweigh an advantage at very high doses. For example, it has been shown that for cocaine to produce a "high", at least 60% of the dopamine transporters must be blocked and this effect should occur and dissipate rapidly [41]. A similar effect would be anticipated for methylphenidate, giving a narrow therapeutic range in which to capitalize on clinical effects without inducing euphoria.

At optimal clinical doses in ADHD adults, methylphenidate has been shown to reverse relative increases in rCBF in the precentral gyrus and left caudate nucleus when compared with the baseline drug-free state [42]. These effects have been correlated with improvements on ADHD symptom ratings, suggesting that at usual clinical doses, methylphenidate produces a meaningful change in brain blood flow and associated motor behavior.

The *in vivo* effects of dexamphetamine administration on the brain are less well studied. Using FDG-PET to study the effects of an intravenous dose of 0.15 mg/kg of dexamphetamine in healthy humans, an increase in glucose utilization in subcortical limbic, frontal and cerebellar regions was observed [43]. Using a similar protocol, these authors noted inconsistent changes in glucose utilization in a small number of ADHD subjects during intravenous administration of dexamphetamine [44]. In healthy humans subjects studied with ^{11}C raclopride PET, a differential effect of amphetamine on striatal D_2 receptor availability has been demonstrated [45]. Amphetamine induced a significantly larger reduction in D_2 receptor availability in limbic and sensorimotor striatum than in other regions. Using SPECT and a specific dopamine transporter ligand, a reduction in availability of the dopamine transporter has been observed following four weeks of low dose (15mg/day) dexamphetamine treatment in ADHD adults [46]. These data suggest that low dose dexamphetamine in healthy subjects and in ADHD adults produces substantial and regionally specific alteration in dopaminergic neurotransmission and glucose utilization.

In summary, the functional neuroimaging data for methylphenidate and dexamphetamine suggests that acute and long-term dosing induces a significant alteration in dopaminergic neurotransmission. In addition, clear effects of low dose stimulants are apparent on cerebral blood flow and glucose metabolism. There is inadequate information to address differential effects of different doses of stimulant on these parameters. However, the evidence suggests a relatively narrow therapeutic window in which a stimulant medication produces beneficial cognitive effects without inducing euphoria. This observation would suggest that modest stimulant dosing should be the goal for the majority of patients.

The Question of Tolerance

Whether tolerance develops to chronic low dose stimulant administration is an important question. If such a phenomenon existed, there may be an argument for dose escalation when these drugs are used long term in clinical practice, or alternatively an argument for extended 'drug holidays'. Tolerance to some actions of stimulant drugs has been demonstrated in animal studies [47, 48] Long-term administration of dexamphetamine induces long-lasting down regulation of D_2 dopamine receptors in monkeys [49]. However, tolerance does not develop to all actions of these drugs [47]. There is experimental evidence that long-term use of dopamine agonists leads to a reduced density of D_2 receptors [50]. It is also possible that chronic stimulant treatment could alter the functional state of both D_1 and D_2 receptors, but the significance of this is not known [32]. Whether long-term changes in dopamine receptors occur when stimulants are used clinically in humans is unknown. Furthermore, the practical implications of any long-term changes in dopaminergic function remain unclear. In clinical practice, in parallel with other forms of psychotropic medication, both dexamphetamine and methylphenidate appear to maintain their effectiveness long-term. This is evidenced by continued effectiveness of medication across the developmental lifespan of children and, where appropriate, through to adulthood [18]. In a recent randomized, double-blind, placebo-controlled study of dexamphetamine treatment in children with ADHD, no evidence of tolerance to therapeutic effect was noted over a period of 15 months [51]. Clearly, such a study is of sufficient length to demonstrate tolerance if it was going to develop. In summary, the empirical basis is weak but clinical experience argues against the need for an escalation of dose with continuing treatment once the therapeutic effect has been established. Furthermore, based on the available data, chronic low dosing rather than an intermittent dose schedule appears to be a reasonable proposition.

Pharmacokinetics

The pharmacokinetic profile of orally administered stimulant medication is important in determining a rationale for dosing regimes. With oral administration, both methylphenidate and dexamphetamine are almost completely absorbed [52] with food having little impact on this process [53, 54]. When administered to adults, methylphenidate has a pharmacokinetic profile similar to that of children [52, 53], reaching a peak concentration in 1.5-2.5 hours and having an elimination half-life of 2-3.5 hours after oral administration of a single dose [52, 53, 55]. Non-linear kinetics have been observed with higher doses of methylphenidate [56, 57] and have also been proposed with repeated doses [58]. A proposed mechanism of the non-linear kinetics is saturation of presystemic metabolism [56] which may itself be stereoselective [59]. In theory, therefore, dose escalation carries the potential for sudden increase in adverse effects. Dexamphetamine typically takes 2-3 hours to reach peak concentration after a single oral dose [52], but with a half-life of approximately 7 hours is considerably longer acting than the equivalent measure for methylphenidate. In adults, as with children, serum concentrations of both stimulants may vary greatly between individuals. For example, one hour serum levels of methylphenidate may show inter-individual variation of up to thirty fold [53]. Peak serum levels of methylphenidate show less but still substantial inter-individual variation of between four to five fold [53, 54, 56]. Such variability may arise from a number of pharmacokinetic factors. Substantial differences in presystemic metabolism have been noted between individuals [56] Considerable inter-individual variability in plasma clearance is seen with both drugs [52]. Contrary to earlier suggestions [60], the latter does not appear to be less likely with methylphenidate. There are no reliable ways to assess individual differences in pharmacokinetics, leaving the clinician in a somewhat difficult situation. However, inter-individual differences in pharmacokinetics may be less dramatic when dose is adjusted for body weight [54]. Therefore, it would seem appropriate to use mg/kg as a general guide for determining maximum dose in individual patients.

Inter-individual variability might provide an argument for high dosing of individuals failing to respond to conventional dosing strategies. However, as with other psychotropics, there may be a number of reasons why an individual fails a particular trial of medication. Many of these reasons do not relate to pharmacokinetic considerations but may relate more to issues of accuracy of diagnosis, expectation of the degree of effect of medication on symptoms, poor compliance, and the experience of distressing side effects such as anxiety which may mask clinical benefit. Furthermore, it remains unclear whether clinical response to stimulant medication is related to peak brain concentration or the rate of increase of the drug in the brain [61]. Therefore, dose escalation purely on the basis of 'inadequate' response cannot be recommended. Whilst there may be an argument for examining the individual pharmacokinetics of stimulants in those patients failing to respond to conventional dosing strategies, this requires ready access to a laboratory with an established assay, and is not feasible in routine clinical practice. Furthermore, earlier data from children suggest that mean serum levels do not differ between drug responders and nonresponders [53]. Clearly, further study of the relationship between serum levels and clinical response to stimulants in adults is necessary in order to progress this issue.

Side Effects

The clinical dose of stimulants is significantly associated with side effects [62, 63], which range from those of mostly nuisance value such as dry mouth to more substantial ones such as psychosis. Examination of the side effect profile of stimulants and particularly the relationship of side effects to dose is an important step in determining whether high dose stimulant treatment caries a substantially higher risk. In this section, major side effects are reviewed and evidence for association with dose examined.

Anorexia and Insomnia

The ability of stimulants to produce anorexia and insomnia is well established. In clinical trials, as the dose of methylphenidate exceeds 0.5 mg/kg, the risk of appetite suppression and insomnia increases [63]. The mechanism of induction of anorexia is by no means clear. However, tolerance to this effect may develop [64] and may be mediated by both dopaminergic and noradrenergic effects [65]. Insomnia is often encountered in clinical practice and is minimised by reducing the dose and ensuring lack of proximity to sleep initiation. At low doses, severe anorexia and insomnia are rarely seen.

Tics

The ability of stimulant medications to induce tics and obsessive compulsive symptoms is widely known. Early concerns [66, 67] that stimulants were highly likely to induce tics have been generally unfounded [68]. Emergent tics are seen in less than 10% of children treated with stimulant medication, with the vast majority being transient in nature [69]. Short term trials of stimulant medication in children with comorbid tic disorder indicate that the risk of exacerbation of tics is low [70, 71] and that abrupt discontinuation of stimulant medications is unlikely to exacerbate tics [72]. Long term follow up of children with comorbid ADHD and tic disorder also suggest that chronic low dose stimulant treatment does not exacerbate tic disorder [72, 73]. A vexing question is whether the ability of stimulants to induce such phenomena is dose dependent. Within a small dose range, this appears to not be the case [74, 70]. However, there have been no studies of the emergence or exacerbation of tics in children given very high doses of stimulant medication. It could be argued that the risk of inducing tics in adults is low, given that the onset of tic disorder in early childhood. However, in treating ADHD adults as with ADHD children, comorbidity with tic disorders should be borne in mind. Low dose stimulant treatment remains the most prudent measure for adults, particularly when treating ADHD adults with comorbid tic disorder.

Cardiovascular Effects

The cardiovascular effects of stimulants, e.g. increases in pulse and blood pressure, have not been well-examined but they cannot be ignored at higher doses. Such effects will be of most importance in adults with pre-existing cardiovascular disease. There are no clear guidelines for managing this risk. However, good clinical practice dictates that cardiovascular parameters are regularly reviewed during stimulant prescription. Furthermore, as the risk is likely to increase with age, an argument can be made for minimising stimulant dose, particularly in at risk individuals (e.g., those with family history of essential hypertension or with personal risk factors for cardiovascular disease).

Effects on Seizure Threshold

Although stimulant medications are commonly believed to lower the seizure threshold, there is no data on the propensity of stimulant medication to induce seizures in adults. In children, the seizure risk in nonepileptic children treated with stimulants appears negligible. However, epileptiform activity on electroencephalography has been observed in approximately 15% of children with ADHD prior to treatment [75]. For children with both epilepsy and ADHD, low dose stimulant medication does not appear to significantly alter seizure control [76, 77]. However, the risk of convulsions may escalate with higher doses [62]. Given the risks associated with seizures, it would be prudent to adopt a low dose strategy to minimise any risk of the seizure induction, particularly in at risk individuals.

Abuse Potential

In adults and adolescents, the therapeutic use of stimulant medication is open to potential abuse. Adults with ADHD are known to have high rates of comorbid disorders, including substance use [5]. It is possible that stimulant medications, as a result of their potential to increased extracellular dopamine concentrations, could be powerfully reinforcing. Furthermore, there are parallels between the effect of stimulant medication and cocaine on the dopamine transporter. Indeed, repeated administration of methylphenidate in adult rats results in decreased latency for the acquisition of cocaine self administration and this effect is dose dependent [78]. Could such an effect encourage abuse of prescribed stimulant medication in humans? Direct evidence regarding the potential for abuse of prescribed stimulants in adults is lacking. Only a handful of case reports in which adults appear to have abused stimulants have been published. The intranasal and intravenous abuse of prescription stimulants (ones own or from a friend) has been reported [79, 80, 81] and oral abuse has also been recognised [82]. A number of factors are likely to determine the reinforcing effects of stimulants. These include the rapidity of rise of dopamine levels together with the extent of dopamine increases, the context in which the drug is taken and individual factors determining sensitivity to the drug [83]. In theory, prescription of large doses of stimulant medication for ADHD, could increase potential for abuse due to the extent of rise of dopamine levels seen with higher doses. Overall, the likelihood of abuse of prescribed stimulant medications is probably reduced by virtue of the pharmacokinetics of orally administered stimulant, regular clinical review of patients, controlled prescription and use of relatively modest doses. It remains unknown whether slow-release stimulant preparations are less likely to be abused in routine clinical practice.

An additional question, also relevant to adults being treated with stimulants is whether previously treated children are more prone to stimulant abuse as a virtue of their exposure to stimulant medication. A number of studies now support the position that stimulant prescription does not increase substance abuse later in life [84]. Furthermore, some longitudinal studies demonstrate reduced rates of substance use disorders in those ADHD subjects previously medicated with stimulants [85, 86, 87]. It is likely that treatment for childhood ADHD minimizes the risk of later development of psychiatric conditions including substance abuse. Whilst the relevance of this observation to adults being treated is unclear, future studies will assist in determining whether adequate treatment of ADHD in adults is associated with a reduction in psychiatric comorbidity, including risk of substance abuse.

Psychosis

Stimulants are recognized to sometimes cause a psychosis characterized by persecutory delusions and auditory and visual hallucinations [88]. The development of psychosis is usually associated with intravenous usage of high doses and has been modeled in an escalating dose 'binge' model of amphetamine psychosis in the rodent [49]. Although psychosis is rarely seen in the context of low-dose prescription stimulants for ADHD, the use of large or very large doses raises this is a distinct possibility. Additionally, there has been recent interest in the overlap between ADHD and bipolar disorder in children [89]. Given the propensity of stimulants to induce psychosis or possible euphoria at higher doses, the purported comorbidity raises concerns about the safety of prescription stimulants in this subgroup, particularly in view of the propensity of some manic episodes to be associated with psychosis.

Central Nervous System (CNS) Toxicity

CNS toxicity of stimulant medications is seen in animals given high dose amphetamine. Behaviours such as extreme vigilance, tracking of non-apparent stimuli, constant checking, hyperresponsiveness and grasping in midair have been reported in non-human primates treated chronically with high dose amphetamine [90]. Other behaviours noted in monkeys include posturing and other catatonic features [91]. Intermittent but escalating doses of amphetamine given to monkeys have been associated with behavioral sensitization, an effect observed even at low doses [92]. While fixed, but low dose chronic treatment may produce similar behaviors at a lesser severity [92], high doses are more likely to cause such behaviors. Although both amphetamine and methylphenidate sensitize stereotypic behaviors in rats, only amphetamine induces locomotor sensitization [93]. The differential effect has been postulated to reflect the different methods by which these two drugs increase synaptic dopamine [93], although the precise mechanism mediating the difference remains obscure. There is increasing interest in elucidating precise alterations in dopamine-stimulated signal transducing mechanisms that may be responsible for different components of behavioural sensitization [94]. Chronic and high dose amphetamine exposure in monkeys and rodents has also been reported to produce nigrostriatal toxicity [90, 95]. This can be prevented if an intermittent low dose schedule is used for amphetamine administration [96]. Of interest is the observation by Yuan et al [97] that methylphenidate appears to lack the dopaminergic neurotoxic effect shown by dexamphetamine in rats when examined 2 weeks after a high dose. The apparent contrast in neurotoxic potential of these two drugs at high doses suggests that dopaminergic efflux may not be the direct mediator of such damage [97]. The human implications of these laboratory findings remain unclear. However, in light of information regarding potential neurotoxic effects of high dose stimulants, careful review and strict justification of chronic stimulant treatment is necessary. In addition, stimulant doses should be restricted to the lowest effective doses.

Summary

In summary, there is clear evidence from studies of both children and adults that chronic low dose stimulant treatment is an appropriate, safe and effective treatment for ADHD. There are significant methodological limitations of the data for adults including the small number of studies in adulthood, lack of direct comparison of the effectiveness of different doses and the lack of high and very high dose studies. Examination of the behavioral pharmacology of stimulants suggests that chronic low stimulant treatment produces reduction in hyperkinesis without inducing euphoria. High doses cannot be justified on the basis of the pharmacokinetics of either methylphenidate or dexamphetamine and the potential to induce euphoria or other adverse effects. Given the chronic nature of stimulant treatment for ADHD, any such treatment must be well tolerated, with the perceived benefits outweighing the long-term risks. As high doses are associated with increased risk of both minor and major adverse events in humans, and behavioral sensitization and CNS toxicity at higher doses, a low dosing strategy should be adopted for ADHD adults. Whilst there is no clear upper limit that should be used in clinical practice, we recommend staying within the upper limits of 1 mg/kg for methylphenidate and 0.5 mg/kg for dexamphetamine. Clearly, this recommendation is not absolute and flexibility of dosing is required in some individuals who appear to only respond to higher doses. We recommend that these doses should be exceeded only after careful consideration and objective documentation of beneficial and adverse consequences. Furthermore, blood levels may be of some value if poor compliance or failure of the dose to produce adequate serum levels are being considered, as there is a direct relationship between blood and brain levels as well as dopamine transporter occupancy.

References

[1] Gittelman R, Mannuzza S, Shenker R, Bonagura N. Hyperactive boys almost grown up. I. Psychiatric status. *Archives of General Psychiatry* 1985; 42(10):937-947.

[2] Mannuzza S, Klein RG, Bonagura N, Malloy P, Giampino TL, Addalli KA. Hyperactive boys almost grown up. V. Replication of psychiatric status. *Archives of General Psychiatry* 1991; 48(1):77-83.

[3] Sachdev P. Attention deficit hyperactivity disorder in adults. [Review] [89 refs]. *Psychological Medicine* 1999; 29(3):507-514.

[4] Spencer T, Biederman J, Wilens T, Faraone SV. Is attention deficit hyperactivity disorder in adults a valid disorder?. [Review] [88 refs]. *Harvard Review of Psychiatry* 1994; 1(6):326-335.

[5] Biederman J, Faraone SV, Spencer T, Wilens T, Norman D, Lapey KA et al. Patterns of psychiatric comorbidity, cognition, and psychosocial functioning in adults with attention deficit hyperactivity disorder. *American Journal of Psychiatry* 1993; 150(12):1792-1798.

[6] Schachter HM, Pham B, King J, Langford S, Moher D. How efficacious and safe is short-acting methylphenidate for the treatment of attention deficit disorder in children

and adolescents? A meta-analysis.[see comment]. *CMAJ Canadian Medical Association Journal* 2001; 165(11):1475-1488.

[7] Wilens TE, Biederman J, Spencer TJ, Prince J. Pharmacotherapy of adult attention deficit/hyperactivity disorder: a review. [Review] [81 refs]. *Journal of Clinical Psychopharmacology* 1995; 15(4):270-279.

[8] Wood DR, Reimherr FW, Wender PH, Johnson GE. Diagnosis and treatment of minimal brain dysfunction in adults: a preliminary report. *Archives of General Psychiatry* 1976; 33(12):1453-1460.

[9] Wender PH, Reimherr FW, Wood DR. Attention deficit disorder ('minimal brain dysfunction') in adults. A replication study of diagnosis and drug treatment. *Archives of General Psychiatry* 1981; 38(4):449-456.

[10] Mattes JA, Boswell L, Oliver H. Methylphenidate effects on symptoms of attention deficit disorder in adults. *Archives of General Psychiatry* 1984; 41(11):1059-1063.

[11] Gualtieri CT, Ondrusek MG, Finley C. Attention deficit disorders in adults. *Clinical Neuropharmacology* 1985; 8(4):343-356.

[12] Spencer T, Wilens T, Biederman J, Faraone SV, Ablon JS, Lapey K. A double-blind, crossover comparison of methylphenidate and placebo in adults with childhood-onset attention deficit hyperactivity disorder. *Archives of General Psychiatry* 1995; 52(6):434-443.

[13] Kessler S. Drug therapy in attention deficit hyperactivity disorder. *Southern Medical Journal* 1996; 89(1):33-38.

[14] Block RW. Medication for attention deficit hyperactivity disorder: balancing art and science. *Southern Medical Journal* 1996; 89(1):95-96.

[15] Bouffard R, Hechtman L, Minde K, Iaboni-Kassab F. The efficacy of 2 different dosages of methylphenidate in treating adults with attention deficit hyperactivity disorder. *Canadian Journal of Psychiatry - Revue Canadienne de Psychiatrie* 2003; 48(8):546-554.

[16] Paterson R, Douglas C, Hallmayer J, Hagan M, Krupenia Z. A randomised, double-blind, placebo-controlled trial of dexamphetamine in adults with attention deficit hyperactivity disorder.[see comment]. *Australian & New Zealand Journal of Psychiatry* 1999; 33(4):494-502.

[17] Wender PH. Attention deficit hyperactivity disorder in adults. New York: *Oxford University Press*, 1995.

[18] Dulcan M. Practice parameters for the assessment and treatment of children, adolescents, and adults with attention deficit/hyperactivity disorder. American Academy of Child and Adolescent Psychiatry. *Journal of the American Academy of Child & Adolescent Psychiatry* 1997; 36(10:Suppl):Suppl-121S.

[19] O'Toole K, Abramowitz A, Morris R, Dulcan M. Effects of methylphenidate on attention and nonverbal learning in children with attention deficit hyperactivity disorder. *Journal of the American Academy of Child & Adolescent Psychiatry* 1997; 36(4):531-538.

[20] Horrigan JP, Barnhill LJ. Low-dose amphetamine salts and adult attention deficit/hyperactivity disorder. *Journal of Clinical Psychiatry* 2000; 61(6):414-417.

[21] Hornykiewicz O. Dopamine (3-hydroxytyramine) and brain function. [Review] [250 refs]. *Pharmacological Reviews* 1966; 18(2):925-964.

[22] Boissier JR, Simon P. [On the potentiation of DOPA effects by monoamine oxidase inhibitors]. [French]. *Psychopharmacologia* 1966; 8(6):428-436.

[23] Helmeste DM, Seeman P. Amphetamine-induced hypolocomotion in mice with more brain D2 dopamine receptors. *Psychiatry Research* 1982; 7(3):351-359.

[24] Carlson JH, Bergstrom DA, Walters JR. Stimulation of both D1 and D2 dopamine receptors appears necessary for full expression of postsynaptic effects of dopamine agonists: a neurophysiological study. *Brain Research* 1987; 400(2):205-218.

[25] Piercey MF, Hyslop DK, Hoffmann WE. Excitation of type II caudate neurons by systemic administration of dopamine agonists. *Brain Research* 1996; 706(2):249-258.

[26] Solanto MV. Neuropsychopharmacological mechanisms of stimulant drug action in attention deficit hyperactivity disorder: a review and integration. [Review] [290 refs]. Behavioural *Brain Research* 1998; 94(1):127-152.

[27] Steiner NO, Delay ER, Isaac W. Effects of drugs, age and illumination on response speed of squirrel monkeys. *Pharmacology, Biochemistry & Behavior* 1986; 24(3):503-506.

[28] Strombom U. Effects of low doses of catecholamine receptor agonists on exploration in mice. *Journal of Neural Transmission* 1975; 37(3):229-235.

[29] Taylor KM, Snyder SH. Differential effects of D- and L-amphetamine on behavior and on catecholamine disposition in dopamine and norepinephrine containing neurons of rat brain. *Brain Research* 1971; 28(2):295-309.

[30] Luthman J, Fredriksson A, Lewander T, Jonsson G, Archer T. Effects of d-amphetamine and methylphenidate on hyperactivity produced by neonatal 6-hydroxydopamine treatment. *Psychopharmacology* 1989; 99(4):550-557.

[31] Ruskin DN, Bergstrom DA, Shenker A, Freeman LE, Baek D, Walters JR. Drugs used in the treatment of attention deficit/hyperactivity disorder affect postsynaptic firing rate and oscillation without preferential dopamine autoreceptor action. *Biological Psychiatry* 2001; 49(4):340-350.

[32] Seeman P, Madras BK. Anti-hyperactivity medication: methylphenidate and amphetamine.[see comment]. [Review] [105 refs]. *Molecular Psychiatry* 1998; 3(5):386-396.

[33] Parsons LH, Justice JB, Jr. Extracellular concentration and in vivo recovery of dopamine in the nucleus accumbens using microdialysis. *Journal of Neurochemistry* 1992; 58(1):212-218.

[34] Wall SC, Gu H, Rudnick G. Biogenic amine flux mediated by cloned transporters stably expressed in cultured cell lines: amphetamine specificity for inhibition and efflux. *Molecular Pharmacology* 1995; 47(3):544-550.

[35] Sharp T, Zetterstrom T, Ljungberg T, Ungerstedt U. A direct comparison of amphetamine-induced behaviours and regional brain dopamine release in the rat using intracerebral dialysis. *Brain Research* 1987; 401(2):322-330.

[36] Kuczenski R, Segal D. Concomitant characterization of behavioral and striatal neurotransmitter response to amphetamine using in vivo microdialysis. *Journal of Neuroscience* 1989; 9(6):2051-2065.

[37] Gonon FG. Nonlinear relationship between impulse flow and dopamine released by rat midbrain dopaminergic neurons as studied by in vivo electrochemistry. *Neuroscience* 1988; 24(1):19-28.

[38] Castellanos FX, Elia J, Kruesi MJ, Marsh WL, Gulotta CS, Potter WZ et al. Cerebrospinal fluid homovanillic acid predicts behavioral response to stimulants in 45 boys with attention deficit/hyperactivity disorder. *Neuropsychopharmacology* 1996; 14(2):125-137.

[39] Volkow ND, Wang G, Fowler JS, Logan J, Gerasimov M, Maynard L et al. Therapeutic doses of oral methylphenidate significantly increase extracellular dopamine in the human brain. *Journal of Neuroscience* 2001; 21(2):RC121.

[40] Volkow ND, Wang GJ, Fowler JS, Gatley SJ, Logan J, Ding YS et al. Dopamine transporter occupancies in the human brain induced by therapeutic doses of oral methylphenidate. *American Journal of Psychiatry* 1998; 155(10):1325-1331.

[41] Volkow ND, Ding YS, Fowler JS, Wang GJ, Logan J, Gatley JS et al. Is methylphenidate like cocaine? Studies on their pharmacokinetics and distribution in the human brain. *Archives of General Psychiatry* 1995; 52(6):456-463.

[42] Schweitzer JB, Lee DO, Hanford RB, Tagamets MA, Hoffman JM, Grafton ST et al. A positron emission tomography study of methylphenidate in adults with ADHD: alterations in resting blood flow and predicting treatment response. *Neuropsychopharmacology* 2003; 28(5):967-973.

[43] Ernst M, Zametkin AJ, Matochik J, Schmidt M, Jons PH, Liebenauer LL et al. Intravenous dextroamphetamine and brain glucose metabolism. *Neuropsychopharmacology* 1997; 17(6):391-401.

[44] Ernst M, Zametkin AJ, Matochik JA, Liebenauer L, Fitzgerald GA, Cohen RM. Effects of intravenous dextroamphetamine on brain metabolism in adults with attention deficit hyperactivity disorder (ADHD). Preliminary findings. *Psychopharmacology Bulletin* 1994; 30(2):219-225.

[45] Martinez D. Imaging human mesolimbic dopamine transmission with positron emission tomography. Part II: amphetamine-induced dopamine release in the functional subdivisions of the striatum. *Journal of Cerebral Blood Flow & Metabolism* 23(3):285-300, 2003 Mar 2003;(3):285-300.

[46] Krause KH, Dresel SH, Krause J, Kung HF, Tatsch K. Increased striatal dopamine transporter in adult patients with attention deficit hyperactivity disorder: effects of methylphenidate as measured by single photon emission computed tomography. *Neuroscience Letters* 2000; 285(2):107-110.

[47] Ginovart N, Farde L, Halldin C, Swahn CG. Changes in striatal D2-receptor density following chronic treatment with amphetamine as assessed with PET in nonhuman primates. *Synapse* 1999; 31(2):154-162.

[48] Persico AM, Schindler CW, O'Hara BF, Brannock MT, Uhl GR. Brain transcription factor expression: effects of acute and chronic amphetamine and injection stress. *Brain Research Molecular Brain Research* 1993; 20(1-2):91-100.

[49] Segal DS, Kuczenski R. An escalating dose "binge" model of amphetamine psychosis: behavioral and neurochemical characteristics. *Journal of Neuroscience* 1997; 17(7):2551-2566.

[50] Seeman P. Brain dopamine receptors. [Review] [999 refs]. *Pharmacological Reviews* 1980; 32(3):229-313.

[51] Gillberg C, Melander H, von Knorring AL, Janols LO, Thernlund G, Hagglof B et al. Long-term stimulant treatment of children with attention deficit hyperactivity disorder symptoms. A randomized, double-blind, placebo-controlled trial.[see comment]. *Archives of General Psychiatry* 1997; 54(9):857-864.

[52] Patrick KS, Markowitz JS. Pharmacology of methylphenidate, amphetamine enantiomers and pemoline in attention deficit hyperactivity disorder. *Human Psychopharmacology* Vol 12(6)()(pp 527-546), 1997 1997;(6):527-546.

[53] Gualtieri CT, Wargin W, Kanoy R, Patrick K, Shen CD, Youngblood W et al. Clinical studies of methylphenidate serum levels in children and adults. *Journal of the American Academy of Child Psychiatry* 1982; 21(1):19-26.

[54] Angrist B, Corwin J, Bartlik B, Cooper T. Early pharmacokinetics and clinical effects of oral D-amphetamine in normal subjects. *Biological Psychiatry* 1987; 22(11):1357-1368.

[55] Wargin W, Patrick K, Kilts C, Gualtieri CT, Ellington K, Mueller RA et al. Pharmacokinetics of methylphenidate in man, rat and monkey. *Journal of Pharmacology & Experimental Therapeutics* 1983; 226(2):382-386.

[56] Aoyama T, Sasaki T, Kotaki H, Sawada Y, Sudoh Y, Honda Y et al. Pharmacokinetics and pharmacodynamics of (+)-threo-methylphenidate enantiomer in patients with hypersomnia. *Clinical Pharmacology & Therapeutics* 1994; 55(3):270-276.

[57] Aoyama T, Kotaki H, Sasaki T, Sawada Y, Honda Y, Iga T. Nonlinear kinetics of threo-methylphenidate enantiomers in a patient with narcolepsy and in healthy volunteers. *European Journal of Clinical Pharmacology* 1993; 44(1):79-84.

[58] Shader RI, Harmatz JS, Oesterheld JR, Parmelee DX, Sallee FR, Greenblatt DJ. Population pharmacokinetics of methylphenidate in children with attention deficit hyperactivity disorder. *Journal of Clinical Pharmacology* 1999; 39(8):775-785.

[59] Srinivas NR, Hubbard JW, Quinn D, Korchinski ED, Midha KK. Extensive and enantioselective presystemic metabolism of dl-threo-methylphenidate in humans. *Progress in Neuro-Psychopharmacology & Biological Psychiatry* 1991; 15(2):213-220.

[60] Hungund BL, Perel JM, Hurwic MJ, Sverd J, Winsberg BG. Pharmacokinetics of methylphenidate in hyperkinetic children. *British Journal of Clinical Pharmacology* 1979; 8(6):571-576.

[61] Birmaher B, Greenhill LL, Cooper TB, Fried J, Maminski B. Sustained release methylphenidate: pharmacokinetic studies in ADDH males. *Journal of the American Academy of Child & Adolescent Psychiatry* 1989; 28(5):768-772.

[62] Wilens TE, Biederman J. The stimulants. [Review] [121 refs]. *Psychiatric Clinics of North America* 1992; 15(1):191-222.

[63] Levy F. Side effects of stimulant use. [Review] [39 refs]. *Journal of Paediatrics & Child Health* 1993; 29(4):250-254.

[64] Heffner TG, Seiden LS. The effect of depletion of brain dopamine by 6-hydroxydopamine on tolerance to the anorexic effect of d-amphetamine and fenfluramine in rats. *Journal of Pharmacology & Experimental Therapeutics* 1979; 208(1):134-143.

[65] Sanghvi IS, Singer G, Friedman E, Gershon S. Anorexigenic effects of d-amphetamine and l-DOPA in the rat. *Pharmacology, Biochemistry & Behavior* 1975; 3(1):81-86.

[66] Lowe TL, Cohen DJ, Detlor J, Kremenitzer MW, Shaywitz BA. Stimulant medications precipitate Tourette's syndrome. JAMA 1982; 247(8):1168-1169.

[67] Golden GS. The relationship between stimulant medication and tics. *Pediatric Annals* 1988; 17(6):405-406.

[68] Kurlan R. Tourette's syndrome: are stimulants safe?. [Review] [35 refs]. *Current Neurology & Neuroscience Reports* 2003; 3(4):285-288.

[69] Lipkin PH, Goldstein IJ, Adesman AR. Tics and dyskinesias associated with stimulant treatment in attention deficit hyperactivity disorder. *Archives of Pediatrics & Adolescent Medicine* 1994; 148(8):859-861.

[70] Gadow KD, Sverd J, Sprafkin J, Nolan EE, Ezor SN. Efficacy of methylphenidate for attention deficit hyperactivity disorder in children with tic disorder.[erratum appears in Arch Gen Psychiatry 1995 Oct;52(10):836]. *Archives of General Psychiatry* 1995; 52(6):444-455.

[71] Castellanos FX, Giedd JN, Elia J, Marsh WL, Ritchie GF, Hamburger SD et al. Controlled stimulant treatment of ADHD and comorbid Tourette's syndrome: effects of stimulant and dose. *Journal of the American Academy of Child & Adolescent Psychiatry* 1997; 36(5):589-596.

[72] Gadow KD, Sverd J, Sprafkin J, Nolan EE, Grossman S. Long-term methylphenidate therapy in children with comorbid attention deficit hyperactivity disorder and chronic multiple tic disorder.[see comment]. *Archives of General Psychiatry* 1999; 56(4):330-336.

[73] Law SF, Schachar RJ. Do typical clinical doses of methylphenidate cause tics in children treated for attention deficit hyperactivity disorder? *Journal of the American Academy of Child & Adolescent Psychiatry* 1999; 38(8):944-951.

[74] Varley CK, Vincent J, Varley P, Calderon R. Emergence of tics in children with attention deficit hyperactivity disorder treated with stimulant medications. *Comprehensive Psychiatry* 2001; 42(3):228-233.

[75] Hemmer SA, Pasternak JF, Zecker SG, Trommer BL. Stimulant therapy and seizure risk in children with ADHD. *Pediatric Neurology* 2001; 24(2):99-102.

[76] Gross-Tsur V, Manor O, van der MJ, Joseph A, Shalev RS. Epilepsy and attention deficit hyperactivity disorder: is methylphenidate safe and effective?[comment][republished from J Pediatr. 1997 Jan;130(1):40-4; PMID: 9003849]. *Journal of Pediatrics* 1997; 130(4):670-674.

[77] Gucuyener K, Erdemoglu AK, Senol S, Serdaroglu A, Soysal S, Kockar AI. Use of methylphenidate for attention deficit hyperactivity disorder in patients with epilepsy or electroencephalographic abnormalities. *Journal of Child Neurology* 2003; 18(2):109-112.

[78] Schenk S, Izenwasser S. Pretreatment with methylphenidate sensitizes rats to the reinforcing effects of cocaine. *Pharmacology, Biochemistry & Behavior* 2002; 72(3):651-657.

[79] Garland EJ. Pharmacotherapy of adolescent attention deficit hyperactivity disorder: challenges, choices and caveats. [Review] [79 refs]. *Journal of Psychopharmacology* 1998; 12(4):385-395.

[80] Jaffe SL. Intranasal abuse of prescribed methylphenidate by an alcohol and drug abusing adolescent with ADHD. *Journal of the American Academy of Child & Adolescent Psychiatry* 1991; 30(5):773-775.

[81] Parran TV, Jr., Jasinski DR. Intravenous methylphenidate abuse. Prototype for prescription drug abuse. *Archives of Internal Medicine* 1991; 151(4):781-783.

[82] Goyer PF, Davis GC, Rapoport JL. Abuse of prescribed stimulant medication by a 13-year-old hyperactive boy. *Journal of the American Academy of Child Psychiatry* 1979; 18(1):170-175.

[83] Volkow ND, Swanson JM. Variables that affect the clinical use and abuse of methylphenidate in the treatment of ADHD. [Review] [60 refs]. *American Journal of Psychiatry* 2003; 160(11):1909-1918.

[84] Barkley RA, Fischer M, Smallish L, Fletcher K. Does the treatment of attention deficit/hyperactivity disorder with stimulants contribute to drug use/abuse? A 13-year prospective study.[see comment]. *Pediatrics* 2003; 111(1):97-109.

[85] Biederman J. Pharmacotherapy for attention deficit/hyperactivity disorder (ADHD) decreases the risk for substance abuse: findings from a longitudinal follow-up of youths with and without ADHD. *Journal of Clinical Psychiatry* 64 Suppl 11:3-8, 2003 2003;3-8.

[86] Mannuzza S, Klein RG, Moulton JL, III. Does stimulant treatment place children at risk for adult substance abuse? A controlled, prospective follow-up study. *Journal of Child & Adolescent Psychopharmacology* 2003; 13(3):273-282.

[87] Wilens T, Pelham W, Stein M, Conners CK, Abikoff H, Atkins M et al. ADHD treatment with once-daily OROS methylphenidate: interim 12-month results from a long-term open-label study. *Journal of the American Academy of Child & Adolescent Psychiatry* 2003; 42(4):424-433.

[88] McConnell H. Catecholamine metabolism in the attention deficit disorder: implications for the use of amino acid precursor therapy. *Medical Hypotheses* 1985; 17(4):305-311.

[89] Kent L, Craddock N. Is there a relationship between attention deficit hyperactivity disorder and bipolar disorder? *Journal of Affective Disorders* 2003; 73(3):211-221.

[90] Ridley RM, Baker HF, Owen F, Cross AJ, Crow TJ. Behavioural and biochemical effects of chronic treatment with amphetamine in the vervet monkey. *Neuropharmacology* 1983; 22(4):551-554.

[91] Ellison G, Morris W. Opposed stages of continuous amphetamine administration: parallel alterations in motor stereotypies and in vivo spiroperidol accumulation. *European Journal of Pharmacology* 1981; 74(2-3):207-214.

[92] Castner SA, Goldman-Rakic PS. Long-lasting psychotomimetic consequences of repeated low-dose amphetamine exposure in rhesus monkeys. *Neuropsychopharmacology* 1999; 20(1):10-28.

[93] McNamara CG, Davidson ES, Schenk S. A comparison of the motor-activating effects of acute and chronic exposure to amphetamine and methylphenidate. *Pharmacology, Biochemistry & Behavior* 1993; 45(3):729-732.

[94] Crawford CA, McDougall SA, Meier TL, Collins RL, Watson JB. Repeated methylphenidate treatment induces behavioral sensitization and decreases protein kinase A and dopamine-stimulated adenylyl cyclase activity in the dorsal striatum. *Psychopharmacology* 1998; 136(1):34-43.

[95] Ellison G, Ratan R. The late stage following continuous amphetamine administration to rats is correlated with altered dopamine but not serotonin metabolism. *Life Sciences* 1982; 31(8):771-777.

[96] Robinson TE, Becker JB. Enduring changes in brain and behavior produced by chronic amphetamine administration: a review and evaluation of animal models of amphetamine psychosis. [Review] [321 refs]. *Brain Research* 1986; 396(2):157-198.

[97] Yuan J, McCann U, Ricaurte G. Methylphenidate and brain dopamine neurotoxicity. *Brain Research* 1997; 767(1):172-175.

Index

A

B

C

D

E

F

G

H

I

J

K

L

M

N

O

P

Q

R

T

U

V

W

Y